Outline of Periodontics

Outline of Periodontics

Third edition

J.D. Manson MChD, PhD, FDSRCS
Formerly Senior Lecturer in Periodontology, Institute of Dental Surgery;
Honorary Consultant, Eastman Dental Hospital, London, UK

B.M. Eley BDS, FDSRCS, PhD
Head, Department of Periodontology and School of Hygiene,
King's College School of Medicine and Dentistry, London;
Honorary Consultant, King's College Hospital, London, UK

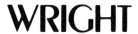

Wright
An imprint of Butterworth-Heinemann Ltd
Linacre House, Jordan Hill, Oxford OX2 8DP

ℛ A member of the Reed Elsevier group

OXFORD   LONDON   BOSTON
MUNICH   NEW DELHI   SINGAPORE   SYDNEY
TOKYO   TORONTO   WELLINGTON

First published 1983
Second edition 1989
Reprinted 1991, 1993
Third edition 1995

British Library Cataloguing in Publication Data
Manson, J. D.
  Outline of Periodontics. – 3Rev.ed
  I. Title II. Eley, B. M.
  617.632

ISBN 0 7236 1018 5

Library of Congress Cataloguing in Publication Data
Manson, J. D. (Julius David)
  Outline of periodontics / J.D. Manson, B.M. Eley. — 3rd ed.
  p. cm.
  Includes bibliographical references and index.
  ISBN 0 7236 1018 5
  1. Periodontics. I. Eley, B. M. (Barry M.) II. Title.
  [DNLM: 1. Periodontal Diseases. 2. Periodontal Diseases—therapy.
  WU 240 M289o 1995]
  RK361.M349 1995
  617.6'32—dc20
  DNLM/DLC   95-7449
  for Library of Congress   CIP

Composition by Scribe Design, Gillingham, Kent
Printed and bound in Great Britain by the Bath Press, Avon

Contents

Preface to the third edition

In the past decade periodontology entered a phase of considerable questioning of old ideas, of speculation, intense research activity, and excitement. Formerly held concepts about the natural history of periodontal diseases have been overthrown, in particular the notion that unless radically controlled, plaque-produced gingival inflammation inexorably progresses to destruction of the tooth-supporting tissues and tooth loss. At the same time, many large-scale epidemiological studies have pointed out the flaws in older methods of data collection and analysis, and have indicated that the prevalence of periodontal diseases is lower than past studies had led us to believe, thus leading to a reappraisal of periodontal disease as a public health problem.

The notion of the 'at risk' individual has been highlighted, and a considerable body of research on the bacteriology and immunology of periodontal diseases have focused on factors which may potentiate the susceptible individual. The identification of such individuals and the definition of prognosis face us with stimulating challenge.

On the clinical side emphasis has been placed on the control of plaque bacteria rather than on the radical elimination of the periodontal lesion, and this conservative approach has been reinforced by real progress in the field of tissue regeneration.

Although we have retained the title *Outline of Periodontics*, in this edition we have tried to provide a comprehensive and up-to-date picture of thinking and activity in both scientific and clinical spheres, so that the text will be useful not only to the undergraduate and general dental practitioner, but also to those engaged in postgraduate studies.

In this endeavour we have been helped by many people, and we would like to acknowledge our debt to the many colleagues who have offered information and opinion, in particular Martin Addy, Paul Batchelor, Harald Löe, Ian Macgregor, Richard Palmer, Taco Pilot, Richard R. Ranney, David Rule and Aubrey Sheiham.

Most particularly, we would like to thank Dr M. Soory for her help with the sections on 'Gingival Hyperplasia' and 'Dental Implants'; Mr C.A. Waterman for his help with Chapter 18 'Mucogingival Problems and their Treatment' and the section on 'Dental Implants'; and Professor R.M. Watson for his help on the section on 'Dental Implants'.

J.D.M.
B.M.E.

Preface to the first edition

There is now a considerable body of knowledge about the aetiology and pathogenesis of periodontal disease. Yet this knowledge is scarcely applied; chronic gingivitis and chronic inflammatory periodontal disease remain universal and tooth loss in the adult is still regarded by many people as an inevitable part of the ageing process. There are several reasons for this sorry state of affairs, including socioeconomic factors beyond the influence of the dental profession. One factor which is wholly dependent upon the profession is the standard of undergraduate teaching. Periodontics still occupies a minor position in the curriculum of many dental schools and is regarded by too many undergraduates and dentists as an esoteric subject peripheral to the main body of conservative dentistry.

This basic text has been written in an attempt to make our understanding of periodontal disease accessible to the undergraduate, to hygienists and to any interested reader. The main emphasis is on the plaque theory and on the prevention and early diagnosis of disease. I have tried to avoid too great an emphasis on surgical techniques. Periodontics is not a surgical discipline; such techniques have to be resorted to only when prevention, early diagnosis and treatment techniques fail.

I am indebted to many of my colleagues, recognized in the text, for providing illustrative material, to Dr Barry Eley for his valuable comments, to Mr James Morgan of the Eastman Dental Hospital and Mr Peter Gordon for help with photography and to Mrs Jenny Halstead for her drawings without which the text would be incomplete.

J.D.M.

1

The periodontal tissues

The masticatory system consists of the mandible and maxilla, the muscles of mastication, the temporomandibular joints and associated ligaments, and the teeth plus the tooth-supporting or periodontal tissues.

It is essential to view this system as a functional unit in which all the parts are interdependent. Breakdown of the dentition may affect other components of the masticatory system; alterations in the functional activity of the muscles of mastication or temporomandibular joints can affect the dental tissues. Like all vital tissues the tissues of the masticatory system are in a state of constant activity. Cells metabolize, reproduce, die and are replaced; non-cellular tissue components, e.g. collagen and ground substance, are synthesized, broken down and replaced. This activity is influenced by age, nutritional and hormonal status and by functional demand. It is also affected by disease.

The periodontium has four components: the gingivae, the alveolar bone, the periodontal ligament and the cementum. Knowledge of the periodontal tissue in health is essential to an understanding of its behaviour in disease.

The gingivae

Introduction

The gingiva is that part of the oral mucosa which surrounds the tooth and covers the alveolar ridge. It is part of the tooth-supporting apparatus, the periodontium, and by forming a connection with the tooth the gingiva protects the underlying tissues of the tooth attachment from the oral environment. The gingiva is tooth dependent; when there are teeth there are gingivae and when teeth are extracted the gingivae disappear.

Like all vital tissues the gingiva can adapt itself to changes in its environment, and the mouth which is the first part of the alimentary tract and the site of the initial preparation of food in digestion may be regarded as a relatively hostile environment. The oral tissues are exposed to an enormous range of stimuli. The temperature and consistency of food and drink, its chemical composition, acidity and alkalinity vary considerably. The number of bacteria in the mouth is immense and their variety beyond exact definition. Add to this the insults and irritations of dental manipulations and one can only be impressed by the sheer resilience of the oral mucosa and the efficiency of gingival defence mechanisms, which include:

1. The salivary flow and saliva contents, e.g. lysozyme, IgA.
2. Cell turnover and surface desquamation.
3. The activity of the immune mechanisms.

The junction between the tooth and the oral mucosa, the dentogingival junction, is unique and peculiarly vulnerable. It is the only attachment in the body between a soft tissue and a calcified tissue which is exposed to the external environment.

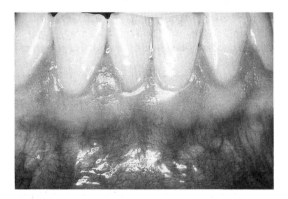

Figure 1.1 Healthy gingivae in a girl of 19 years

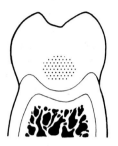

Figure 1.3 The interdental gingiva in the shape of a 'col' reflects the contours of the tooth contact area

This junction is a highly dynamic tissue with its own battery of protective mechanisms.

Healthy gingiva is pink, firm, knife-edged and scalloped to conform to the contour of the teeth (*Figure 1.1*). Its colour may vary with the amount of melanin pigmentation in the epithelium, the degree of keratinization of the epithelium and the vascularity and fibrous nature of the underlying connective tissue. In the Caucasian individual pigmentation is minimal; in patients of African or Asian origin brown or blue-black areas of pigmentation may cover a great part of the gingiva; in Mediterranean peoples occasional patches of pigmentation are found. It is important to distinguish physiological pigmentation from that which occurs in some diseases and with metal contamination.

The gingiva is divided into two zones: the marginal gingiva and attached gingiva (*Figure 1.2*).

The gingival margin

The marginal gingiva forms a cuff 1–2 mm wide around the neck of the tooth and is the external wall of the gingival crevice which is 0–2 mm deep. This cuff can be separated from the tooth by careful manipulation of a blunt probe. Between the teeth the margin forms a cone-shaped gingival papilla, the labial surface of which is frequently indented by a groove called a 'sluice-way'. The papilla fills the space in the interdental embrasure apical to the contact point and its facial-lingual shape conforms to the curvature of the cemento-enamel junction to form the interdental col (*Figure 1.3*).

The surface of the gingival margin is smooth in contrast to that of the attached gingiva, from which it is demarcated by an indentation called the 'free gingival' groove (*see Figure 1.2*).

Attached gingiva

The attached gingiva or 'functional mucosa' extends from the free gingival groove to the mucogingival junction where it meets the alveolar mucosa (*see Figure 1.2*). The attached gingiva is a mucoperiosteum which is tightly bound to the underlying alveolar bone. At the mucogingival junction the mucoperiosteum splits so that the alveolar mucosa is separated from the periosteum by a loose, highly vascular, connective tissue. Thus the alveolar mucosa is a relatively loose and mobile tissue, deep red, in marked contrast to the pale pink attached gingiva (*see Figure 1.1*). The surface of the attached gingiva is stippled like orange peel. This stippling varies considerably. It is most prominent on facial surfaces and often

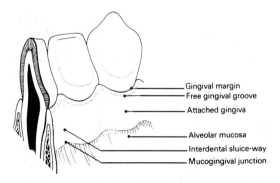

Gingival margin
Free gingival groove
Attached gingiva
Alveolar mucosa
Interdental sluice-way
Mucogingival junction

Figure 1.2 Diagram illustrating anatomical features of the gingiva

disappears in old age. There is some doubt about the cause of the stippling but it appears to coincide with epithelial rete pegs.

The width of the attached gingiva can vary from about zero to 9 mm. It is usually widest in the incisor region (3–5 mm) and narrowest over mandibular canines and premolars. In the past it has been assumed that some attached gingiva is necessary to maintain the health of the gingival margin by separating the stable margin from the mobile alveolar mucosa, but this does not appear to be the case in the clean mouth. This variation in width has given rise to controversy about what form of anatomy is compatible with health and techniques have been devised to widen areas of attached gingiva considered to be too narrow irrespective of whether disease is present or not. Any width, even a zero width, is acceptable if the tissue is healthy.

Microscopic features of the gingiva

The gingival margin consists of a core of fibrous connective tissue covered by stratified squamous epithelium which, like all squamous epithelium, undergoes constant renewal by continuous cell reproduction in its deepest layers and shedding of the superficial layers. The two activities are held in balance so that the thickness of the epithelium remains constant. It has the characteristic layers of squamous epithelium:

1. The basal or formative cells layers of columnar or cuboidal cells.
2. The prickle-cells or spinous layer (stratum spinosum) of polygonal cells.
3. The granular layer (stratum granulosum) in which the cells are flatter and contain many particles of keratohyaline.
4. The cornified layer (stratum corneum) in which the cells have become flat and shrunken, and keratinized or parakeratinized.

The mitotic rate of oral epithelium varies from place to place, with age and also from one animal to another. Turnover times in the experimental animal are said to be: palate, tongue and cheek 5–6 days, gingiva 10–12 days.

Like all epithelial cells gingival epithelium cells are connected to each other and to the underlying connective tissue corium by thick-enings on the periphery of the cells called hemidesmosomes. The epithelium is joined to the underlying corium by a thin basal lamina made of a protein-polysaccharide complex which is permeable to fluid. Seen by electron microscopy it can be resolved into two layers, the lamina lucida and the lamina densa.

The epithelium of the outer or oral surface of the gingival margin is keratinized or para-keratinized while the epithelium of the inner or crevicular surface is thinner and not keratinized. Contrary to popular opinion non-keratinized oral epithelium is not necessarily always more permeable than keratinized epithelium. Intact epithelium is an effective barrier against microorganisms which can breach damaged epithelium, but intact epithelium is permeable to many smaller substances such as the molecules of skin antiseptics, topical anaesthetics and vasodilators, e.g. glyceryl trinitrate.

Pigmentation is produced by pigment-forming melanocytes. However, variation in pigmentation is not produced by variation in the number of these cells but by genetically determined variation in their pigment-producing capacity. The ratio of melanocytes to the keratin-producing epithelial cells is relatively constant at 1:36 cells.

The gingival connective tissue is made up of a mesh of collagen fibre bundles running in a ground substance which contains fibroblasts, histiocytes, blood vessels, nerves, lymphocytes, plasma cells and other cells of the defence system, which are more numerous near the junctional epithelium, where immune activity is maintained.

The ground substance

Connective-tissue cells and fibres, together with vessels and nerves, are embedded in an amorphous, non-fibrous and non-cellular matrix made up of glycosaminoglycans (GAGs), proteoglycans and glycoproteins. All the components of the matrix are synthesized and secreted by fibroblasts. The most common GAG is hyaluronic acid, large amounts of which are found in gingiva.

The GAGs linked to protein to form proteoglycans include heparin sulphate and dermatan sulphate. GAGs are long unbranched polysaccharides which can bind large amounts of water. As a result of this tissues containing large amounts of GAG resist compressive forces well. GAG also facilitates the transport of nutrients through the extracellular spaces. The matrix also transports metabolic products, cells and chemical messengers known as cytokines which moderate cellular function.

One of the most important glycoproteins is fibronectin. This is a large protein which binds to cells, collagen and proteoglycans. It is important in promoting the adhesion of fibroblasts to the extracellular matrix, and also plays a role in the alignment of collagen fibres.

The gingival fibres (*Figure 1. 4*)

The connective tissue of the gingiva is organized to keep the gingival margin tight around the neck of the tooth and to maintain the integrity of the dentogingival attachment.

The arrangement of these fibres is complicated but they have been described as being divided into several discernible groups of collagen fibre bundles:

1. *Dentogingival* or free gingival fibres which are attached to cementum and fan out into the gingiva and over the alveolar margin to merge with the periosteum of the attached gingiva.
2. *Alveolar-gingival* or alveolar crest fibres which arise from the alveolar crest and run coronally into the gingiva.
3. *Circular* 'fibres' which encircle the tooth.
4. *Trans-septal* fibres which run from tooth to tooth coronally to the alveolar septum.

There is a great deal of interlinking between fibre groups and special stains are needed to define the fibres.

Collagen is synthesized by fibroblasts and is secreted in an inactive form, procollagen, which is then converted into tropocollagen. In the extracellular space, tropocollagen is polymerized into collagen fibrils which are then aggregated into collagen bundles by the formation of cross linkages. Different forms of collagen may be secreted and each is based on variations in the composition of the basic tropocollagen molecule. The most common form found in the gingiva is Type I collagen which forms the major fibre bundles and the loose collagenous fibres. Some Type III and V collagens are also present. Type VI collagen is present in the basement membranes of blood vessels and the overlying epithelium.

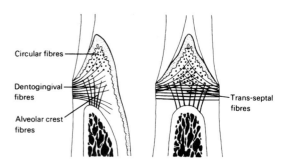

Figure 1.4 Gingival fibre groups: dentogingival, circular, alveolar crest and trans-septal fibres

Gingival blood, lymph and nerve supply

The gingiva has a rich blood supply derived from three sources: supraperiosteal and periodontal ligament vessels plus alveolar vessels which emerge from the alveolar crest (*Figure 1.5*). These link in the gingiva to form capillary loops in the connective-tissue papillae between the epithelial rete pegs. Lymphatic drainage starts in connective-tissue papillae and drains into regional lymph nodes: from the mandibular gingiva into the cervical, submandibular and submental nodes; from the maxillary gingiva into the deep cervical lymph nodes.

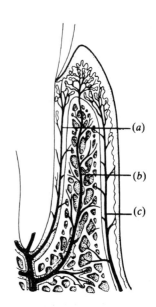

Figure 1.5 The rich gingival blood supply derives from: (*a*) periodontal ligament, (*b*) alveolar bone and (*c*) supraperiosteal vessels

The nerve supply is derived from branches of the trigeminal nerve. A number of nerve endings have been identified in the gingival connective tissue as tactile corpuscles, and temperature and pain receptors.

The interdental gingiva

The gingiva between the teeth is concave and has been described as a 'col' which joins the facial and lingual papillae (*see Figure 1.3*). Where teeth make contact the cols conform to the shape of the teeth apical to the contact area. Where neighbouring teeth do not contact there is no col and the interdental gingiva is flat or convex.

The epithelium of the col is very thin, not keratinized, and made up of only a few cell layers. Its structure probably reflects its sheltered position. Turnover of interdental epithelial cells is the same as that of the rest of the gingiva.

The interdental region is of special importance as it is the site of the most persistent bacterial stagnation and its structure makes it especially vulnerable. *It is the site of the initial lesion in gingivitis.*

The dentogingival junction

It is possible to define three zones of gingival epithelium (*Figure 1.6*). Oral epithelium extends from the mucogingival junction to the gingival margin where crevicular (or sulcular) epithelium lines the gingival crevice (or sulcus). At the base of the crevice the connection between the gingiva and the tooth is mediated by a special kind of epithelium called junctional epithelium.

In health the junctional epithelium lies against enamel and extends to the cemento-enamel junction. If there is gingival recession the junctional epithelium lies on cementum. Thus the base of the gingival crevice is the free surface of the junctional epithelium. It is said that in perfect health the depth of the crevice is zero so that there is no crevicular epithelium and oral epithelium therefore merges directly into the junctional epithelium. This does not occur in humans.

At an ultrastructural level a very thin basement lamina lies between the junctional epithelial cells and the connective-tissue corium, and between the junctional epithelium

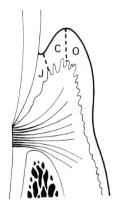

Figure 1.6 The dentogingival junction. There are three zones of gingival epithelium: oral epithelium (O), crevicular (or sulcus) epithelium (C) and the junctional epithelium (J)

and the tooth surface. The latter basement lamina and related hemidesmosomes form the 'epithelial attachment', which is a product of epithelial cells. If gingivectomy is carried out and the junctional epithelium is completely removed, on healing a new gingival margin plus new junctional epithelium are formed whether the gingiva is on enamel, dentine or cementum.

The junctional epithelium is very fragile and does not form a barrier against probing. Its cells are larger than those of oral epithelium and loosely connected together, indeed the cell-to-cell connection is more fragile than the attachment to the tooth surface. Unlike keratinized epithelial cells of the crevice, the cells of the junctional epithelium can attach via hemidesmosomes to tooth surface.

The junctional epithelium in adults is about 40 cells long from apex to crevicular surface but varies from 0.25 to 1.35 mm; in the young it is a narrow sleeve as thin as 3–4 cells, in the adult it is 10–20 cells wide. Although it undergoes constant renewal, with cell division taking place throughout its structure, the junctional epithelium is homogeneous and without any pattern of cell differentiation. Although the turnover time for human junctional epithelium is not known, in other primates it is said to be approximately 4–6 days, i.e. half that of oral epithelium which is roughly 10–12 days. Desquamation of the junctional epithelium takes place through the small free area at the base of the gingival crevice. Listgarten (1972) has calculated that the rate of cellular exfoliation from a unit surface of junctional epithelium is 50–100 times as fast as that from a unit of oral gingival epithelium. A small number of leucocytes (neutrophils) are often found within the junctional epithelium.

In contrast to oral gingival epithelium and crevicular epithelium the junctional epithelium is relatively permeable and allows a two-way movement of a variety of substances:

1. From corium into the crevice. Gingival fluid exudate, polymorphonuclear leucocytes, various cells of the immune system plus immunoglobulins and complement. It is the exit point for most of the leucocytes found in saliva. In inflammation the movement of fluid and cells increases and as the population of leucocytes increases the junctional epithelium may degenerate and become even more permeable. Some research workers believe that in perfect health there is no passage of gingival fluid into the crevice.
2. From crevice into the corium. Foreign materials such as carbon particles, trypan blue (mol. wt 960) and many other substances inserted into the gingival crevice are found subsequently in the gingival corium and the bloodstream. *Microorganisms cannot penetrate junctional epithelium* but a large number of substances, some of them with high molecular weights, have been shown to pass through the intercellular spaces of the junctional epithelium. This is an extremely important finding as it is believed that gingival inflammation is initiated by bacterial enzymes, and metabolic products, which diffuse from the crevice through the junctional epithelium into the gingival connective tissue.

Because of the permeability of junctional epithelium it is inevitable that the tissue defence mechanisms should be in a constant state of alertness and this is manifest by an infiltration of inflammatory cells, lymphocytes and plasma cells in the underlying corium. This used to be interpreted as a sign of disease but indicates the constant presence in health of the defence mechanisms.

Formation of the dentogingival attachment

There has been some controversy about the origin and structure of the attachment tissues but using electron microscope findings and the results of autoradiographic studies of cellular activity a consensus seems to have been achieved.

When enamel formation is complete the reduced enamel epithelium is attached to enamel by a basal lamina and hemidesmosomes. As the tooth penetrates the oral mucosa the reduced enamel epithelium unites with the oral epithelium and with continuing eruption this epithelium condenses along the crown. Ameloblasts gradually atrophy and are replaced by squamous epithelium, i.e. the junctional epithelium which forms a collar around the fully erupted tooth. As already described, junctional epithelium, like all squamous epithelium, is a constantly renewing structure with epithelial cells moving coronally to be shed at the free surface into the bottom of the crevice.

Gingival crevicular fluid

If a filter paper strip is inserted into the gingival crevice it will absorb fluid already in the crevice and may also provoke an outward flow of fluid. This also happens in mastication, on tooth brushing and with any other stimulation of the gingivae; the flow is greatly increased when the gingivae are inflamed. Sex hormones, oestrogen and progesterone appear to increase the flow, perhaps by causing increased permeability of gingival blood vessels. Certain chemotactic factors found in plaque may also increase the flow. This fluid is an inflammatory exudate and carries polymorphonuclear leucocytes and other antimicrobial substances. It forms part of the defence mechanism of the dentogingival junction. If a patient is on systemic tetracyclines the drug finds its way via gingival blood vessels, connective tissue and junctional epithelium into the gingival crevice. In summary, the fluid performs the following functions:

1. It washes the crevice, carrying out shed epithelial cells, leucocytes, bacteria and other debris.
2. The plasma proteins may influence the epithelial attachment to the tooth.
3. It contains antimicrobial agents, e.g. lysozyme.
4. It carries polymorphonuclear leucocytes and macrophages, which are capable of phagocytosing bacteria. It also transports

immunoglobulins IgG, IgA, IgM and other factors of the immune system.

The amount of gingival crevicular fluid can be measured and used as an index of gingival inflammation. Its composition may also be determined by a variety of biochemical and immunocytochemical techniques, and it may relate to the severity of the underlying periodontal pathology.

The periodontal ligament

A ligament is a bond, usually linking two bones together. The root of the tooth is connected to its socket in alveolar bone by a connective-tissue structure which can be regarded as a ligament. The periodontal ligament not only connects the tooth to the jaw bone but also supports the tooth in the socket and absorbs loads imposed on the tooth thus protecting the tooth especially at the apex. The cells of the ligament maintain and repair alveolar bone and cementum. Thus the ligament is a reservoir from which bone cells and cementum cells are derived; precursor cells are formed from stem cells in the bone marrow, and from there migrate into the periodontal ligament.

The proprioceptor nerve endings in the ligament form part of the extremely refined neurological control of mastication. The mechanoreceptors in the periodontal ligament monitor changes in pressure within the ligament space, and as forces increase greater numbers of mechanoreceptors are stimulated. This results in increasing numbers of impulses passing via the sensory nerves to the trigeminal nuclei. This in turn results in inhibitory impulses passing to the motor nucleus which reduces the number of motor impulses to the muscle fibres, reducing or stopping masticatory forces. A similar reflex arc passes from the muscle spindle receptors which monitor muscle stretch. The loads in mastication, swallowing and speaking vary considerably in amount, frequency, duration and direction, and in normal function the structure of the ligament usually absorbs these effectively and transmits them to the supporting bone.

Structure

The thickness of the ligament varies from about 0.3 to 0.1 mm. It is widest at the mouth

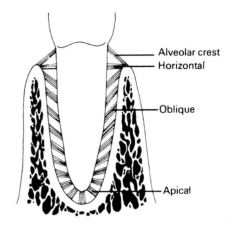

Figure 1.7 Periodontal ligament fibre bundles

of the socket and at the apex, and narrowest at the level of the axis of rotation of the tooth, which is slightly apical to the middle of the root. In health there is a normal range of tooth mobility. Incisors are more mobile than posterior teeth, mobility is greatest on wakening and reduces through the day. As for other parts of the skeleton functional stresses are essential to the maintenance of the integrity of the periodontal ligament. When functional stresses are heavy the ligament is thicker and when a tooth is functionless the ligament can become as thin as 0.06 mm. With ageing the ligament becomes thinner.

The ligament consists of well-organized collagen fibre bundles about 5 μm in diameter, in a ground substance matrix through which vessels and nerves course. The fibre bundles, which are inserted at one end into cementum and at the other into the socket wall as Sharpey's fibres, are usually described in identifiable groups according to their predominant orientation (*Figure 1. 7*):

1. Alveolar crest fibres run from the cementum at the neck of the tooth to the alveolar crest.
2. Horizontal fibres run from cementum to alveolar crest.
3. Oblique fibres form the main component of the ligament and run from the bone in a slightly apical direction to be inserted in the cementum so that they appear to be suspending the tooth in its socket.
4. Apical fibres radiate from the apex to the base of the socket. One can also include the

inter-radicular fibres which are found in the furcation of multirooted teeth and like trans-septal fibres run from root to root coronal to the alveolar crest.

These fibre bundles appear to follow a wavy course and a single bundle cannot be traced from tooth to bone. An intermediate plexus is seen in the midsection of the ligament during eruption, after which it disappears.

Apart from these major fibre bundles there are less regular collagen fibre bundles and 'oxytalan' fibres which may be immature elastic fibres. Fibroblasts are aligned along the collagen fibres; cementoblasts line the cementum; bone cells, osteoblasts and osteoclasts are present on the bone surfaces.

Fibroblasts are the most abundant cell type in the periodontal ligament. Because of the high turnover of collagen and proteoglycan within the ligament these cells are actually engaged in protein synthesis and appear plump with abundant cytoplasm. They are also responsible for collagen degradation within the ligament.

Cementoblasts on the cementum surface and osteoblasts on the endosteal and periosteal surfaces of alveolar bone are only conspicuous when active deposition of bone and cementum is taking place, at which time these cells also appear plumper. Multinucleated cells (osteoclasts and cementoclasts) appear on bone and cementum surfaces when resorption is taking place, and indeed there appears to be no reason to differentiate between them since they both resorb mineralized tissue. All of these cell types derive from stem and precursor cells in the ligament and/or bone marrow. Osteoclasts derive from bloodborne precursors of marrow origin, which originate from mononuclear phagocyte cell precursors.

Groups of epithelial cells, the 'epithelial rests of Malassez', which are remnants of the Hertwig root sheath, are found close to the cementum. They may play a part in the formation of dental cysts.

It is important to recognize that these collagen structures undergo constant remodelling, i.e. resorption of old fibres and formation of new ones, and the fibroblasts are involved in both processes. Autoradiographic studies demonstrate a high rate of collagen turnover which is greatest at the alveolar crest and at the apex. The turnover of collagen in the periodontal ligament is said to be faster than in any other connective tissue. This probably reflects the constant functional demand placed on teeth.

As in the gingiva, the main collagen types present in the ligament are Types I, III and V. Most major fibres are composed of Type I collagen. However, Type III collagen is present in similar proportions to those found in embryonic tissues, and this probably reflects the high turnover rate within the ligament. Type III is more fibrillar and extensible than Type I and may be important in maintaining the integrity of the ligament during the small vertical and horizontal movements which occur during chewing.

The ligament ground substance is an amorphous matrix of GAGs, proteoglycans and glycoproteins, and plays an extremely important role in the absorption of functional stresses. Its composition is similar to that of gingival ground substance; hyaluronic acid, heparin sulphate, chondroitin-4- and chondroitin-6-sulphates and dermatan sulphate are all present. These molecules turn over at an even faster rate than collagen. They are important in binding water and may thus act as a hydraulic cushion in the periodontal ligament. This cushioning effect is probably more important in resisting the forces of mastication than traction on the ligament fibres.

The ligament has a rich network of blood vessels from apical arteries and from vessels penetrating the alveolar bone. Veins within the ligament do not usually accompany the arteries. There is considerable anastomosis with the gingival blood vessels. Nerve bundles from the trigeminal nerve follow the blood vessels from the apex and through the alveolar bone to supply the ligament with tactile, pressure and pain receptors. The nerves appear to terminate as free nerve endings or spindle-shaped structures associated with proprioceptive activity which is central to the control of the masticatory system in chewing, swallowing and talking.

The nerve and blood supply, the ground substance and collagen bundles all take part in the absorption of functional stresses and their transmission to the bones. There is some debate about the exact mechanism but the system described by Parfitt (1967) appears to explain the observed behaviour of a tooth in function. He describes the vascular-ground substance complex as a shock absorbing system and the fibre-bundle system as a suspensory system limiting tooth movement and transmitting strain to the supporting bone. Thus, when a force is applied to a tooth a series of events follow:

1. The initial displacement of the tooth is associated with intravascular and extravascular fluid movement through blood vessels and through bone spaces.
2. As the load increases the collagen fibre bundles take the strain and become extended. They are not elastic and they do not stretch.
3. With further pressure the alveolar process distorts.
4. If the load is sufficiently powerful and prolonged the tooth substance itself, i.e. the dentine, distorts.

This has been described as a viscoelastic system in which the vascular, tissue fluid and ground substance components provide the viscous response while the fibrous tissue and bone provide elasticity. When an axial load is applied to a tooth there appears to be a biphasic response, the elastic phase preceding the viscous phase. It is an extremely versatile and resilient system which can cope with the variable loads imposed on the tissues by the mastication of a heterogenous diet. However, it can break down when subject to abnormal loads or when involved in inflammation.

Axial forces are absorbed most readily. On loading, the wavy principal fibres assume their full length and the tooth is depressed in the socket. Lateral and rotational forces are absorbed less easily. On the tension side fibres extend; on the pressure side fibres are compressed. Further compression results in bone resorption and further tension bone deposition.

All teeth are slightly mobile and that mobility is influenced by:

1. The quantity and duration of the applied load.
2. Length and shape of the root or roots and therefore the position of the axis of rotation. Inevitably mobility of the lower incisor with a relatively short and conical root is easier to elicit than that of the multi-rooted upper first molar with its large root base.

3. The status of the supporting tissues, i.e. thickness of collagen fibre bundles and proportion of mature collagen (the erupting tooth is more mobile than the fully erupted tooth); the state of aggregation of the ground substance, thus in pregnancy some increase in tooth mobility is caused by hormone-induced disaggregation.

Cementum

Cementum is the calcified connective tissue which covers the root dentine and into which periodontal fibre bundles are inserted. It can be regarded as a 'bone of attachment' and is the only specifically dental tissue of the periodontal tissues. It is pale yellow and softer than dentine, and in some animals is present on the crowns of the teeth as an adaptation to a herbivorous diet. On the root its relationship to the enamel margin varies, it may abut on or overlap enamel but it may be separated from the enamel by a thin band of exposed dentine. The thickness of cementum varies considerably; the coronal third may be only 16–60 μm and the very thin layer of cervical cementum can be easily removed by the toothbrush or dental instrumentation so that the very sensitive dentine is exposed. The apical third can be 200 μm or even thicker. Cementum is formed slowly throughout life, a layer of uncalcified matrix, the precementum, being laid down first. It can triple its thickness throughout life. It is avascular and without enervation, more permeable than dentine, but this permeability decreases with age.

Like other calcified tissues, bone and dentine, it consists of collagen fibres embedded in a calcified organic matrix. Its inorganic content, hydroxyapatite, is less than that of bone, i.e. about 45% (bone 65o, dentine 70%, enamel 97%).

There are two main types of cementum: cellular and acellular. The former contains cementocytes in lacunae which, like osteocytes in bone, communicate with each other through a network of canaliculi. Acellular cementum forms a thin surface layer, often confined to cervical portions of the root. It does not contain cementocytes within its substance but as cementoblasts populate its surface the term 'acellular' may not be appropriate.

There are two arrangements of collagen fibrils in cementum. The principal fibrils are those of the periodontal ligament embedded as Sharpey's fibres in the calcified matrix and incorporated in the cementum as it is laid down. They are arranged at right angles to the cementum surface. The other fibrils form a dense and irregular meshwork within the matrix. In acellular cementum the Sharpey's fibres are closely packed and largely calcified; in cellular cementum they are more widely spaced and partly calcified. Unlike bone there is no evidence of cementum remodelling, i.e. of internal resorption and deposition; however, there is continuous apposition of surface cementum as cementoblast activity continues at a low level throughout life. Cementoid or precementum is the name given to the cementum matrix prior to calcification. During calcification hydroxyapatite crystals are deposited within collagen fibrils parallel to their surface, then on their surface and finally within the cementoid matrix. The cementum surface is formed into conical projections about single fibrils or bundles.

The greatest thickness of cementum is formed at the apex and in furcation areas. With attrition, i.e. wear of the occlusal surface of the tooth, compensatory deposition of apical cementum takes place which, together with bone deposition at the alveolar crest and at the socket fundus, maintains the vertical dimension of the face. At the tooth apex the cementum forms a constriction so that the root canal exit is very narrow.

Excessive formation of cementum, hypercementosis, may follow pulp disease or occlusal stress. A generalized hypercementosis involving all teeth may be hereditary; it also occurs in Paget's disease. Occasionally cementicles, small spherical masses of cementum may be found attached to the cementum surface or free in the periodontal ligament. Cementum resorption can be a consequence of excessive occlusal stress or orthodontic movements, pressure from tumours or cysts or deficiencies of calcium or vitamins A and D. It is also found in metabolic diseases but the pathogenesis is obscure. Deposition of cementum can follow resorption when the cause is removed. Occasionally ankylosis of the cementum and socket bone takes place. Root fracture may be followed by the formation of a cementum callus, but this repair process does not demonstrate the highly organized remodelling capacity of bone.

Alveolar bone

The alveolar process is that part of the jaw bone which supports the teeth. It is partly tooth dependent and after tooth extraction some bone resorption follows. It is absent in anodontia. The bone of the alveolar process is in no fundamental way different from bone in any other part of the body. It has facial and lingual plates of compact bone between which is cancellous trabeculation. This cancellous bone is oriented around the tooth to form the tooth socket wall or cribriform plate. As the name implies the cribriform plate is perforated like a sieve so that a large number of vascular and neural connections can be made between the periodontal ligament and the trabecular spaces. The collagen fibres of the periodontal ligament are inserted into the socket wall, into what is called 'bundle bone'. The periodontal ligament fibres embedded in bone are called Sharpey's fibres.

Like all bone, alveolar bone undergoes constant remodelling as a response to mechanical stress and to metabolic need for calcium and phosphorus ions. In health the remodelling process maintains the total volume of bone and its overall anatomy relatively stable. In the primate the teeth drift mesially as interproximal tooth surface wear takes place, together with resorption on the mesial and deposition on the distal surfaces of the socket wall.

The shape of the jaws and the morphology of the alveolar processes vary between individuals and the size, shape and thickness of cortical plates and interdental septa vary in different parts of the same jaw. The margin of the alveolar crest usually runs parallel to the amelocemental junction at a remarkably constant distance of 1–2 mm, but this relationship may vary with the alignment of the tooth and the contour of the root surface. Where a tooth is displaced out of the arch the overlying alveolar plate may be very thin or even perforated so that fenestrations (circumscribed defects) or dehiscence (splits) are formed. These defects occur more frequently in facial than in lingual bone and are more common over anterior than posterior teeth, although they are seen over the palatal root of the upper first molar if the roots are very divergent. These defects are very important clinically because where they occur the root of the tooth is covered only by mucoperiosteum, i.e. periosteum and the overlying gingiva which may atrophy under irritation and thus expose the root. Where tooth roots approximate, interdental bone may be absent.

Regulation of tissue turnover in the periodontium

Epithelium

Stratified squamous epithelium continually renews itself by division of cells in the basal layer and shedding of keratinocytes from the surface. The turnover time for skin is 12–75 days, oral epithelium 8–40 days and junctional epithelium 4–11 days. Systemic hormones influence this, with oestrogen stimulating cell division and corticosteroids inhibiting it. Local factors appear to play a more important role in its regulation. There is a negative feedback control system on keratinocytes by substances known as chalones. The precise nature of these is unknown but their function could be due to one or more cytokines. They act on cells in the basal layer and inhibit their division. Epithelial turnover is also affected by at least three cytokines. Epithelial growth factor (EGF) and transforming growth factors alpha (TGFα) and beta (TGFβ). EGF and TGFα stimulate cell proliferation whilst TGFβ appears to have an inhibitory effect.

The differentiation of epithelium is also profoundly affected by the underlying connective tissue lamina propria. The nature of the connective tissue or chemical messages from it determines the nature of the overlying epithelium for instance whether it is keratinized or not. Thus, in the free gingival graft it is the nature of the underlying connective tissue which determines the epithelium which forms.

Periodontal ligament

The periodontal ligament is constantly breaking down and renewing its constituent tissues. In health, this process is carefully controlled and is in balance. The tooth responds to functional demands and rates of turnover reflect increases or decreases in function.

Connective tissue turnover in the periodontium is 5 times higher than alveolar bone and 15 times higher than the dermis of normal skin. Fibroblasts are responsible for both the synthesis (*see p. 4*) and degradation of all components of the extracellular matrix. They secrete collagenolytic enzymes (collagenases) and these are part of a family of metalloproteinases which require the presence of metallic cations such as magnesium and calcium for their activity. Other proteinases in this group include a proteoglycanase known as stromolysin and gelatinases which degrade proteoglycans and other non-collagenous components. This process of collagen degradation is carefully controlled. Collagenase is secreted as an inactive enzyme known as procollagenase and this needs to be activated by other proteinases. A number of serine proteinases can do this but the most likely one in health is plasmin. This is generated from blood plasminogen by the action of plasminogen activating factor secreted by macrophages. Another important regulator is known as tissue inhibitor of metalloproteinases (TIMP) and this is secreted by fibroblasts. This inhibitor binds and inhibits metalloproteinases including collagenase and protects against excessive matrix degradation.

Active collagenase cleaves collagen at a specific site and separates small segments of fibrils from the fibre bundle. These small collagen segments are then phagocytosed by fibroblasts and degraded intracellularly by lysosomal enzymes.

The mechanisms controlling connective tissue turnover are only partly understood. Some cytokines stimulate collagen, fibronectin and proteoglycan synthesis and secretion and these include fibroblast growth factor (FGF), platelet-derived growth factor (PDGF) and transforming growth factor alpha (TGFα). Other cytokines such as interleukin-1 (IL-1) and interferon gamma (IFNγ) can stimulate collagenase secretion. However, the control mechanisms governing the secretion of these cytokines is not fully understood.

Bone

Bone turnover takes place continually throughout life with bone deposition mediated by osteoblasts which is linked to bone resorption largely mediated by osteoclasts.

Osteoblasts are responsible for the synthesis of the bone matrix and its subsequent calcification. Initially, uncalcified matrix or osteoid is formed and this mineralized as a result of deposition of crystals of hydroxyapapite.

Osteoclasts are only formed at bone surfaces undergoing resorption. However, bone resorption cannot take place unless both osteoclasts and osteoblasts are present (Dziak, 1993). Osteoblasts control the functions of osteoclasts through regulating hormones and local messengers (*see Chapter 5, pp. 59–66*). Stimulated osteoblasts secrete procollagenase which removes the non-mineralized collagenous surface of bone. Osteoclasts then spread over the bone surface and beneath the ruffled border secrete acid which dissolves the mineral phase (*see Figure 5.4*). It also secretes lysosomal cysteine proteinases such as cathepsins B and L which are active at acid pHs and these are responsible for removing the collagenous matrix.

This process is regulated by systemic hormones such as parathyroid hormone (PTH), vitamin D_3 and calcitonin and local produced factors such as prostaglandin E_2 (PGE_2), leukotrienes and cytokines such as IL-2, TNFα and β, TGFβ, PDGF, IL-3 and IL-6 (*see Figure 5.3*).

Radiographic appearance of the periodontal tissues

The radiographic image represents the product of the radiodensity of the various tissues which lie in the path of the X-ray beam so that only the most radiodense tissues may be discernible. Thus, interdental bone registers while buccal and lingual plates of bone may be almost completely obscured by the image of the tooth (*Figure 1.8*).

The discernible anatomical features on the radiograph are as follows:

The socket walls and crest of the interdental septa register as linear radio-opacities, the white line of the lamina dura outlining the socket (*Figure 1. 9*). The presence and clarity of these features reflect the contour of the alveolar crest and of the tooth socket, and variations in the thickness of these white lines, or their complete absence, do not necessarily mean that disease is present.

Because the facial-lingual width of the interdental septum between molars is substantial

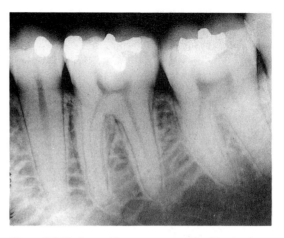

Figure 1.8 Radiographic appearance of healthy tooth-supporting tissue. The alveolar crest and sockets are delineated by a radio-opaque line. The images of buccal and lingual plates of bone are obscured by the image of the tooth

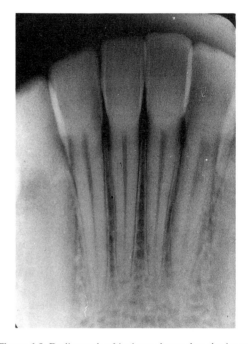

Figure 1.9 Radiograph of incisors shows that the image of the crest of alveolar septa is less well defined than between molars

the image of the crest is well delineated. The interdental septa between premolars and incisors are much narrower, therefore they are more radiolucent and the images of the crests tend to be less well defined (*Figure 1.9*).

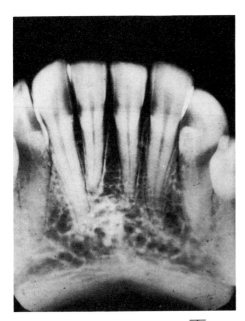

Figure 1.10 Widened periodontal space at 1|1 indicating thickened ligament as a response to increased occlusal stress

The periodontal space between the calcified structures is extremely narrow and shows as a thin dark line around the root. Where the proximal tooth surface is wide this line is likely to be clearer than where the interproximal dimension is narrow and in some cases it may not be discernible at all. Increased functional stress produces a thickened periodontal ligament which is reflected on the radiographic film (*Figure 1.10*). A composite image of the cancellous bone trabeculation is projected on to the radiograph and the image density reflects the density of the bone.

Cementum is discernible only when hypercementosis has taken place.

As the radiographic image can be distorted easily by alterations in beam angle and variation in exposure time and developing time, it is essential to use a completely standardized procedure. Lack of standardization makes comparison impossible and misdiagnosis possible.

Age changes in the periodontium

Because destructive periodontal disease tends to manifest itself most frequently in early middle age and is more advanced in the older individual, it was regarded as part of the ageing process. This is not the case. Age changes do take place in the healthy periodontal tissues; periodontal disease is not one of them. It is important to distinguish true age changes from the effects of trauma and disease which may accompany age.

The vasculature, the gingiva, periodontal ligament, cementum and alveolar bone demonstrate age changes and it is possible that the vascular changes, e.g. thickening of vessel walls, narrowing of the lumen, even arteriosclerosis, are central to changes in the tissues generally. Briefly, these consist of loss of cellularity and increasing fibrosis. There may also be loss of ground substance and thickening of basement membranes.

In the periodontal ligament, fibre bundles are thicker and less distinct. Cementum, especially in the apical area, is thicker largely as a compensation for attrition of occlusal tooth surfaces.

The alveolar bone becomes less vascular and many haversian systems are closed. Some osteoporosis may be evident but this is not usually as severe as in the long bones.

Wound healing may be slower.

References

Dziak, R. (1993) Biochemical and molecular mediators of bone metabolism. *Journal of Periodontology* **64**, 407–415

Listgarten, M. A. (1972) Normal development, structure, physiology and repair of the gingival epithelium. *Oral Science Review* **1**, 3–67

Parfitt, G. J. (1967) The physical analysis of the tooth-supporting structures. In: Anderson, D. J. *et al.* (eds) *The Mechanisms of Tooth Support*. Bristol: Wright, pp. 154–160

Further reading

Berkowitz, B.M.B., Moxham, B.J. and Newman, H.N. (1982) *Periodontal Ligament in Health and Disease*. Oxford: Pergamon Press

Williams, D.M., Hughes, F.J., Odell, E.W. and Farthing, P.M. (1992) The normal periodontium. In: *Pathology of Periodontal Disease*. Oxford: Oxford Medical Press, pp. 17–31

2

The oral environment in health and disease

The oral mucosa is bathed in saliva and exposed to the passage of food, the oral flora and stimulus or injury from toothbrushes and other oral hygiene aids, as well as other objects that people put in their mouths such as cigarettes, pipes, hair-grips and so. Considering the variety of such factors, the variations in temperature, pH values, range of textures and the diversity of oral habits, the oral mucosa demonstrates remarkable adaptability and resistance.

The tooth surface which is also exposed to these factors may become covered wholly or in part by a number of deposits, pellicle, plaque, food debris, calculus, materia alba and stains.

Saliva

Saliva plays a vital role in maintaining the integrity of the oral tissues, in food digestion and in speech. As every clinician knows there is considerable variation in the rate of secretion from the several salivary glands. This is influenced by neurotransmission mechanisms in response to olfactory, gustatory and masticatory stimuli, and even the thought of food can increase secretion. The average unstimulated or resting flow rate is about 0.3–0.4 ml/min but in some people can reach about 2 ml/min. The stimulated flow rate can vary between 0.2–6.0 ml/min.

Composition

Saliva is 99.5% water plus 0.5% organic and inorganic substances. The organic fraction contains both large and small molecules, the former is mainly protein in the form of glycoproteins together with some gammaglobulins, serum albumin and enzymes; the latter include glucose, urea and creatinine. The inorganic fraction consists of calcium, phosphorus, sodium, potassium and magnesium as well as dissolved carbon dioxide, oxygen and nitrogen. The main salivary enzyme is amylase but in disease many enzymes produced by bacteria and leucocytes are found. Most of the organic fraction is produced by the salivary gland cells, the remainder is transported into saliva from the blood. Among the compounds transported from the blood are the electrolytes, albumin, immunoglobulins G, A and M, and vitamins, drugs and hormones. Indeed there is a good correlation between plasma and salivary levels of hormones and medications.

Function

Saliva has a number of functions:

1. In the digestive process it helps to form the food bolus and provides amylase for the digestion of starch.
2. The flow of viscous fluid helps to remove bacterial and food debris.

3. Bicarbonates and phosphates buffer food and bacterial acids.
4. Salivary mucin and other constituents protect the oral mucosa and tooth surfaces in a variety of ways:
    (a) Salivary glycoproteins cover and lubricate the mucosa. This protective action becomes more obvious when it is removed, as in xerostomia (dry mouth) caused by pathology of the salivary glands. The oral mucosa becomes dry and red, bleeds readily and is prone to infection.
    (b) The antibacterial enzyme lysozyme acts by splitting bacterial cell walls and acting as a scavenger.
    (c) Antibacterial gammaglobulin (antibody), mostly immunoglobulin A (IgA), appears to have two forms of protective action:
        (i) It prevents the attachment of bacteria and viruses to the tooth surface and oral mucosa.
        (ii) It reacts with food antigens to neutralize their effect.
    (d) Leucocytes: Saliva contains a large number of leucocytes which migrate through the junctional epithelium and, as stated, the number of salivary leucocytes increases when there is gingival inflammation.
    (e) The enzyme sialoperoxidase has antibacterial activity, especially against lactobacilli and streptococci.
    (f) The mineral components, in particular calcium and phosphorus ions, act to maintain tooth integrity by modulating ion diffusion and preventing the loss of mineral ions from the tooth tissue. The interchange of minerals between tooth structure and saliva goes on constantly and decalcification of enamel may be remineralized.
5. The water and mucin (glycoprotein) form the lubricant essential to speech in making smooth the movements and contacts of the lips, and the tongue against the teeth and palate which enable us to form consonants.

Oral bacteria

At birth the mouth is sterile but within a few hours microorganisms appear, mainly *Streptococcus salivarius*. By the time the deciduous teeth erupt a complex flora is present.

Bacteria are present in saliva, on the tongue and cheeks, on tooth surfaces, especially in fissures, and in the gingival crevice. The number of bacteria in saliva can be measured in thousands of millions per millilitre but the largest population of bacteria is found on the dorsum of the tongue. Even the healthy gingival crevice contains more bacteria than are free in saliva, and in periodontal disease the crevicular population multiplies.

One can regard the various parts of the mouth, i.e. tongue, cheeks, tooth fissures, saliva, gingival crevices, as consisting of different ecosystems in which different varieties of bacteria are found in balance with one another and with the tissues. The dominant organisms are streptococci. The number and variety vary from person to person, from one part of the mouth to another, even on different surfaces of the same tooth, before and after eating or toothbrushing. Age, diet, composition of saliva and its rate of flow as well as systemic factors influence the oral flora (see pp. 15–17, 19–22 and Chapters 3, 4 and 5).

Tooth deposits

Acquired salivary pellicle

Within seconds of tooth cleaning a thin layer of salivary protein, largely glycoprotein, is deposited on to the tooth surface (as well as on to restorations and dentures). This layer, called pellicle, is thin (0.5 μm), smooth, colourless and translucent. It adheres firmly to the tooth surface and can be removed only by positive friction. There appears to be an electrostatic affinity between hydroxyapatite and glycoprotein. Initially it is bacteria free.

The function of salivary pellicle is protective. Salivary glycoproteins and salivary calcium phosphate are adsorbed on to the enamel surface and help to reduce tooth wear. Pellicle also restricts the diffusion of acid products of sugar breakdown. It can bind various inorganic ions, e.g. calcium, phosphate and fluoride, and contains antibacterial factors including IgG, IgA, IgM, complement and lysozyme.

Dental plaque

Very soon, indeed within minutes, after the pellicle has been deposited it is populated by

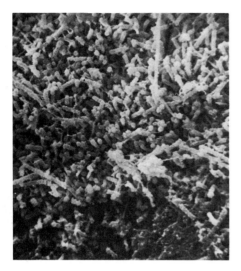

Figure 2.1 Scanning electron micrograph of organisms in mature plaque (× 1400). (Courtesy of Dr H. N. Newman and the publishers of the *British Dental Journal*)

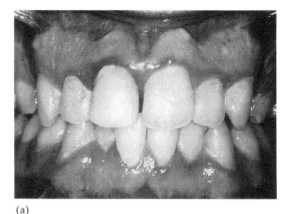

(a)

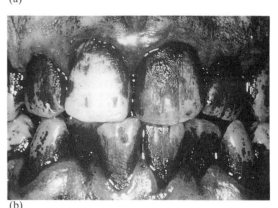

(b)

Figure 2.2 (a) Plaque deposits seen prior to the use of a disclosing agent; (b) as revealed by disclosing agent

bacteria. Bacteria may deposit directly on to enamel but usually they attach to pellicle and the bacterial aggregates may be coated in salivary glycoprotein. In primitive peoples on a 'natural' diet of hard and fibrous food occlusal surfaces and contact areas are subject to considerable wear so that bacterial deposition is minimal. When a soft 'civilized' diet is used tooth wear is slight or absent and bacterial deposition is encouraged. Accumulations are greatest in sites sheltered from functional friction and tongue movement. The interdental region below the contact area is the site of greatest plaque thickness.

Plaque formation

Within the first few hours species of *Streptococcus* and a little later *Actinomyces* attach to the pellicle. During the first few days this bacterial population grows along and spreads out from the tooth surface so that under electron microscope one can see palisades of organisms rather like skyscrapers, one layer on top of another radiating from the surface. Plaque grows by internal multiplication and surface deposition. Different varieties of bacteria attach to these columns and multiply so that after 3–4 weeks a complex microflora is established which represents a balanced equilibrium of organisms or microbial ecosystem on the tooth surface (*Figure 2.1*).

Supragingival plaque formation is pioneered by bacteria with an ability to form extracellular polysaccharides which allow them to adhere to the tooth and each other. The first colonizing bacteria are *Streptococcus mitior, S. sanguis, Actinomyces viscosus* and *A. naeslundii*. If these bacteria grow unchecked for a few days gingival inflammation will develop. During this process the environmental conditions will gradually change causing a selective overgrowth. This results in a shift in the bacterial composition and after 2–3 weeks of uninhibited growth a complex flora develops including Gram negative anaerobes, motile bacteria and spirochaetes. Moore *et al.* (1982) have isolated 166 bacterial species from supragingival plaque.

At a clinical level dental plaque is a soft, non-calcified layer of bacteria which accumulates on and adheres to teeth and other objects in the mouth, e.g. restorations, dentures and calculus. In thin layers it is scarcely visible and can be revealed only by the use of a disclosing agent (*Figure 2.2*). In thick layers it can be seen as a yellowish or grey deposit which *cannot* be removed with mouthwash or by irrigation but can be brushed off. It is unusual to find it on the masticatory surface of the tooth unless that tooth is out of function, when gross deposits may form.

Composition of mature plaque

Approximately 70% of plaque is microbial and the rest represents extracellular products of plaque bacteria, cell remnants and glycoprotein derivatives. Protein, carbohydrate and lipids are found. The most common carbohydrate is bacteria-produced dextran; there is also some levan and galactose. The principal inorganic components are calcium, phosphorus, traces of magnesium, potassium and sodium. The inorganic salt content is highest on the lingual surface of the lower incisors. Calcium ions may actually aid adhesion between bacteria and between bacteria and the pellicle.

Plaque deposition and food intake

Plaque will form in patients and animals fed by stomach tube, although in diminished amounts. There is some debate as to whether the frequency of meals or the amount of food eaten influences the amount of plaque deposited. However, plaque bacteria do use nutrients which can diffuse easily into the plaque, e.g. soluble sugars, sucrose, fructose, glucose, maltose and lactose. Starches may also serve as a bacterial substrate.

Dextran is the most important extracellular bacterial product because of its relative insolubility and adhesive properties. It can be produced from sucrose in the diet and influences plaque deposition and metabolism. Plaque forms more rapidly during sleep than following meals because the mechanical action of eating plus the stimulated salivary flow deters plaque deposition. Eating hard, coarse and fibrous food deters plaque formation and this fact is used in the experimental production

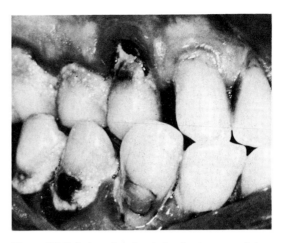

Figure 2.3 Soft deposits of materia alba in a very dirty mouth. Deposits of plaque and subgingival calculus are also present

of plaque. Gingivitis in the dog can be produced by feeding a soft diet for as short a time as 4 days.

Although some debate still lingers about the benefits of finishing meals with apples, celery and carrots, these are preferable to the usual very sweet dessert offerings. Certainly vigorous mastication which produces natural tooth wear on both occlusal and interproximal surfaces minimizes plaque deposition.

Materia alba (*Figure 2.3*)

This is a yellowish or whitish, soft, loose deposit found in neglected mouths. It consists of a mass of microorganisms, desquamated epithelial cells, food debris, leucocytes plus salivary deposits. Its structure is amorphous and unlike plaque it can be removed easily and washed away with a water spray.

Dental calculus (tartar)

Calculus, the 'stony crust' that forms on teeth, has long been associated with periodontal disease. Along with other pathological calcifications, e.g. kidney stones and gallstones, dental calculus is described in ancient medical writings. Calculus is a calcified mass which forms on and adheres to the surface of teeth and other solid objects in the mouth, e.g. restorations and dentures, which are not

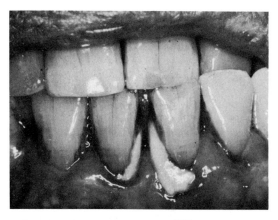

Figure 2.4 Supragingival calculus on 1̅|̅1̅

exposed to friction. *Calculus is calcified plaque.* Stages in its formation can be studied by collection on plastic veneers attached to teeth or dentures.

Calculus is rarely found on deciduous teeth and is not common on the permanent teeth of young children. However, by the age of 9 it is found frequently and it is present in virtually all adult mouths.

Deposits are classified according to their relationship to the gingival margin, i.e. they are either supragingival or subgingival.

Supragingival calculus (*Figure 2.4*)

By definition this is found coronal to the gingival margin. It is deposited first on tooth surfaces opposite salivary ducts, on the lingual surfaces of lower incisors and the buccal surfaces of upper molars, but it may be deposited on any tooth or denture not adequately cleaned, as for example the occlusal surface of an unopposed tooth. It is light yellow unless stained by other factors (e.g. tobacco, wine, betel nut), fairly hard, brittle and easily detached from the tooth by a suitable instrument.

Subgingival calculus

This is attached to root surface and its distribution is not related to the salivary glands but to the presence of gingival inflammation and pocketing, a fact reflected by its old name 'seruminal calculus'. It is dark green or black,

much harder than supragingival calculus and more tightly adherent to the tooth surface. It may be found on roots close to the apical limit of a deep pocket, in severe cases as far down as the apex of the tooth. It can be difficult to detect on clinical examination. Sometimes its presence can be seen as a darkening of the thin overlying layer of gingiva, and its presence can be revealed directly by detaching the gingiva with a carefully directed blast of warm air. Cautious probing along the root surface with a fine probe will reveal deposits; if thick enough these may be seen on radiographs.

Composition of calculus

The composition of calculus varies slightly with the age of the deposit, its position in the mouth and even the geographical location of the individual.

It consists of 80% inorganic matter, some water and an organic matrix of protein and carbohydrate which includes desquamated epithelial cells, Gram positive filamentous bacteria, cocci and leucocytes. The proportion of filamentous forms in calculus is greater than in the rest of the mouth. The inorganic fraction consists mainly of calcium phosphate as hydroxyapatite, brushite, whitlockite and octacalcium phosphate. There are also small amounts of calcium carbonate, magnesium phosphate and fluoride. The fluoride content of calculus is many times higher than in plaque.

The surface of calculus is covered by bacterial plaque but the centre of thick deposits may be sterile.

The obvious differences in appearance and distribution of supragingival and subgingival calculus suggest that their composition and mode of deposition may be different.

The composition of subgingival calculus is very similar to that of supragingival calculus except that its Ca/P ratio is higher and its sodium content greater. Salivary proteins are not found in subgingival calculus, indicating a non-salivary source for this deposit.

The deposition of calculus

Calculus is mineralized bacterial plaque but not all plaque mineralizes. Supragingival calculus is rarely seen on the facial surface of lower molars but commonly on facial surfaces of upper molars which are opposite the mouth of the parotid ducts. Perhaps 90% of all supragingival calculus on a dentition is on the lower incisors which are bathed in saliva directly from the submandibular and sublingual salivary glands. Precipitation of mineral salts into plaque may be seen only hours after plaque deposition but is more usual 2–14 days after plaque is formed. Mineral in supragingival calculus derives from saliva, that in subgingival calculus from gingival fluid exudate. In early plaque, concentrations of calcium and phosphorus ions are high; indeed the concentration of calcium in plaque is about twenty times that in saliva, but no apatite crystals are present. Furthermore, there is no evidence that hydroxyapatite crystals form spontaneously in saliva. Some trigger appears to be necessary and it is generally believed that some element in plaque acts as a seeding or nucleation site where crystallization can start. Electron microscope studies suggest that apatite crystals are formed either in or on filamentous microorganisms but as calculus can be formed in germ-free animals it is likely that other factors can act as a seed. Once calcification is started it can continue by crystal growth.

Various theories have been put forward for the mechanism of initial mineralization:

1. Saliva can be regarded as an unstable supersaturated solution of calcium phosphate. As CO_2 tension is relatively low in the mouth CO_2 can be lost from saliva with deposition of insoluble calcium phosphate.
2. During sleep salivary flow is reduced and ammonia is formed from salivary urea, producing a rise of pH which favours precipitation of calcium phosphate.
3. Protein may hold calcium in high concentrations but when saliva contacts the teeth the protein comes out of solution leading to precipitation of calcium and phosphate ions.

Whichever of these mechanisms operates the calcified deposit fixes the plaque in position against the tooth and gingiva. Calculus is attached to pellicle, to irregularities in the tooth surface or via filamentous organisms which penetrate the surface of cementum.

Tooth stains

Many substances form stains which are tenaciously fixed to the tooth surface and require professional cleaning for removal. Tobacco, wine, metal salts, chlorhexidine mouthwash, etc. produce characteristic stains. A green stain is found on children's teeth which may be the pigmentation of salivary pellicle by chromogenic bacteria.

Stains are unsightly but there is no evidence that they cause gingival irritation or act as a focus for plaque deposition.

The subgingival flora

Subgingival bacterial colonization only occurs if supragingival plaque and gingivitis are present. It does not occur as a simple apical downgrowth of plaque but rather by the slow apical movement of pioneer bacteria which may be attracted by nutrient and oxygen tension gradients (Newman, 1977). This initial pioneering growth is followed by progressive colonization by other indigenous bacteria and multiplication of those species that are particularly well adapted to the subgingival conditions, such as Gram negative rods and spirochaetes. This is partly due to the environment but also to symbiotic relationships between different bacterial species and selective inhibition of some species by others. Anaerobic *Actinomyces* species are associated with the root surface, forming discrete colonies or continuous layers. Other bacteria remain unattached and free within the protected environment of the pocket which provides them with many of the trace substances that they require. The subgingival flora is a very complex community of many different species.

Methods of investigating subgingival flora

The composition of dental plaque and the identification of individual bacterial species can be partially or fully determined in a number of ways. These are dark ground or phase contrast microscopy (Listgarten, 1986), culture techniques, immunological techniques including immunofluorescence (Zambon *et al.*, 1985; Zambon *et al.*, 1986) or enzyme linked immunosorbent assay (ELISA) (Ebersole *et al.*, 1984), DNA probes (French *et al.*, 1986) and other molecular biological techniques and enzyme-based assays (Loesche, 1986). These are more fully described in Chapter 13, pp. 145–146. Precise speciation of bacteria in culture can be carried out with a variety of laboratory-based methods including selective sub-cultures, biochemical tests, SDS PAGE, gene probes, ribotyping, DNA fingerprinting and cell wall long chain fatty acid analysis (Genco *et al.*, 1986; Greenstein, 1988).

However, it must be realized that whatever methods are used to determine the bacteria present in the subgingival flora the picture will always be incomplete and sometimes can be very misleading. It will also depend on the methods used for collection. The flora contains either facultative or strict anaerobic bacteria and many bacteria will only be preserved if strict anaerobic conditions are adhered to during both collection and culture. Furthermore, it is estimated that less than 50% of the bacteria in the subgingival flora are culturable even with special selective culture conditions. The best examples of this are the spirochaetes which may account for between 40–60% of the total flora. In addition, a considerable number of both Gram positive and negative bacterial species can only be cultured with difficulty using very selective techniques. Also, some Gram positive bacteria may appear as Gram negative when grown in poor cultural conditions.

The latest molecular techniques which detect bacteria on the basis of their genetic composition have yielded very different compositions to cultural techniques using the same sample. Thus, the composition of the subgingival flora is still incomplete and may appear different as these new techniques yield information.

Finally, DNA and RNA probes and monoclonal antibodies are available for some subgingival bacteria and can detect these species when they are present. They are very specific and can only detect the species to which they are directed and will thus only detect bacteria already suspected to be present.

Nomenclature of anaerobic rods in the subgingival flora

The nomenclature of oral black-pigmented Gram negative anaerobic rods has recently changed as a result of extensive investigations of these bacteria. The principal changes have been reviewed by van Steenbergen *et al.* (1991) and are shown in *Table 2.1*.

Table 2.1 The nomenclature of black pigmented anaerobes

Former name	New name
Black-pigmented Bacteroides	Black-pigmented anaerobic rods
Bacteroides gingivalis	*Porphyromonas gingivalis*
Bacteroides endodontalis	*Porphyromonas endodontalis*
Bacteroides intermedius	*Prevotella intermedia*
Bacteroides corporis	*Prevotella corporis*
Bacteroides melaninogenicus	*Prevotella melaninogenica*
Bacteroides denticola	*Prevotella denticola*
Bacteroides loescheii	*Prevotella loescheii*

For the moment *Bacteroides forsythus* retains its present name but *Wolinella recta* has been renamed *Campylobacter recta*. Subdivision of some current species will probably occur soon as our knowledge increases and the next likely division will probably affect *Fusobacterium nucleatum*.

Several new species with very fastidious growth requirements making them difficult to cultivate routinely are beginning to be reported from subgingival plaque samples (Tanner, 1991). These include Gram positive bacteria such as *Eubacterium* species including *E. timidum*, *E. brachy* and *E. nodatum* (Holdeman *et al.*, 1980), *Streptococcus oralis* and *S. gordonii* (Kilian *et al.*, 1989) and *Actinomyces georgiae*, *A. genencseriae* (Johnson *et al.*, 1990). Fastidious Gram negative bacteria reported include *Fusobacterium alocis* and *F. sulci* (Cato *et al.*, 1985), *Mitsuokella dentalis*, a motile Selenomonas (Moore *et al.*, 1987), *Treponema socranskii* sub-species (Smibert *et al.*, 1984) and *B. forsythus* (Tanner *et al.*, 1986).

Subgingival flora in health and disease

Dark ground and phase contrast microscopy studies have shown that in periodontal health there is a very scant subgingival flora consisting of non-motile rods and cocci (Listgarten and Hellden, 1978). In gingivitis there is a marked decrease in the proportion of cocci and a parallel increase in motile rods and spirochaetes. In chronic adult periodontitis the number of motile rods and spirochaetes show further increases. There is also evidence that the numbers of spirochaetes and motile rods are greater in pockets with recurrent periodontitis than those that remain inactive (Listgarten *et al.*, 1984).

Table 2.2 Bacterial species associated with health

Gram positive rods
    Actinomyces israelii   *Rothia dentocariosa*
    Actinomyces naeslundii   *Actinomyces gerencseriae*
    Actinomyces odontolyticus
Gram positive cocci
    Streptococcus mitis   *Streptococcus sanguis*
    Streptococcus oralis   *Streptococcus gordonii*
    Peptostreptococcus micros
Gram negative rods
    Selenomonas sputigena   *Prevotella intermedia*
    Capnocytophaga gingivalis   *Fusobacterium nucleatum* subsp. *vincentii*

Table 2.3 Bacterial species associated with gingivitis

Similar proportions in health, gingivitis and periodontitis	Elevated in gingivitis	Elevated in gingivitis and periodontitis
Actinomyces gerencseriae	*Actinomyces naeslundii* III	*Prevotella intermedia*
Actinomyces naeslundii	*Campylobacter concisus*	*Eubacterium timidum*
Bacteroides gracilis	*Streptococcus anginosis*	*Fusobacterium nucleatum*
Capnocytophaga ochracea	*Streptococcus sanguis*	*Campylobacter recta*
Haemophilus aphrophilus		
Proprionibacter acnes		
Gamella (Streptococcus) morbillorula		
Veillonella parvula		

Cultural studies have identified about 300 bacterial species in the periodontal pocket, some of which occur infrequently and in low numbers (Slots and Listgarten, 1988). The healthy gingival sulcus contains a scant microflora dominated by Gram positive facultative species of *Streptococcus* and *Actinomyces* and a similar flora is found in successfully treated periodontal pockets. In chronic gingivitis Gram negative anaerobic bacteria make up about 45% of the culturable flora (Slots, 1979). The predominating bacteria are *Actinomyces* species, *Streptococcus* species, *Fusobacterium nucleatum, Prevotella intermedia* and various non-pigmenting *Bacteroides* species. In advancing adult periodontitis the proportions of these bacteria continue to increase until Gram negative bacteria form about 75% and anaerobic and facultative bacteria about 90% of the cultural flora. Common Gram negative bacteria in chronic adult periodontitis include *P. gingivalis, P. intermedia, F. nucleatum, Capnocytophaga* species, *Campylobacter* (formerly *Wolinella*) *recta, Eikenella corrodens* and *Actinobacillus actinomycetemcomitans*, seen in cultural studies (Slots, 1979; Slots and Genco, 1984),

and spirochaetes seen by dark ground microscopy.

The description of the precise bacterial species present in the subgingival flora associated with health, gingivitis and progressive

Table 2.4 Bacterial species associated with progressive periodontitis

Gram positive rods	Gram positive cocci
Eubacterium brachy	*Peptostreptococcccus micros*
Eubacterium nodatum	*Peptostreptococcus anaerobius*
Eubacterium timidum	*Peptostreptococcus acnes*
Proprionibacter acnes	
Lactobacillus minutus	
Gram negative rods	**Gram negative spirochaetes**
Porphyromonas gingivalis	*Borrelia vincentii*
Prevotella intermedia	*Treponema denticola*
Prevotella denticola	*Treponema macrodentium*
Prevotella oralis	*Treponema oralis*
Bacteroides forsythus	*Treponema socranskii*
Actinobacillus actino-	
mycetemcomitans	
Eikenella corrodens	
Campylobacter recta	
Fusobacterium nucleatum	
subsp. *nucleatum*	
Fusobacterium alocis	
Selenomonas sputigena	
Selenomonas flueggei	

periodontitis has been refined as the speciation of the flora has developed in recent years. These bacterial species have recently been reviewed and described by Tanner (1991) and are listed in *Tables 2.2, 2.3* and *2.4*.

The composition of the pocket flora may vary from one individual to another and from one tooth site to another. The predominance of certain bacteria in the pocket does not necessarily indicate that these bacteria are exclusive pathogens since all the different bacterial species which predominate the pocket flora in various proportions and frequencies originate from the normal oral flora (Theilade, 1986).

References

Cato, E.P., Moore, L.V.H. and Moore, W.E.C. (1985) *Fusobacterium alocis* sp. nov. and *Fusobacterium sulci* sp. nov. from the human gingival sulcus. *International Journal of Systematic Bacteriology* **35**, 475–477

Ebersole, J.L., Frey, D.E., Taubman, M.A. *et al.* (1984) Serological identification of oral *Bacteroides* sp. by enzyme-linked immunosorbent assay. *Journal of Clinical Microbiology* **19**, 639–644

French, C.K., Savitt, E.D., Simon, S.L. *et al.* (1986) DNA probe detection of periodontal pathogens. *Oral Microbiology and Immunology* **1**, 58–62

Genco, R.J., Zambon, J.J. and Christersson, L.A. (1986) Use and interpretation of microbiological assays in periodontal disease. *Oral Microbiology and Immunology* **1**, 73–79

Greenstein, G. (1988) Microbiological assessments to enhance periodontal disease diagnosis. *Journal of Periodontology* **59**, 508–515

Holdeman, V., Cato, E.P., Burnmeister, J.A. and Moore, W.E.C. (1980) Description of *Eubacterium timidum* sp. nov., *Eubacterium brachy* sp. nov. and *Eubacterium nodatum* sp. nov. isolated from human periodontitis. *International Journal of Systematic Bacteriology* **30**, 163–169

Johnson, J.L., Moore, L.V.H., Kaneko, B. and Moore W.E.C. (1990) *Actinomyces georgiae* sp. nov., *Actinomyces genencseriae* sp. nov., designation of two genospecies of *Actinomyces naeslundii*, and inclusion of *A. naeslundii* serotypes II and III and *Actinomyces viscosus* serotype II in *A. naeslundii* genospecies II. *International Journal of Systematic Bacteriology* **40**, 273–286

Kilian, M., Mikkelson, L. and Henrichsen, J. (1989) Taxonomic study of viridans streptococci: description of *Streptococccus gordonii* sp. nov. and embedded description of *Streptococcus sanguis* (White and Niven, 1946), *Streptococcus oralis* (Bridge and Neath, 1982) and *Streptococcus mitis* (Andrews and Horder, 1996). *International Journal of Systematic Bacteriology* **39**, 471–484

Listgarten, M. A. (1984) Subgingival microbiological differences between periodontally healthy sites and diseased sites prior to and after treatment. *International Journal of Periodontics and Restorative Dentistry* **4**, 27

Listgarten, M.A. (1986) Direct microscopy of periodontal pathogens. *Oral Microbiology and Immunology* **1**, 31–36

Listgarten, M.A. (1992) Microbial testing in the diagnosis of periodontal disease. *Journal of Periodontology* **63**, 332–337

Listgarten, M. A. and Hellden, L. (1978) Relative distribution of bacteria at clinically healthy and periodontally diseased sites in humans. *Journal of Clinical Periodontology* **5**, 115–132

Listgarten, M. A., Levin, S., Schifter, C.C. el al. (1984) Comparative differential dark-field microscopy of subgingival bacteria from tooth surfaces with recent evidence of recurring periodontitis and from non-affected sites. *Journal of Periodontology* **55**, 398–401

Loesche, W.J. (1986) The identification of bacteria associated with periodontal disease and dental caries by enzymatic methods. *Oral Microbiology and Immunology* **1**, 65–70

Moore, W.E.C., Holdeman, L.V., Smibert, R.M. *et al.* (1982) Bacteriology of experimental gingivitis in young adult humans. *Infection and Immunity* **38**, 651–667

Moore, L.V.H., Johnson, J.L. and Moore, W.E.C. (1987) *Selenomonas noxia* sp. nov., *Selenomonas flueggei* sp. nov., *Selenomonas infelix* sp. nov., *Selenomonas dianae* sp. nov. and *Selenomonas artemidis* sp. nov. from human gingival crevice. *International Journal of Systematic Bacteriology* **36**, 271–280

Newman, H.N. (1977) Ultrastructure of the apical border of dental plaque. In: Lehner, T. (ed.) *The Borderland between Caries and Periodontal Disease*. London: Academic Press, pp. 79–103

Slots, J. (1979) Subgingival microflora and periodontal disease. *Journal of Clinical Periodontology* **6**, 351–352

Slots, J. and Genco, R.J. (1984) Black-pigmented *Bacteroides* species, *Capnocytophaga* species and *Actinobacillus actinomycetemcomitans* in human periodontal disease: virulence factors, colonization, survival and tissue destruction. *Journal of Dental Research* **63**, 412–421

Slots, J. and Listgarten, M.A. (1988) *Bacteroides gingivalis*, *Baceroides intermedius* and *Actinobacillus actinomycetemcomitans* in human periodontal diseases. *Journal of Clinical Periodontology* **15**, 85–93

Smibert, R.M., Johnson, J.L. and Ranney, R.R. (1984) *Treponema socranskii* subsp. *socranskii* subsp. nov., *Treponema socranskii* subsp. *buccule* subsp. nov. and *Treponema socranskii* subsp. *paerdis* subsp. nov. isolated from human periodontitis. *International Journal of Systematic Bacteriology* **34**, 457–462

Tanner, A.C.R. (1991) Microbial succession in the development of periodontal disease. In: Hamada, S., Holt, S.C. and McGhee, J.R. (eds) *Periodontal Disease: Pathogens and Host Immune Responses*. Quintessence Publishing Co. Ltd, Tokyo, pp. 13–25

Tanner, A.C.R., Listgarten, M.A., Ebersole, J.L. and Strzempko, M.N. (1986) *Bacteriodes forsythus* sp. nov., a slow-growing fusiform *Bacteroides* sp. from the human oral cavity. *International Journal of Systematic Bacteriology* **36**, 213–221

Theilade, E. (1986) The non-specific theory in microbial etiology of inflammatory periodontal diseases. *Journal of Clinical Periodontology* **13**, 905–911

van Steenbergen, T.J.M., van Winkelhoff, A.J. and de Graaff, J. (1991) Black-pigmented oral anaerobic rods: Classification and role in periodontal disease. In: Hamada, S., Holt, S.C. and McGhee, J.R. (eds) *Periodontal Disease: Pathogens and Host Immune Responses*. Quintessence Publishing Co. Ltd, Tokyo, pp. 41–52

Zambon, J.J., Reynolds, H.S., Chen, P. and Genco, R.J. (1985) Rapid identification of periodontal pathogens in subgingival dental plaque. Comparison of indirect immunofluorescence microscopy with bacterial culture for detection of *Bacteroides gingivalis. Journal of Periodontology* **56** (Special Issue), 32–40

Zambon, J.J., Bochacki, V. and Genco, R.J. (1986) Immunological assays for putative periodontal pathogens. *Oral Microbiology and Immunology* **1**, 39–44

3

Host–parasite interaction

The description of periodontal anatomy in Chapter 1 provides little idea of the continuous activity of living tissue. Health is not a static condition; it is a dynamic state in which the living and functioning organism or tissue remains in balance with a constantly changing environment. These changes in the environment provoke corresponding alterations in tissue activity so that normal function can continue. This constant process of readjustment to maintain normal tissue activity, normal function and ultimately the continuity of life is known as homeostasis. If an environmental change is so great that homeostasis cannot be maintained the activity of the tissues becomes abnormal, normal function cannot be continued and the change in tissue activity is perceived as disease.

Bacteria constitute an important part of our environment; indeed life without bacteria would be impossible. Usually all external surfaces in nature including those of living tissues are covered by bacteria. The skin and the gut are no exceptions and the oral mucosa as part of the gut is covered by many species of bacteria, the oral flora. Bacteria attach themselves to surfaces by a number of means: by the microscopic roughness of the surface, by hairlike extensions on the surface of the bacteria and by natural glues made of proteins and polysaccharides, as in the glycoprotein of the salivary pellicle described in Chapter 2.

Where different life forms exist together there is competition for existence, therefore mechanisms have evolved which help one form

to protect itself from another. As the tissues of the body have evolved together with their microorganisms over millions of years one would expect that these defence mechanisms would have been perfected and that a state of harmony or balance between the host and its bacteria would have been achieved. If such a balance had not been established, as explained by Darwin's theory of natural selection, at least one of the species involved would have died out. In fact we live quite happily in a state of partnership (symbiosis) with most of the bacteria on our bodies and only under certain circumstances do we suffer from their presence. For example, both dental caries and periodontal disease are caused by bacteria which are normally resident in our mouths. In primitive man and in so-called 'primitive' communities today the prevalence of dental disease is very low, and bacterial plaque occurs in much smaller quantities and only rarely apical to the tooth-contact area. By contrast in 'civilized' man bacterial plaque may be found on almost all tooth surfaces and dental disease is rampant. The change in texture of our diet and its large component of refined and easily fermentable carbohydrate have altered the oral environment in such a way that bacterial stagnation takes place around the teeth and gum margin, with resultant imbalance in the bacteria–tissue relationship and the production of substances which have the capacity for damaging the tissues. This is amply demonstrated in animals which do not normally suffer from dental diseases and which develop periodontal disease and caries when fed on a soft, sticky diet rich in carbohydrate.

Defence mechanisms

A number of mechanisms operate to protect the body from attack by foreign bodies and toxins, including infection by bacteria (*Figure 3.1*). These mechanisms can be classed as:

1. Non-specific mechanisms.
2. Mechanisms specific to invading foreign proteins called antigens which stimulate the immune system.

Non-specific protection mechanisms

There are five non-specific protection mechanisms.

1. Bacterial balance

The mouth as a whole and various zones in the mouth, including what has been called the 'crevicular domain', can be viewed as ecosystems in which a balance exists between the different species of microorganisms and between this flora and the tissues. Upset in this balance is most commonly seen after prolonged use of antibiotics which suppress some types of bacteria and allow others to flourish to the detriment of the tissues, e.g. the production of the fungal infection, *Candida* (thrush) after the use of some antibiotics.

2. Surface integrity

The surface integrity of skin and mucous membrane barriers, including the gingiva, is maintained by the continuing renewal of the epithelium from its base and desquamation of the surface layers. These two activities balance so that the thickness of the epithelium remains constant. The efficiency of the surface barrier is enhanced by keratinization and parakeratinization. The junctional epithelium, although semipermeable, has a very high rate of cell turnover.

3. Surface fluid and enzymes

All vital surfaces are washed by fluids which are the products of surface glands and which

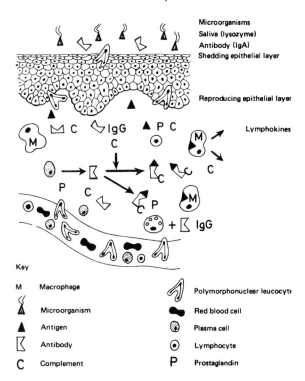

Key

M	Macrophage		Polymorphonuclear leucocyte
	Microorganism		Red blood cell
	Antigen		Plasma cell
	Antibody		Lymphocyte
C	Complement	P	Prostaglandin

Figure 3.1 Diagram to show the multiplicity of factors which take part in the tissue defence system

contain substances capable of attacking foreign material, e.g. gastric acid, lysozyme in tears washing the eyeball, and sebum from skin hair follicles. Saliva bathes the oral mucosa and contains antibacterial substances. The gingival fluid exudate flows through the junctional epithelium into the gingival crevice and this fluid contains phagocytic leucocytes and their enzymes.

4. Phagocytosis

Certain cells in the bloodstream and in the tissues are capable of engulfing and digesting foreign material. The two most important phagocytic cells are the polymorphonuclear leucocyte and the macrophage (Greek: big eater) (M in *Figure 3.1*).

Polymorphonuclear leucocytes (PMNs, neutrophils)

PMNs are the most common of the white blood cells. Produced in the bone marrow they are the most important blood cell for protecting the body against acute invasion by bacteria. Because they possess an amoeba-like ability to change shape and move rapidly they can pass through the walls of capillaries and move through the tissues, including gingival connective tissue and junctional epithelium. The direction in which they move is determined by chemical substances, mainly derived from bacteria or the complement cascade. These attract PMNs to the site of damage where foreign particles are engulfed and digested. While their role is primarily defensive PMNs can also produce proteolytic enzymes which can destroy the surrounding tissue.

Macrophages (monocytes)

The macrophage is an indiscriminate scavenger of foreign material. It starts life as a monocyte which moves into the tissues and matures to become the extremely efficient phagocyte, the macrophage, which is capable of digesting large foreign particles. If a bacterial disease lasts more than a few days the number of monocytes in the tissues increase until there may be as many monocytes as PMNs. Unlike PMNs, monocytes are capable of several divisions within the tissues which progressively increase the number of macrophages.

While PMNs are the main line of defence in acute infection the monocytes are more important in long-term chronic infection. The macrophages also take up antigens from the circulating fluid for processing and presentation to the lymphocytes.

Phagocytosis is aided by a battery of nine related proteins known as 'complement'. The complement cascade is initiated by the combination of immunoglobulin and the C1 component. The final product of the cascade is an esterase which damages cell membranes and leads to bacteriolysis. Two intermediary products, C3a and C5a, are produced which attach to receptor sites on mast cells and inflammatory cells. They release histamine and other substances from mast cells and prostaglandins from inflammatory cells, and these released substances increase vascular permeability. They are also chemotactic to PMNs. C3a also aids phagocytosis by attaching the antigen to the phagocyte via the C3 receptor on the surface of PMNs and macrophages (monocytes).

In addition, after detecting infection macrophages can secrete interleukin (IL)-6 (*see Table 3.1*) which can stimulate hepatocytes in the liver to secrete a mannose-binding protein which can bind to some bacterial capsules resistant to complement binding (Janaway, 1993). After binding it can activate the complement cascade.

There are diseases in which leucocyte-forming tissues become deficient and the number of PMNs may fall to almost zero (leucopenia).

5. *The inflammatory reaction*

The inflammatory reaction is stimulated by tissue injury and infection, and leads to changes in the local microcirculation. This produces hyperaemia, increased vascular permeability and the formation of a fluid and cellular exudate. In this way serum proteins and phagocytic cells accumulate around the irritant.

Innate immunity cannot protect against all infections as microbes evolve rapidly enabling them to devise means of evading these defence mechanisms. To counter these changes, vertebrates have developed a unique system of adaptive immunity which enables the body to recognize, remember and respond to any bacteria, virus or cancer cell even if it has never faced it before.

Specific protective mechanisms

The adaptive immune system

The unique surveillance and attack system developed to the full by mammals has three main characteristics:

1. It can distinguish between itself and the enemy, i.e. between 'self' and 'non-self' so that it does not attack parts of itself. This recognition system can go wrong and in certain diseases known as autoimmune diseases the defence system attacks pieces of its own body.
2. The defences contain elements specific against any given antigen. This is possible because each antigen contains specific amino acid sequences or 'flags' which the immune system uses to recognize 'non-self'. Antigens are proteins and because of their novelty the body does not resist the

invasion on the first attack of bacteria or viruses containing them, but within a few days or weeks the immune system will have developed specific 'answers' to each antigen. Certain non-protein substances, known as haptens, can become antigenic by associating with proteins.

3. The system has a memory. The first contact with the antigen produces a primary response in which the uneducated or virgin lymphocytes (the main cell in the immune system) proliferate and mature, and the antigen is memorized so that further contact provokes a ready secondary response.

Overview

The adaptive immune system is brought about by the actions of an array of cells which take up, process, present and react to foreign proteins known as antigens (Nossal, 1993). Antigen presenting cells such as macrophages roam the body ingesting the antigen they find and fragmenting it into antigenic peptides. Within the cell these species of peptide are joined to the major histocompatibility complex (MHC) molecules and displayed on the surface of the cell. Thymus-dependent (T) lymphocytes have antigenic surface receptors which recognize the specific antigenic peptide-MHC combinations. The T lymphocytes are activated by that process and divide to produce memory and effector cells. The effector cells secrete chemical signals (lymphokines) which mobilize other components of the immune system. One set of cells that respond to these signals are B lymphocytes which also have specific receptor molecules on their surface but unlike T lymphocytes can recognize parts of the whole antigen free in solution. When activated they differentiate into plasma cells that secrete specific antibodies which are soluble forms of their receptors. By binding to antigen the antibodies can neutralize them or precipitate their destruction by activating the complement cascade or enabling phagocytic cells to destroy them. Some B lymphocytes also persist as memory cells.

Development of immune cells

It is known that the cells concerned with immunity all develop from stem cells in the bone marrow (Weissman and Cooper, 1993). One group of these cells, T lymphocytes, is dependent on the thymus gland for its development and if this gland is removed in a foetal animal T-cell immunity does not develop. In birds another group of cells is similarly dependent on a sac in the hind gut known as the bursa of Fabricius and are known as bursal dependent or B lymphocytes. In mammals B lymphocyte development takes place in the bone marrow.

Cells destined to become T lymphocytes migrate early in foetal life to the thymus where they divide and differentiate. They give rise to successive bands of cells which migrate to the lining epithelia of body orifices and later to the lymphoid organs. The first cells going to the epithelia develop T-cell receptors (TCR) with gamma delta chains whereas the later ones going to the lymphoid organs develop TCRs with alpha-beta chains and will develop into helper (T4) and killer (T8) lymphocytes.

B lymphocytes develop under the influence of the stromal cells which produce factors needed for their growth and development. They develop interleukin (IL)-7 receptors which are stimulated by IL-7 from the stromal cells. They then progressively develop and express specific antibody receptors. They form the heavy chain first, then add the light chain and ultimately express the complete specific immunoglobulin (Ig) receptor. They produce additional Ig alpha and beta chains which associate with the Ig molecule to produce the complete receptor. If the developing B lymphocytes react with large amounts of self antigens then they are signalled to undergo programmed death (apoptosis). The clones that survive this process migrate to the lymphoid organs.

The T lymphocyte pathway is more complex and they pass through a number of challenges in their development. As they develop they make and express either CD4 or CD8 receptors. CD4 cells react with Class II MHC and become T4 helper cells and CD8 cells react with Class I MHC and become T8 killer cells. Following this the cells make and express the specific TCR. They are first tested to see whether they detect antigens presented by other cells, an essential feature of T cells. Cells which react with self MHC survive and those which do not undergo apoptosis. They also die if they react with large amounts of self antigen.

The surviving T lymphocytes migrate to the lymphoid organs and these are the cells which can recognize both foreign peptides and self-MHC.

Development of the specific receptors

There is tremendous diversity of both the TCR and Ig receptors on T and B cells respectively (Janaway, 1993; Marrak and Kappler, 1993). This is determined during their development in a unique way. Both the antibody and TCR genes are inherited as gene fragments known as mini genes which are functional only after they join together to form complete genes. This process only occurs in individual lymphocytes as they develop. The order in which they join and the joining process itself produce immense diversity. Immunoglobulins consist of heavy and light chains joined together to form a Y shape. Each cell produces one type of heavy and one type of light chain to produce together the unique Ig receptor. Each chain consists of combinations of the products of mini genes which are shuffled to produce a myriad of different combinations. Diversity springs from the size of the mini gene families which are divided into variable (V) of which there are more than 100, Diversity (D) of which there are 12 and Joining (J) of which there are 4. There are also constant (C) mini genes which only vary slightly to affect the function of the antibody and not its specificity. During development the shuffling of these mini genes into different VDJC combinations produces 4800 different heavy chains and 400 VDJ combinations in the light chains making 1 920 000 antibody genes. In addition, special enzymes insert a few extra DNA coding units at VD or DJ junctions which further increases diversity.

The alpha-beta or gamma-delta chains of the TCR of T lymphocytes are constructed in a similar way producing similar levels of diversity.

Lymphoid tissues

Nearly all the T lymphocytes in the lymphoid organs and over 90% of those in the blood have alpha-beta TCRs whereas virtually all such cells associated with epithelia have gamma-delta TCRs (Lydyard and Grossi, 1993). In the lymphoid organs T and B cells which have matured but are not associated with immune responses reside in separate domains. After stimulation by antigen the cells which will participate in antibody production form new structures known as germinal centres. Three types of cells, T4 helper lymphocytes, B lymphocytes and dendritic cells, which are types of antigen presenting cell, preominate in the interface between B and T cell domains.

Lymphocyte circulation

Lymphocytes constantly circulate around the body to provide each lymphoid organ a rapid sampling of all the lymphocytes that may possess receptor for foreign antigens already attracting the body's attention (Weissman and Cooper, 1993). They pass into the lymphoid organs through a specialized blood vessel known as a high endothelial venule (HEV). Only lymphocytes expressing homing receptors that match the receptors on the HEV can pass through. There are two types of receptors, one which matches lymph nodes and one which matches lymphoid organs of the GI tract. When T and B cells become activated they stop producing these homing markers and produce another integrin VCAM-1 which matches receptors on blood vessels so that they pass through inflamed vessels into infected tissues.

The immune response and function (*Figure 3.2*)

Antigens are first taken up by antigen presenting cells (Janaway, 1993; Marrak and Kappler, 1993; Paul, 1993). These include macrophages throughout the body, follicular dendritic cells in lymphoid organs and dendritic and Langerhans cells present throughout the mucosal surfaces. All these cells carry the CD4 surface marker. Antigens usually in the form of infecting organisms are phagocytosed by these cells and broken down within phagolysosomes into their constituent peptides. A Class II MHC molecule made in the endoplasmic reticulum (ER) is transported to the vesicle. A covering protein chain keeps the molecule inactive until it reaches the antigenic peptide within its processing vesicle. In this vehicle the chain falls away enabling the MHC molecule to bind to any antigenic peptides there. The

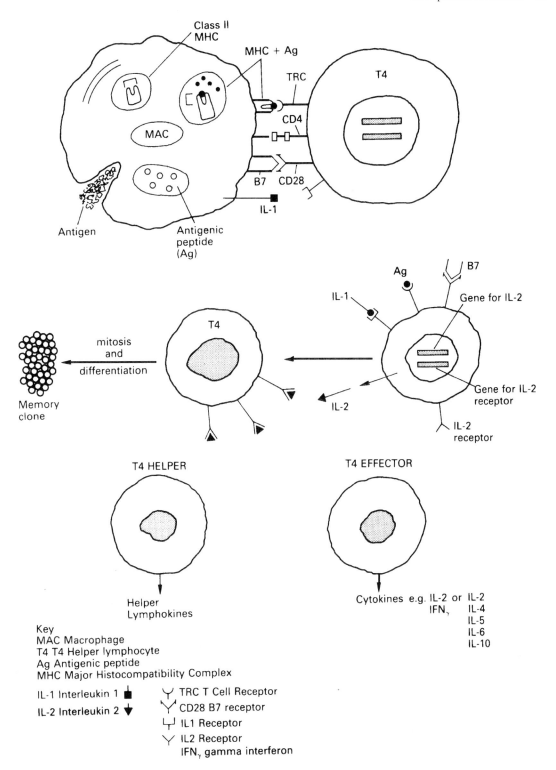

Figure 3.2 Diagram to show primary stages in the immune reaction

Table 3.1 Lymphokines and cytokines

Cytokines	Cell source(s)	Main cell target(s)	Main actions
IFNγ	T cells NK cells	Lymphocytes Macrophages Tissue cells	Immunoregulation B cell differentiation Some antiviral action
IL-1α IL-1β	Macrophages Dendritic cells Some B cells Fibroblasts Epithelial cells Endothelium Astrocytes	Thymocytes Neutrophils T and B cells	Immunoregulation Inflammation Fever Protein synthesis
IL-2	T cells NK cells	T cells, B cells Macrophages	Proliferation Activation
IL-3	T cells	Stem cells Progenitors	Pan-specific colony-stimulating factor
IL-4	T cells	B cells T cells	Division and differentiation
IL-5	T cells	B cells Eosinophils	Differentiation
IL-6	T cells Macrophages Fibroblasts Some B cells	T cells, B cells Thymocytes Hepatocytes	Differentiation Acute phase protein synthesis
IL-8 (family)	Macrophages Skin cells	Granulocytes T cells	Chemotaxis
IL-10	T cells	Macrophages T cells	Inhibits antigen presentation, production of INFγ and macrophage production of IL-1, IL-6 and TNFα
TNFα TNFβ (lymphotoxin)	Macrophages Lymphocytes	Fibroblasts Endothelium	Inflammation catabolism, fibrosis, production of other cytokines (IL-1, IL-6, GM-CSF) and adhesion molecules

complex then moves to the cell surface where it is presented so that it can be detected by T and B cells with the appropriate specific antigen receptor.

Antigenic peptides held in the groove of the Class II MHC molecule are recognized by T4 helper lymphocytes carrying CD4 marker and the appropriate TCR. The binding of the antigen to the receptor interacts with the biochemical message system in the T4 cell which will tell the cell to divide, grow, differentiate and produce its products. The lymphocyte must also receive a second message at the same time for these events to occur and if this is not received the cell will be programmed to die rather than develop. A molecule known as B7 serves this purpose and is presented at the same time by the antigen presenting cell and reacts with a CD28 receptor on the T-helper cell. B7 is only produced by infected cells and thus protects against stimulation by auto-antigens.

During this process IL-1 is also produced by the macrophage (*Table 3.1*) and reacts with its receptor on the T4 cell (Rook, 1993). This activates the appropriate genes in the T4 cell to produce IL-2 and IL-2 receptor. Stimulation by IL-2 and other cytokines causes cell division and results in the production of a clone of memory T4 cells and effector T4 cells. The effector T4 helper lymphocytes produce helper lymphokines which stimulate T4, T8 and B-lymphocytes reacting to the same antigen.

T4 immunity controlling intracellular parasites (*Figure 3.2*)

Effector T4 lymphocytes produce lymphokines which activate macrophages containing the antigens to destroy the material within their vesicles (Paul, 1993). This response occurs with intracellular bacterial or protozoan infections such as tuberculosis, leprosy, Leishmania etc. The T4 cells consist of two subsets of cells and one (TH1) secretes predominantly IL-2 and gamma interferon (IFNγ) and the other (TH2) IL-2, IL-4, IL-5, IL-6 and IL-10 (*Table 3.1*). The type of T4 response may affect the outcome. IFNγ induces macrophages to produce tumour necrosis factors (TNF) and chemicals such as nitric oxide and toxic forms of oxygen which lead to microbial destruction in the phagosome. The other response activates B lymphocytes.

Humoral immunity (*Figure 3.3*)

The antibody receptor on the surface of a B lymphocyte can recognize foreign antigens in the blood stream and binds to it (Paul, 1993). The antigen is taken into the cell and placed with a vesicle inside the cell. Class II MHC molecules made in the ER are delivered to the vesicle as previously described. It is then presented on the cell surface where it is detected by the appropriate clone of T4 helper lymphocytes. The TCR and CD4 bind to the antigen and MHC respectively. B cells also need a second signal from the T-helper cell. This comes from the production and presentation of CD40 by the helper cell which binds to the CD40 receptor on the B cell. The T4 cell produces helper lymphokines which then switch on the signal system which results in division, differentiation to plasma cells and antibody production. These helper lymphokines (*Table 3.1*) include IL-2, IL-4, IL-5, IL-6 and IFNγ (Feldmann, 1993).

When differentiation of B lymphocytes begins they cease to display their antibody receptor molecule and prepare for antibody production. The antibodies produced by the cell are the same as those which are presented by the cell as antigen receptors. Different kinds of antibody are made each with the same specificity by a different variation of the antibody molecule during development. This is done by altering the so-called constant part of the heavy chain, again by gene rearrangement. This creates different receptor areas on this part of the molecule enabling the antibodies to go to different parts of the body. After binding to antigens on the microbe these different antibody types can activate complement, promote phagocytosis (opsonization) or activate mast cells.

All antibody molecules have the same basic structure with 2 specific antigen-combining sites and a single receptor-binding site. There are 5 types of antibody molecule each made by a separate group of plasma cells. These are: IgG, IgM, IgA, IgE and IgD. IgG and IgM are found mainly in blood and inflammatory exudates. IgG is the most abundant and is a single Ig molecule with a receptor area for the C3 and Ig gamma receptors on macrophages and polymorphs. IgM is a polymer of 5 Ig molecules with the same receptors as IgG. IgA is a dimer and has a secretory piece added between the 2 molecules by cells in secretory glands which allows it to pass through glandular epithelium into the secretion where it binds to the surface of mucous membranes. IgE binds to receptors on mast cells and basophils and causes a release of mediators.

The main function of these antibody types is as follows:

IgG
- Antitoxin
- Opsonin
- Complement activation
- Neutralizes virus in blood

IgM
- Opsonin
- Bacterial agglutination

IgA
- Prevents viral attachment
- Neutralizes virus on mucous membrane
- Prevents bacterial adherence on mucous membrane
- Antitoxin

IgE
- Degranulates mast cells
  - promotes inflammation
  - some factors may be lethal to parasites
- Attaches to macrophages and may bind parasites

IgD
- Possible role in B cell function.

T8 immunity controlling viral infection (*Figure 3.4*)

Class I MHC molecules are manufactured by practically all body cells in their ER and they bind to peptides that originate from proteins in the cytosolic compartment of the cell (Paul,

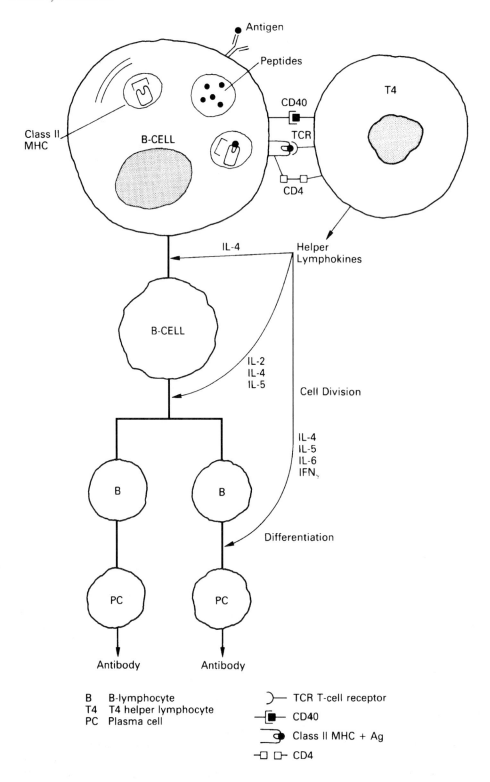

Figure 3.3 Diagram to show the principal events in humoral immunity

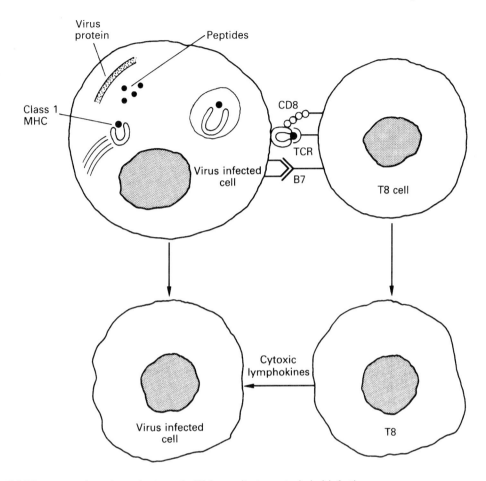

Figure 3.4 Diagram to show the main stages in T8 immunity to control viral infections

1993). Viruses infect this area of the cell and some of the viral proteins are broken down to peptides. They are pumped by a transport system into the ER. There the Class I MHC molecules are synthesized as long chains of amino acids which shape themselves around the antigenic peptide to form the complete molecule. This signals for it to be transported to the surface in a vesicle to be displayed on the surface of the cell. Here it can be detected by a killer T8 lymphocyte which expresses the CD8 protein. Again two stimuli are needed to activate the cell, one from the Class I MHC and antigen and the other from B7 which is synthesized and expressed by the body cell when it presents a foreign peptide. This links to the CD28 receptor on the T8 cell.

When activated, the killer T8 lymphocyte acts directly and indirectly to kill the infected cells. They secrete perforin and other proteins that disrupt the cellular membrane and may also release molecules that promote programmed cell death or apoptosis. They also release IFNγ and TNF (*Table 3.1*) which limit viral multiplication inside a cell and also attract macrophages and other phagocytes which can destroy the cell.

Hypersensitivity

Although the activity of the immune system has the primary function of defending the body, once set in motion its activity can become excessive and lead to gross tissue damage. This excessive activity is called hypersensitivity (Lichtenstein, 1993). There are four main types of hypersensitivity. Types I, II and III are called immediate reactions and depend on antibody-antigen reactions. Type I is related to the production of IgE antibodies which attach to receptors on mast cells and basophils resulting in the release of the contents of their granules and membranes which mediate the allergic responses. The granular mediators are histamine and platelet activating factor and the lipid mediators are leukotrienes and prostaglandin D. These dilate and increase the permeability of blood vessels, stimulate mucous production and constrict bronchial smooth muscle. Conditions caused by these reactions include hay fever, asthma, urticaria and anaphylaxis. Type II reactions involve the production of IgG antibody which activates complement on cell surfaces harbouring the antigen and cause cell damage. Type III (Arthus) reactions involve IgG antibody-antigen complexes reacting within blood vessel walls. The resulting activation of complement damages the vessel wall. Type IV hypersensitivity is termed delayed and is essentially the cell-mediated immune reaction described in the last section.

Periodontal pathology

The periodontal tissues are subject to two types of environmental factor:

1. A mechanical system in which the varying stresses of mastication demand constant modulation of the periodontal ligament, alveolar bone and cementum.
2. Those oral factors described in Chapter 2, in particular the bacterial ecosystem of the gingival crevice.

In health the periodontal tissues metabolize and function normally in harmony with these two milieux, and because of the adaptability of vital tissues a balance can be maintained within broad environmental limits.

The periodontal tissues may undergo a variety of pathological changes, inflammatory, degenerative and neoplastic. They may also be involved in autoimmune diseases. Inflammation is by far the most common form of periodontal pathology. This may be restricted to the gingivae, that is gingivitis, or involve the deeper periodontal tissues, i.e. periodontitis. Inflammation may be acute or chronic. By definition, acute inflammation comes on suddenly, is painful and is of short duration. Chronic inflammation comes on

slowly, is rarely painful and is of long duration. Acute gingivitis is usually caused by specific infection or injury. Acute periodontitis may follow a blow to a tooth or develop as a complication of chronic periodontitis. Chronic gingivitis and chronic periodontitis are successive stages in chronic inflammatory periodontal disease, and although gingival inflammation is the essential precursor to chronic periodontitis this progression is not inevitable.

Epidemiological studies indicate that this progression seems to take place in a much smaller proportion of individuals than was previously believed. Unfortunately, we cannot yet predict in which individual the progression from gingivitis to periodontitis will take place, and much current research is directed to trying to define the person who is 'at risk'. A great deal of epidemiological and clinical research in the past decade has highlighted considerable variation in clinical features and rates of disease progression, and although all periodontitis involves loss of connective tissue attachment to the root surface in the presence of gingival inflammation (Proceedings of the World Workshop in Clinical Periodontics, 1989), it is now usual practice to speak of periodontal diseases in the plural. This is not only because of the considerable variation in most features of the disease, even in the otherwise healthy individual, but also because this variation in the periodontal lesion does not appear to bear a clear and simple relationship to the causal agent, the quantity of related bacterial plaque or the types of bacteria in the plaque.

These variables are in:

1. The distribution, extent and severity of gingival inflammation.
2. The presence or absence of gingival ulceration.
3. The quantity of plaque and its bacterial constituents.
4. The extent and distribution of areas of loss of periodontal attachment, i.e. periodontitis.
5. The rapidity of loss of attachment and alveolar bone.
6. The form of the bone lesion.
7. The humoral and cellular component of the lesion described above.

This variation is further confused in the presence of systemic factors, genetic, hormonal, nutritional, haematological and pharmaceutical, as described in Chapter 6.

On classifications

Many forms of classification have been devised in attempting to provide the clinician with some rationale for making a differential diagnosis, and arriving at a reasonable prediction of how the tissues will respond to treatment. Some classifications have used variation in clinical presentation as parameters; others in trying to provide some understanding of the causes of disease have included both aetiological factors and clinical features. The results have been confusion rather than clarification.

A classification should be a systematic arrangement of groups (plants, animals, diseases etc.) that possess common attributes. This arrangement should provide insight into the relationship between groups, and between members of the same group. This requires some form of homogeneity within the group and clear delineation between groups. A very simple example of this process is to put dogs and cats in different animal groups because dogs of all kinds can interbreed but cannot mate with cats of any kind.

In the host–parasite interaction which results in periodontal pathology many factors enter the equation to produce a variety of tissue changes and therefore clinical features. On one side lie the rich oral flora plus any 'secondary' factors described in subsequent chapters; on the other side of the equation are a multiplicity of host or systemic factors. Also there are wide quantitative variations rather than a simple present or absent situation in the different parameters connected with periodontal diseases. Thus,

clear correlations between the severity of periodontal tissue destruction and, for example, specific bacterial species, or deficiencies in neutrophil activity, or even oral hygiene status, become difficult to define. Establishing a simple cause and effect relationship is impossible, and drawing the lines that a classification demands becomes a matter of approximation, and therefore of probable confusion. Given our present knowledge this would not help to bring rationality to bear on our clinical problems.

References

Feldmann, M. (1993) Cell cooperation in the antibody response. In: Roitt, I., Brostoff, J. and Male, D. (eds.) *Immunology*, 3rd edn. St. Louis: C.V. Mosby, pp. 7.1–7.16

Janaway, C.A. (1993) How the immune system recognizes invaders. *Scientific American* (Sept.) pp. 41–47

Lichenstein, L.M. (1993) Allergy and the immune system. *Scientific American* (Sept.) pp. 85–91

Lydyard, P. and Grossi, C. (1993) Cells involved in the immune response. In: Roitt, I., Brostoff, J. and Male, D. (eds.) *Immunology*, 3rd edn. St. Louis: C.V. Mosby, pp. 2.1–2.20

Marrak, P. and Kappler, J.W. (1993) How the immune system recognizes the body. *Scientific American* (Sept.) pp. 49–55

Nossal, G.V.A. (1993) Life, death and the immune system. *Scientific American* (Sept.) pp. 21–30

Paul, W. (1993) Infectious disease and the immune system. *Scientific American* (Sept.) pp. 57–63

Rook, R. (1993) Cell-mediated immune reactions. In: Roitt, I., Brostoff, J. and Male, D. (eds.) *Immunology*, 3rd edn. St. Louis: C.V. Mosby, pp. 2.1–2.20

Weissman, I.L. and Cooper, M.D. (1993) How the immune system develops. *Scientific American* (Sept.) pp. 33–39

4

The aetiology of periodontal disease

Primary factors

The primary cause of periodontal disease is bacterial irritation. However, small amounts of plaque are compatible with gingival and periodontal health (Lang *et al.*, 1973) and some patients can resist larger amounts of plaque for long periods without developing destructive periodontitis although they exhibit gingivitis.

A number of other factors, local and systemic, predispose towards plaque accumulation or alter the gingival response to plaque. These may be regarded as secondary aetiological factors.

The plaque theory

A relationship between oral hygiene and gingival disease is described in ancient writings. Today a great deal of evidence has been amassed to support this idea.

The evidence stems from clinical observation, epidemiological studies, clinical and microbiological research and, most recently, immunological investigations. This evidence can be summarized as follows:

1. The number of bacteria in the inflamed gingival crevice or periodontal pocket is greater than in a healthy crevice.
2. In the presence of gingival inflammation or periodontal pocketing the number of organisms in the mouth increases.
3. Injection of human oral bacteria into guinea-pigs produces abscess formation, i.e. these bacteria can be pathogenic.
4. Epidemiological studies of many population groups in different parts of the world demonstrate a direct correlation between the amount of bacterial deposit as measured by oral hygiene indices (see Chapter 9) and the severity of gingival inflammation.
5. Epidemiological data show a direct correlation between oral hygiene status and the degree of periodontal destruction as indicated by radiographic evidence of alveolar bone loss.
6. The experimental production of gingival inflammation by the withdrawal of all forms of oral hygiene. Löe *et al.* (1965) showed that when 12 students stopped cleaning their teeth, thus allowing plaque to accumulate around the gingival margin, gingival inflammation always appeared. When tooth cleaning was resumed and the plaque removed the inflammation disappeared (*Figure 4.1*).
7. The above experiment when repeated in Beagle dogs produced the same result. Indeed, feeding experimental animals on a soft, sticky diet is sufficient to produce periodontal disease.
8. Epidemiological studies demonstrated that oral hygiene control reduced the incidence of gingivitis.
9. Gingival inflammation produced by the withdrawal of oral hygiene measures can

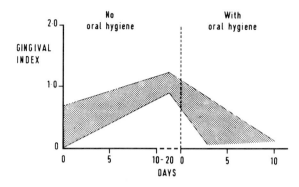

Figure 4.1 The development of gingival inflammation with the withdrawal of oral hygiene measures, followed by resolution of inflammation as plaque control is resumed. (Courtesy of Dr H. Löe)

be prevented by the use of non-specific antiseptic mouthwashes, e.g. chlorhexidine gluconate, in both man and experimental animals (Chapter 15).

10. Topical or systemic antibiotics will reduce gingival inflammation (Chapter 15).

11. Mechanical irritants, such as rough or overhanging filling margins, do not produce persistent gingival inflammation unless the fillings are covered by bacterial plaque.

12. In germ-free animals mechanical abuse of the gingivae by placing silk ligatures between the teeth does not appear to produce gingival inflammation or alveolar bone loss. When bacteria are introduced both gingival inflammation and bone loss result.

13. Cultures of bacteria from human periodontal pockets can produce enzymes which can degrade gingival and periodontal connective tissue (*see* Chapter 5).

14. In periodontal disease there is a raised antibody titre to plaque bacteria. These antibodies can be detected in blood and crevicular fluid.

15. Lymphocytes and immunoglobulin-producing plasma cells are present in gingival connective tissue and gingival fluid, and increase in amount where there is evidence of gingival inflammation.

16. *In vitro* lymphocytes are activated by plaque deposits and there is a direct correlation between the severity of periodontal disease and lymphocyte transformation.

17. When healthy young adults abstained from oral hygiene measures for 28 days the resultant accumulation of bacterial plaque and associated gingival inflammation were correlated with an increase in lymphocyte transformation and release of migration inhibition factor. These cellular responses returned to base-line values 28 days after plaque was removed (Lehner *et al.*, 1974).

Although each piece of evidence taken by itself might be questioned the aggregate provides powerful support for the plaque theory. A further conclusion from the evidence is that it takes a certain minimum amount of time for plaque products to produce inflammation. Lang *et al.* (1973) showed that if teeth are cleaned at intervals of 48 hours no gingivitis results but if cleaning is delayed for 72 hours gingival inflammation is produced.

Specific and non-specific bacterial theories of the aetiology of periodontal disease

Recently it has become popular to speak of different periodontal diseases with possible different causes. However, only three inflammatory periodontal diseases – adult chronic periodontitis (Chapter 8), juvenile periodontitis (Chapter 20) and acute ulcerative gingivitis (Chapter 21) – can be recognized as distinctive. Chronic periodontal disease includes conditions which range from gingivitis to advanced periodontitis with varying rates of progression and a diversity of clinical forms. The condition may or may not progress and when it does it may go through periods of progression, inactivity and regression (Goodson *et al.*, 1982). The controversy between the specific and non-specific theories of the microbial aetiology of inflammatory periodontal disease has continued for nearly 100 years and is discussed below.

Specific theory

According to the pure specific theory a single specific pathogen is the cause of inflammatory periodontal disease, as in the case of the well-known exogenous bacterial infections of man, such as pneumococcal pneumonia, typhoid, tuberculosis and syphilis. If this were the case, treatment would be directed towards the elimination of the specific pathogen from the mouth with the appropriate narrow-spectrum antibiotic. Following this, plaque control would no longer be necessary since plaque without the specific pathogen would be non-pathogenic (Theilade, 1986). However, no one single pathogen has been found and many suspected periodontal pathogens have been suggested, including *Actinomycetes*, spiro-chaetes and a number of Gram negative anaer-obic rods (Socransky *et al.*, 1982). Much recent work has centred around three bacterial species – *Porphyromonas gingivalis*, *Prevotella intermedia* and *Actinobacillus actinomycetem-comitans* (Slots, 1986) and spirochaetes (Listgarten and Levin, 1981; Loesche, 1988). However, none of these bacteria are foreign invaders since they are all members of the normal oral flora. Although they often make up a larger proportion of the subgingival flora in diseased sites with recent evidence of progression, they are also present in smaller numbers in non-progressive pockets and in the absence of disease (Chapter 2). Several of these organisms fulfil some of the criteria set up by Socransky (1979) to indicate pathogenic-ity, including quantitative association with disease, altered immune response, animal pathogenicity and the possession of virulence factors. However, none have yet been shown to fulfil Socransky's other criteria that disease should be cured by eliminating the suspected species without otherwise changing plaque. Such specific treatment is not effective and even the strongest supporters of the specific theory advocate (Goodson *et al.*, 1979) non-specific plaque control with subgingival scaling supplemented by the most broad-spectrum antibiotic, tetracycline (Chapter 15). It should also be noted that over 50% of the subgingi-val flora cannot be cultivated, and modern genetic methods of detecting bacteria have yielded different compositions from cultural techniques (Chapter 2). Thus the bacteria detected from any given site at any given time depend on the methods used to collect and detect them.

Studies of the bacteria associated with active stages of chronic periodontitis are hampered by the fact that the disease is a dynamic condi-tion and may have short periods of active disease progression and long periods of inactivity (Goodson *et al.*, 1982). The chances of taking a bacterial sample from the right place at the right time, coinciding with active

disease, are therefore very small and probably have never been achieved.

Non-specific theory

According to pure non-specific theory the indigenous oral bacteria colonize the gingival crevice to form plaque in the absence of effec-tive oral hygiene (Theilade, 1986). Inflammatory periodontal disease develops when bacterial proliferation exceeds the threshold of host resistance and is caused by the effects of the total plaque flora. All plaque bacteria are thought to have some virulence factors causing gingival inflammation and periodontal destruction. It is implied that plaque will cause disease regardless of its composition. Total plaque control is therefore considered necessary in the prevention and treatment of inflammatory periodontal diseases. This traditional measure, combined where necessary with subgingival scaling and root planing, has proved effective. However, the pure non-specific theory does not consider that variations in the composition of the subgingival flora may have implications for its pathogenic potential. Moreover, it does not explain why some patients or tooth sites have lifelong contained gingivitis, whereas others experience slowly or rapidly progressive periodontitis. This may, however, be due to differences in the general or local host resis-tance rather than changes in the bacterial flora.

It seems likely, therefore, that a modern theory of the microbial aetiology of periodon-tal diseases should be a compromise between the extreme versions of the specific and non-specific theories.

Unified theory of the bacterial aetiology of chronic periodontitis

The modern version of the specific theory (Socransky, 1979) has abandoned the idea of a single periodontal pathogen and states that periodontal disease can be initiated by any of a number of different pathogens. It states that 6–12 bacterial species may be responsible for the majority of cases of destructive periodon-titis and additional species may be responsible for a small number of other cases. On the other hand, the supporters of the non-specific theory agree that some indigenous bacteria are more commonly associated with disease than others and possess important virulence factors. The modern versions of two theories therefore appear to have much in common and a unified theory is possible (Theilade, 1986).

All bacterial plaque may contribute to the pathogenic potential of the subgingival flora to a greater or lesser degree by its ability to colonize and evade host defences and provoke inflammation and tissue damage. Any composition of plaque in sufficient quantity in the gingival crevice causes gingivitis but only in some cases does it lead to destructive periodontitis.

Different combinations of bacteria may be present in individual lesions and together produce the necessary virulence factors. As over 300 species of bacteria make up the oral flora, it is not surprising that different indigenous bacteria predominate in different stages of disease and in different persons and different sites within the same mouth. The increased virulence of the subgingival flora seems to be due to the emergence of a plaque ecology unfavourable to the host but favourable to the growth of bacteria with pathogenic potential (Theilade, 1986).

Over the last 25 years a selected number of bacteria from the subgingival flora have been shown to relate positively to periodontal disease progression (Socransky, 1970; van Palenstein Heldermann, 1981; Genco *et al.*, 1988; Loesche, 1988; Socransky and Haffajee, 1990; Zambon, 1990). They showed positive correlation between their presence and numbers and signs of disease such as inflammation, increased probing depth and loss of attachment. However, such correlations do not distinguish between bacteria which may be pathogenic and non-pathogens which have proliferated because of disease associated tissue change such as deepened pockets, increased serum factors from exudate and blood or bacterial shifts that may have promoted their growth (Listgarten, 1992). Unfortunately at this time it is not possible to determine in any particular patient which of the many bacteria colonizing their pockets are pathogenic or contributing to disease. Furthermore, the pathogenicity of bacterial species may differ at different stages of periodontal disease and a sequence of different bacteria may succeed one another.

Some researchers (Slots *et al.*, 1986; Bragd *et al.*, 1987) have postulated that some bacterial species may act as markers for disease since they are often associated with clinical signs of disease (Chapter 13). In this regard some retrospective studies relating bacterial species numbers to periodontal progression have shown correlations with numbers of *Porphyromonas gingivalis, Prevotella intermedia* and *Actinobacillus actinomycetemcomitans.* They have suggested that critical levels of these bacteria might be predictive for a site at risk for periodontal breakdown. Other retrospective studies using the BANA test have shown that higher numbers of *Treponema denticola, Porphyromonas gingivalis* and *Bacteroides forsythus* correlate with periodontal progression (Schmidt *et al.*, 1988). However, the retrospective nature of the correlations in these studies cannot be related to prospective disease activity.

In a prospective study (Listgarten and Levin, 1981) of a population on maintenance following treatment for periodontitis, the percentage of spirochaetes and motile rods were shown to be predictive of future pocket formation over a year. In a further 3-year prospective study (Listgarten *et al.*, 1986) similar findings were found for patients receiving irregular widely spaced maintenance visits but not for a control group receiving regular 3-monthly maintenance. Similar lack of reliability was found in attempting to predict future episodes of periodontal breakdown using *Porphyromonas gingivalis, Prevotella intermedia* and *Actinobacillus actinomycetemcomitans* as indicators in a 3-year prospective study of patients on regular maintenance following treatment of periodontitis (Listgarten *et al.*, 1991).

Having outlined the theories of bacterial involvement it needs to be emphasized that disease is produced by the interaction of oral bacteria with the tissue defences, i.e. host factors (Chapter 6).

Secondary factors

Secondary factors may be local or systemic. A number of local factors, in the gingival environment, predispose towards the accumulation of plaque deposits and prevent their removal. These are called plaque-retention factors. The systemic or host factors modify the response of the gingivae to local irritation.

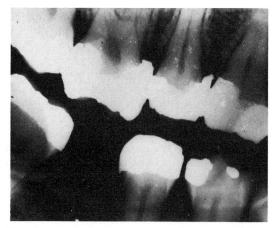

(a)

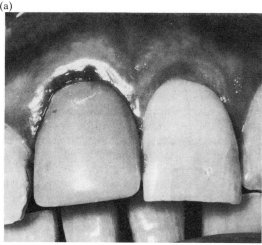

(b)

Figure 4.2 (*a*) Overhanging restoration margins. (*b*) Gingival inflammation in relation to edge of crown on 1|

Local factors

These are:

1. Faulty restorations
2. Carious cavities
3. Food impaction
4. Badly designed partial dentures
5. Orthodontic appliances
6. Malalignment of teeth
7. Lack of lip-seal or mouth-breathing
8. Tobacco smoking
9. Developmental grooves on cervical enamel or root surface

Faulty restorations are probably the most common factor favouring plaque retention.

Overhanging filling margins are extremely frequent and result from careless use of matrix bands and the failure to polish margins (*Figure 4.2*). At one time it was assumed that rough filling margins in proximity to the gingival margin actually irritated the tissue but there is no evidence for this. If there is no plaque accumulation on the restoration margin inflammation does not occur.

Badly contoured restorations, particularly overcontoured and bulbous crowns and fillings, may impede effective toothbrushing.

Carious cavities, particularly those close to the gingival margin, encourage plaque stagnation.

Food impaction is the forceful wedging of food against the gingiva between teeth. Where teeth have drifted apart food wedging can take place, especially in the presence of an opposing 'plunger cusp'. It is questionable whether actual physical trauma occurs but food impaction sites are usually sites of plaque stagnation.

Badly designed partial dentures. Dentures are foreign bodies which can cause tissue irritation in a number of ways. Ill fitting or inadequately polished dentures will tend to act as foci for plaque collection. Dentures which are tissue borne frequently sink into the mucosa and compress the gingival margins causing inflammation and tissue destruction. These effects are compounded when the dentures are inadequately cleaned and worn during sleep. A further consequence of the badly designed partial denture is excessive occlusal stress on abutment teeth, and this together with plaque-induced gingival inflamation is an extremely common cause of tooth loss.

Orthodontic appliances are worn both at night and by day and unless the patient is instructed in cleaning the appliance plaque accumulation is inevitable. As most orthodontic patients are young, a severe inflammation with gingival swelling can occur.

Tooth malalignment predisposes to plaque retention and makes plaque removal difficult (*Figure 4.3*). Unless the patient's oral hygiene technique is very thorough tooth malalignment is frequently accompanied by gingival inflammation and may provide a case for orthodontic treatment. However, it is important to be certain that orthodontic movement is justified. If a patient's oral hygiene is poor it may be just as bad if the teeth are straight. On the other

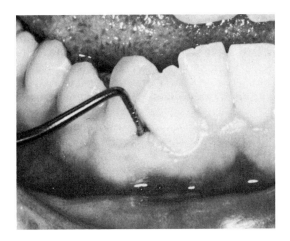

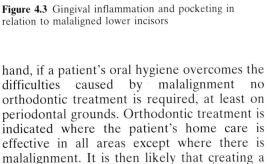

Figure 4.3 Gingival inflammation and pocketing in relation to malaligned lower incisors

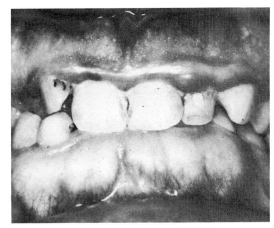

Figure 4.4 Hyperplastic gingivitis in relation to plaque deposits and lack of lip-seal

hand, if a patient's oral hygiene overcomes the difficulties caused by malalignment no orthodontic treatment is required, at least on periodontal grounds. Orthodontic treatment is indicated where the patient's home care is effective in all areas except where there is malalignment. It is then likely that creating a good alignment will also be followed by gingival health.

Other discrepancies in tooth and jaw relationship may also produce gingival inflammation. In a very deep overbite upper incisors may impinge on lower labial gingiva or lower incisors on upper palatal gingiva, causing inflammation and tissue destruction in the presence of plaque.

Failure to replace a missing tooth may result in plaque and calculus accumulations on the non-functional opposing teeth.

Lack of lip-seal. There is some uncertainty about the influence of lip posture on gingival health but a commonly occurring clinical phenomenon is a hyperplastic gingivitis in anterior segments, usually the upper incisor regions, where there is lack of lip-seal. Indeed, in many cases the area of hyperplasia is clearly delineated by the lip line (*Figure 4.4*). Although lack of lip-seal is frequently associated with mouth-breathing, inadequate lip-seal may be present, even when the patient breathes through the nose. With the lips apart the gingivae in the front of the mouth are not bathed in saliva. This seems to have two effects: (i) the normal cleansing action of saliva

is diminished so that plaque accumulation is encouraged; (ii) dehydration of the tissues may impair their resistance.

Tobacco smoking. The most obvious effect of tobacco smoking is tooth staining, but a large number of studies have shown that tobacco smoking has an influence on the prevalence and severity of periodontal diseases, gingivitis, periodontitis and acute ulcerative gingivitis. The effect of smoking on plaque and calculus deposition, gingival inflammation and bleeding, pocket depth and bone loss, as well as the bacteriology of plaque and features of the tissue response, have been investigated. Pindborg (1947) found that smokers had more calculus than non-smokers, and this was confirmed by many other studies such as those by Ainamo (1971) and Sheiham (1971), who also found that plaque deposits were greater in smokers. These early studies showed that the standard of oral hygiene in smokers was significantly poorer than in non-smokers, and Macgregor (1984, 1985) found that smokers spend less time brushing their teeth than non-smokers.

Young smokers appear to have the same degree of, or slightly more gingival inflammation than non-smokers, but in older age groups signs of inflammation are less in smokers. Bergstrom and Floderus-Myrhed (1983) and other workers have found less gingival bleeding in smokers than non-smokers, a finding which Palmer (1987) suggests could be due to vasoconstriction of gingival vessels, but may also be attributable to the heavier keratinization of the gingivae in smokers. The gingivae of smokers contain an increased number of keratinized cells (Calonius, 1962). Pocket depth is greater in smokers (Feldman *et al.*, 1983; Stoltenberg *et al.*, 1993) and, alveolar bone loss is also greater in smokers (Arno *et al.*, 1959; Bergstrom *et al.*, 1991). A study of 70-year-old Swedes demonstrated that toothlessness was higher in smokers and former smokers than in non-smokers (Osterberg and Mellstrom, 1986). Further, the occurrence of refractory periodontitis, i.e. where there has been persistent failure of periodontal treatment, is found more commonly in smokers than in non-smokers (MacFarlane *et al.*, 1992).

The relationship between smoking and poor oral hygiene and its consequences is well established, but where smokers and non-smokers with comparable levels of oral hygiene are studied it is found that smoking *per se* has a marginal but significant harmful effect on the periodontal tissues. Ismail *et al.* (1983) looked at data from epidemiological studies of 3000 individuals in the USA, adjusting the data for age, sex, race, socio-economic status, oral hygiene and frequency of toothbrushing, and found that smokers had a higher Periodontal Index score in all age groups, and they suggest that although the strongest correlation is with poor oral hygiene, smoking has a weaker but independent direct relation to periodontal disease. Bergstrom *et al.* (1991) examined alveolar bone loss in 210 subjects aged 24–60 years, smokers, former smokers and non-smokers, and found a correlation between bone loss and smoking which was not plaque related.

Several investigations have been made into the nature of this direct effect, into possible changes in plaque and pocket flora, and into various components of the tissue reaction. Bacteriological studies (Bastiaan and Waite, 1978; Bardell, 1981) have produced rather unclear results about differences in the make-up of plaque flora or in the rate of plaque formation, in smokers and non-smokers. However, several changes in the tissue response have been noted.

Smoking appears to produce vasoconstriction of the gingival vasculature, and as Palmer (1987) points out, a 'reduction in the vascular component of the inflammatory response may reduce the availability of serum-derived protective factors such as antibodies and a decrease in the passage of leucocytes into the periodontal tissues.' McLaughlin *et al.* (1993) found that smoking produces a marked but transient initial increase in gingival fluid flow rate which they felt might reflect changes in the blood flow known to be produced by nicotine. In a study of the toxicity of nicotine from cigarettes Armitage *et al.* (1975) showed a 50% or more inhibition of function of oral neutrophils. In an earlier study, Eichel and Shahrick (1969) reported that tobacco smoke produced 50–100% inhibition of oral leucocytes due to loss of motility, which they ascribed to such substances as acrolein and cyanide in tobacco smoke.

In the study of refractory periodontitis by MacFarlane (*ibid*) abnormal PMN phagocytosis was found. Both motility and chemotactic ability of PMNs can be impaired, even by small amouts of tobacco smoke (Bridges *et al.*, 1977), and Peacock *et al.* (1993) have shown that in tissue cultures of human gingival fibroblasts continuous nicotine exposure enhances attachment of the fibroblasts, and at low concentrations of nicotine cell replication is stimulated.

The role of smoking in the aetiology of acute ulcerative gingivitis has been much speculated upon. When this form of periodontal disease was very common many studies found a relationship between the prevalence and severity of AUG (or ANUG, Vincent's disease, trench mouth, etc., *see* Chapter 22) and smoking. Stammers (1944) examined 1017 cases of AUG and found that almost all of them were smokers, and in looking at 3880 naval recruits aged 17–21 years, Ludwick and Massler (1952) found 20 cases of AUG, 19 of them smokers, a finding more recently confirmed in an Edinburgh study in which Kowolik and Nisbet (1983) found that 98 out of 100 indivduals with AUG were smokers. No mechanism has so far been defined to explain this relationship, but there is little doubt that smoking has multiple deleterious effects on the tissues, on vascularity and on the immune system. In a study of the effects of cigarette smoking on healing following periodontal surgery Preber and Bergstrom (1990) suggest that smoking may impair the outcome of surgical treatment.

Developmental grooves. Grooves on the root surface or the cervical crown lead to plaque accumulation and are impossible to clean. This may result in local areas of gingivitis and pocketing, most commonly seen palatal to the upper incisors. The canine fossa on the mesial surface of the upper first premolar may also act in this way.

Host factors

These are described in Chapter 6.

References

Ainamo, J. (1971) The seeming effect of tobacco consumption on the occurrence of periodontal disease and caries. *Suomen Hammaslaakariseeuran Toimituksia*, **67**, 87–94

Armitage, A.K., Dollery, C.T., George, C.F. *et al.* (1975) Absorption and metabolism of nicotine from cigarettes. *British Medical Journal*, **4**, 313

Arno, A., Schei, O., Lovdal, A. and Waerhaug, J. (1959) Alveolar bone loss as a function of tobacco consumption. *Acta Odontologica Scandinavica*, **17**, 3–10

Bardell, D. (1981) Viability of six species of normal oropharyngeal bacteria to cigarette smoke *in vitro*. *Microbios*, **32**, 7

Bastiaan, R.J. and Waite, I.M. (1978) Effects of tobacco smoking on plaque development and gingivitis. *Journal of Periodontology*, **49**, 480–482

Bergstrom, J., Eliasson, S. and Preber, H. (1991) Cigarette smoking and periodontal bone loss. *Journal of Periodontology*, **62**, 242–246

Bergstrom, J. and Floderus-Myrhed, B. (1983) Co-twin study of the relationship between smoking and some periodontal disease factors. *Community Dentistry and Oral Epidemiology*, **11**, 113–116

Bragd, L., Dahlén, G., Wikström, M. and Slots, J. (1987) The capability of *Actinobacillus actinomycetemcomitans*, *Bacteroides gingivalis* and *Bacteroides intermedius* to indicate progressive periodontitis. *Journal of Clinical Periodontology*, **14**, 95–99

Bridges, R.B., Kraal, J.H., Huang, L.J.T. and Chancellor, M.B. (1977) The effects of tobacco smoke on chemotaxis and glucose metabolism of polymorphonuclear leucocytes. *Infection and Immunology*, **15**, 115–123

Calonius, P.E.B. (1962) A cytological study on the variation of keratinization in the normal oral mucosa of young males. *Journal of the Western Society of Periodontology*, **10**, 69

Eichel, G. and Shahrick, H.A. (1969) Tobacco smoke toxicity: loss of human oral leocyte function and fluid cell metabolism. *Science*, **166**, 1424–1428

Feldman, R.S., Bravacos, J.S. and Rose, C.L. (1983) Association between smoking different tobacco products and periodontal disease indexes. *Journal of Periodontology*, **54**, 481

Genco, R.J., Zambon, J.J. and Christersson, L.A. (1988) The role of specific bacteria in periodontal disease: The origin of periodontal infections. *Advances in Dental Research*, **2**, 245–259

Goodson, J.M., Haffajee, A.D. and Socransky, S.S. (1979) Periodontal therapy by local delivery of tetracycline. *Journal of Clinical Periodontology* **6**, 83–9

Goodson, J.M., Tanner, A.C.R., Haffajee, A.D. *et al.* (1982) Patterns of progression and regression of advanced destructive periodontal disease. *Journal of Clinical Periodontology* **9**, 472–481

Ismail, A I., Burt, B.A. and Eklund, S.A. (1983) Epidemiologic patterns of smoking and periodontal disease in the United States. *Journal of the American Dental Association*, **106**, 617

Kowolik, M.J. and Nisbet, T. (1983) Smoking and acute ulcerative gingivitis. *British Dental Journal*, **154**, 241–242

Lang, N.P., Cumming, B.R. and Löe, H. (1973) Toothbrushing frequency as it relates to plaque development and gingival health. *Journal of Periodontology* **44**, 396–405

Lehner, T., Wilton, J.M.A., Challacombe, S. *et al.* (1974) Sequential cell mediated immune responses in experimental gingivitis in man. *Clinical and Experimental Immunology* **16**, 481–492

Listgarten, M.A. (1992) Microbial testing in the diagnosis of periodontal disease. *Journal of Periodontology*, **63**, 332–337

Listgarten, M.A. and Levin, S. (1981) Positive correlation between proportions of subgingival spirochaetes and motile bacteria and susceptibility of human subjects to periodontal deterioration. *Journal of Clinical Periodontology*, **8**, 122–138

Listgarten, M.A., Schifter, C.C., Sulivan, P. *et al.* (1986) Failure of a microbial assay to reliably predict disease recurrence in a treated periodontitis population receiving regularly scheduled prophylaxes. *Journal of Clinical Periodontology*, **13**, 768–773

Listgarten, M.A., Slots, J., Nowotny, A.H. *et al.* (1991) Incidence of periodontitis recurrence in treated patients with and without cultivable *Actinobacillus actinomycetemcomitans*, *Porphyromonas gingivalis* and *Prevotella intermedia*: a prospective study. *Journal of Periodontology*, **62**, 377–386

Löe, H., Theilade, E. and Jensen, S.B. (1965) Experimental gingivitis in man. *Journal of Periodontology*, **36**, 177–187

Loesche, W.J. (1988) The role of spirochaetes in periodontal disease. *Advances in Dental Research*, **2**, 275–283

Ludwick, W. and Massler, M. (1952) Relation of dental caries experience and gingivitis to cigarette smoking in males 17 to 21 years old. *Journal of Dental Research*, **31**, 319–322

MacFarlane, G.D., Herzberg, M.C., Wolff, L.F. and Hardie, N.A. (1992) Refractory periodontitis associated with abnormal polymorphonuclear leucocyte phagocytosis and cigarette smoking. *Journal of Periodontology*, **63**, 908–913

Macgregor, I.D.M. (1984) Toothbrushing efficiency in smokers and non-smokers. *Journal of Clinical Periodontology*, **11**, 313–320

Macgregor, I.D.M. (1985) Survey of toothbrushing habits in smokers and non-smokers. *Clinical Preventive Dentistry*, **7**, 27–30

McLaughlin, W.S., Lovat, F.M., Macgregor, I.D.M. and Kelly, P.J. (1993) The immediate effects of smoking on gingival fluid flow. *Journal of Clinical Periodontology*, **20**, 448–451

Osterberg, T. and Mellstrom, D. (1986) Tobacco smoking: a major risk factor for loss of teeth in three 70-year-old cohorts. *Community Dentistry and Oral Epidemiology*, **14**, 367–370

Palmer, R.M. (1987) *Tobacco Smoking and Oral Health*. Health Education Authority. Occasional Paper No. 6

Peacock, M.E., Sutherland, D.E., Schuster, G.S. *et al.* (1993) The effect of nicotine on reproduction and attachment of human gingival fibroblasts *in vitro*. *Journal of Periodontology*, **64**, 658–665

Pindborg, J.J. (1947) Tobacco and gingivitis. *Journal of Dental Research*, **26**, 261–264

Preber, H. and Bergstrom, J. (1990) Effect of cigarette smoking on periodontal healing following surgical therapy. *Journal of Clinical Periodontology*, **17**, 324–328

Schmidt, E.F., Bretz, W.A., Hutchinson, R.A. and Loesche, W.J. (1988) Correlation of the hydrolysis of benzoyl-arginine-naphthylamide (BANA) by plaque with clinical parameters and subgingival levels spirochaetes in periodontal patients. *Journal of Dental Research*, **67**, 1505–1509

Sheiham, A. (1971) Periodontal disease and oral cleanliness in tobacco smokers. *Journal of Periodontology*, **42**, 259–263

Slots, J. (1986) Bacterial specificity in adult periodontitis. A summary of recent work. *Journal of Clinical Periodontology*, **13**, 912–917

Slots, J., Bragd, L., Wikström, M. and Dahlén, G. (1986) The occurrence of *Actinobacillus actinomycetemcomitans, Bacteroides gingivalis* and *Bacteroides intermedius* in destructive periodontal disease in adults. *Journal of Clinical Periodontology*, **13**, 570–577

Slots, J. and Listgarten, M.A. (1988) *Bacteroides gingivalis, Bacteroides intermedius* and *Actinobacillus actinomycetemcomitans* in human periodontal disease. *Journal of Clinical Periodontology*, **15**, 85–93

Socransky, S.S. (1970) Relationship of bacteria to the aetiology of periodontal disease. *Journal of Dental Research*, **49**, 203–222

Socransky, S.S. (1979) Criteria for infectious agents in dental caries and periodontal disease. *Journal of Clinical Periodontology*, **6**, 16–21

Socransky, S.S., Tanner, A.C.R., Haffajee, A.D. *et al.* (1982) Present status of studies on the microbial etiology of periodontal diseases. In: Genco, R. J. and Mergenhagen, S.E. (eds). *Host-Parasite Interactions in Periodontal Diseases*. Washington DC: American Society for Microbiology, pp. 1–12

Stammers, A. (1944) Vincent's infection: observations and conclusions regarding the aetiology and treatment of 1,017 civilian cases. *British Dental Journal*, **76**, 147–155

Stoltenberg, J.L., Osborn, J.B., Philstrom, B.L. *et al.* (1993) Association between cigarette smoking, bacterial pathogens and periodontal status. *Journal of Periodontology*, **64**, 1225–1230

Theilade, E. (1986) The non-specific theory in microbial etiology of inflammatory periodontal diseases. *Journal of Clinical Periodontology*, **13**, 905–911

Van Palenstein Helderman, W.H. (1981) Microbial etiology of periodontal disease. *Journal of Clinical Periodontology*, **8**, 261–280

Zambon, J.J. (1990) Microbial risk factors in human periodontal disease. In: Bader, J.D. (ed.) *Risk Assessment in Dentistry*. Chapel-Hill: University of North Carolina. pp. 91–93

5

Mechanisms of disease production

Bacteria are the primary cause of periodontal disease but are rarely found in the tissues in chronic periodontitis except during abscess formation. Only in acute necrotizing ulcerative gingivitis are spirochaetes seen to invade the tissues on a regular basis and then only penetrate superficially. Intact crevicular epithelium is not permeable to bacteria but is permeable to bacterial antigens, metabolites and enzymes. It is assumed that inflammation and tissue destruction are brought about by these products.

Plaque bacteria produce a number of factors which may operate on the tissues directly or indirectly by stimulating the immune and inflammatory reactions.

Direct effects of bacteria

In order to cause damage bacteria must:

- Colonize the gingival crevice by evading host defences
- Damage the crevicular epithelial barrier
- Produce substances which can either directly or indirectly cause tissue damage.

These will be discussed separately below:

Evasion of host defences

A number of the putative periodontal pathogens possess potent mechanisms of evading or damaging host defences, including the following:

Direct damage to PMNs and macrophages

The leucotoxin (*see* Chapter 20) produced by some strains of *Actinobacillus actinomycetemcomitans* can damage PMNs and macrophages (Tsai *et al.*, 1979).

Reduced PMN chemotaxis

A number of bacterial species, including *Porphyromonas gingivalis, Actinobacillus actinomycetemcomitans* and *Capnocytophaga* species, can reduce PMN chemotaxis and decrease phagocytosis and intracellular killing (Slots and Genco, 1984).

Degradation of immunoglobulins

A number of Gram negative, black pigmented anaerobes and *Capnocytophaga* species produce proteases which can degrade IgG and IgA (Slots and Genco, 1984).

Degradation of fibrin

Some Gram negative, black pigmented anaerobes possess fibrinolytic activity (Slots and Genco, 1984), which will reduce the trapping of bacteria by fibrin for surface phagocytosis.

Altered lymphocyte function

A number of Gram negative bacteria and spirochaetes in the subgingival flora can alter lymphocyte function and produce immunosuppression (Schenker, 1987). It has been suggested that these mechanisms could

Table 5.1 Bacterial protease

Bacteria	AminoP	DPP	Elastase	Trypsin	ChymoT	Collagenase
P. gingivalis	–	++	–	++++	–	++++
P. intermedia	–	++	–	±	–	±
A. actino	–	–	–	–	–	+
C. gingivalis	++	++	±	++	+	–
C. ochracea	++	+	±	+	±	±
C. sputigena	++	+	+	+	±	–
T. denticola	+	±	–	++	++	+
F. nucleatum	–	–	–	–	–	–
C. recta	+	–	–	–	–	–
E. corrodens	–	–	–	–	–	–

A. actino	–	*Actinobacillus actinomycetemcomitans*	
AminoP	–	Aminopeptidase	
DPP	–	Dipeptidyl peptidase	
ChymoT	–	Chymotrypsin-like protease	
Trypsin	–	Trypsin-like protease	
Elastase	–	Elastase-like protease	

++++	Strong activity	
++	Moderate activity	
+	Weak activity	
±	Very weak activity	
–	No activity	

produce a temporary delay in the local immune response which might lead to enhanced colonization, possible invasion and tissue injury and account for the episodic nature of periodontal disease progression.

Damage to crevicular epithelium

Many bacteria in the subgingival flora seem capable of directly or indirectly damaging crevicular epithelium. Factors directly toxic to epithelium are produced by *P. gingivalis*, *Prevotella intermedia*, *A. actinomycetemcomitans*, *Treponema denticola* and *Capnocytophaga* species (Slots and Genco, 1984). This would increase the permeability of the crevicular epithelium to bacterial products and possibly to the bacteria themselves.

Degradation of periodontal tissues by bacterial enzymes

A number of the putative pathogens in the subgingival flora produce enzymes which can degrade components of the periodontal tissues and proteins essential to the defence system and these are described below.

Proteolytic enzymes from putative periodontal pathogens

A number of the putative periodontal pathogens have been shown to produce proteases which are capable of degrading periodontal tissues. The main structural proteins of gingival connective tissue and periodontal ligament are collagen and proteoglycans. An early and persistent feature of periodontal disease is breakdown of connective tissue composed of these proteins (Page and Schroeder, 1976) which can be attacked by proteases of bacterial or host origin. The bacteria associated with periodontal disease produce a variety of proteolytic enzymes which may participate in tissue breakdown. These include collagenases mainly from *Porphyromonas gingivalis* but also from *Actinobacillus actinomycetemcomitans* and spirochaetes (Robertson *et al.*, 1982); an elastase-like enzyme from spirochaetes (Uitto *et al.*, 1986) and *Capnocytophaga* species (Gazi *et al.*, 1995); trypsin-like enzymes from *P. gingivalis*, *Bacteroides forsythus*, *Treponema denticola* and other spirochaetes (Suido *et al.*, 1986), chymotrypsin-like enzymes from *T. denticola* and *Capnocytophaga* species (Uitto *et al.*, 1988), aminopeptidases from *Capnocytophaga* species (Suido *et al.*, 1986) and *Treponema denticola* (Mäkinen *et al.*, 1986) and dipeptidyl peptidases from *P. gingivalis*, *P. intermedia* and *Capnocytophaga* species (Cox *et al.*, 1993), (*Table 5.1*).

The amount of enzyme produced by each bacterial species varies considerably. A recent study has investigated the bacterial proteases from cell sonicates of putative periodontal pathogens using selective peptide substrates with appropriate inhibitors and activators

(Cox *et al.*, 1993; Gazi *et al.*, 1994; Gazi *et al.*, 1995). Strong trypsin-like activity was found in *P. gingivalis*, moderate activity from *T. denticola* and *C. gingivalis* and weak activity from *C. ochracea*, and *C. sputigena* and *Prevotella intermedia*. The activity from *P. gingivalis* and *P. intermedia* had the characteristics of a cysteine proteinase and in the case of *P. gingivalis* there appeared to be two separate cysteine proteinases, one cleaving arginine substrates and one lysine substrates (Gazi *et al.*, 1994) (*see below*). Weak chymotrypsin-like activity was found in *C. gingivalis*, *C. ochracea* and *T. denticola* (Gazi *et al.*, 1995). Weak elastase-like activity was only found in *C. sputigena* and very weak activity in *C. gingivalis* and *C. ochracea* (Gazi *et al.*, 1995). Moderate DPP-like activity was found in *P. gingivalis*, *P. intermedia* and *C. gingivalis* and weak activity in *C. ochracea*, *C. sputigena* and *T. denticola* (Cox *et al.*, 1993) (*Table 5.1*).

These proteases can degrade all the elements of periodontal connective tissue including Type I collagen, basement membrane Type IV collagen, elastin, proteoglycans and fibronectin. They can also degrade components of the host defence systems such as immunoglobulin and complement (*see previous section and below*), inactivate key components of the plasma proteinase cascade systems involved in the inflammatory response and blood clotting (*see below*) and degrade the serum proteinase inhibitor α_1-antiproteinase and α_2-macroglobulin (*see below*). Furthermore, some bacteria have fibrinolytic activity and some can also degrade haemoglobin (*see below*).

Other hydrolytic enzymes from putative periodontal pathogens

These bacteria also produce enzymes capable of degrading the non-proteinaceous elements of the periodontal connective tissue. Hyaluronidase and chondroitinase activities are produced by *C. ochracea*, *F. nucleatum*, *P. gingivalis* and *T. denticola* (Steffan and Hengtes, 1981; Tipler and Embery, 1985; Fiehn, 1986; Seddon and Shah, 1989). These could hydrolyse the glycosaminoglycan components of proteoglycans in the extracellular matrix. Neuraminidase (sialidase) activity, which is found in *B. forsythus*, *P. melaninogenicus* and *P. gingivalis* (Moncla *et al.*, 1990), might attack sialoproteins in the epithelium, thereby increasing its permeability to bacterial products. Damage to the surface of epithelial and other cells could result from the action of phospholipases from *Porphyromonas*, *Prevotella* and *Bacteroides* species (Bulkacz *et al.*, 1979, 1985). Finally, strong acid and alkaline phosphatase activities are present in *Porphyromonas*, *Prevotella*, *Bacteroides* and *Capnocytophaga* species (Slots, 1981; Laughton *et al.*, 1982a). These could contribute to alveolar bone breakdown, but probably only if bacterial invasion advances to this site.

The proteolytic and hydrolytic enzymes from individual putative periodontal pathogens are described in more detail below.

Porphyromonas gingivalis

Proteolytic enzymes

P. gingivalis produces by far the greatest proteolytic activity of any periodontal bacteria. It produces a variety of proteases which differ in size, pH optima, sensitivity to inhibitors, ability to hydrolyse specific substrates and location within or on the surface of the bacterial cell (Lawson and Meyer, 1992). When separated by gel electrophoresis, a total of eight distinct bands of proteolytic activity are seen, each with different properties (Grenier, Chao and McBride, 1989). All these proteases are produced in large quantities by this bacteria and are recognized as important factors because of their potential to favour bacterial growth and cause damage to host tissues (Loesche *et al*, 1985). A number of important proteins are hydrolysed by proteases from this bacteria. These include collagen (Toda *et al.*, 1984; Birkedal-Hansen *et al.*, 1988), fibronectin (Uitto *et al.*, 1989b; Lantz *et al.*, 1991b), immunoglobulins A1, A2 and G (Kilian, 1981; Mortensen and Kilian, 1984; Sato *et al.*, 1987; Grenier, Mayrand and McBride, 1989), complement factors (Sundqvist *et al.*, 1985; Schenkein, 1988), iron-binding proteins (Carlsson, Hofling and Sundqvist, 1984), plasma proteinase inhibitors, α_1-proteinase inhibitor and α_2-macroglobulin (Carlsson *et al.*, 1984), some key factors in the plasma proteinase cascade systems (Nilsson, Carlsson and Sundqvist, 1985) and sailvary lysozyme (Endo *et al.*, 1989).

These proteinases are produced in cell associated and secretory forms (Grenier and McBride, 1987). They could play an important role in periodontal pathology as they have the potential to degrade connective tissues and basement membrane and to interfere with host defences by degrading immunoglobulins and complement and degrading or activating inflammatory proteins (Sojar *et al.*, 1993).

Nakamura *et al.* (1991) separated the proteases in supernatants from *P. gingivalis* cultures into four separate activities which they called proteases A, B and C and a Gly-Pro dipeptidyl peptidase. Proteases B and C were thiol-dependent cysteine proteinases and had trypsin-like activity. Protease A was neither a cysteine proteinase nor had trypsin-like activity. Protease C was the most abundant and had a large molecular size. They felt that it could have represented a mixture of 2 or 3 enzymes. All the collagenolytic activity was present in this fraction. However, they stated that it could well result from a separate enzyme or enzymes from the trypsin-like proteinase.

Trypsin-like proteinases

In surveys of the proteolytic activity of oral bacteria *P. gingivalis* was found to have a particular ability to cleave peptide substrates with arginine terminal groups such as benzoyl-arginine-2-naphthylamide (BANA) or benzoyl-arginine-p-nitroanilide (BAPNA) and this activity was termed trypsin-like (Slots, 1981; Laughton *et al.*, 1982b). In cultures of *P. gingivalis* the relative amount of trypsin-like activity in bacterial cells and medium depends on the stage of growth and growth rate. During high growth rates the enzyme is mainly associated with the cells, but as the culture ages or at low growth rates the proportion of activity in the medium increases (Suido *et al.*, 1987; Tsutsui *et al.*, 1987; Fujimura and Nakamura, 1989; Minhas and Greenman, 1989). Most of the activity is associated with bacterial membranes (Yoshimura *et al.*, 1984; Tsutsui *et al.*, 1987; Fujimura and Nakamura, 1989) and the enzymes are located at the inner membrane and cell surface (Lantz *et al.*, 1993). Activity has also been found in extracellular outer membrane vesicles (Grenier and Mayrand, 1987; Smalley and Birss, 1987) with the relative amount varying in similar way to that in the supernatant (Minhas and Greenman, 1989).

The purified enzyme is inhibited by thiol blocking agents and enhanced by sulphydryl compounds (Yoshimura *et al.*, 1984; Fujimura and Nakamura, 1987; Otsuka *et al.*, 1987; Smalley and Birss, 1987; Sorsa *et al.*, 1987; Suida *et al.*, 1987; Sundqvist *et al.*, 1987; Tsutsui *et al.*, 1987; Shah *et al.*, 1991; Lantz *et al.*, 1993). It is similar in its actions to other cysteine proteinases like papain and by analogy it has been proposed that it is either known as gingivain or gingipain (*see below*).

There have also been some conflicting reports on other properties of the trypsin-like activities. Some workers have found them sensitive to the serine protease inhibitors (Sorsa *et al.*, 1987; Suido *et al.*, 1987; Sundqvist *et al.*, 1987; Tsutsui *et al.*, 1987) whilst others have not (Fujimura and Nakamura, 1987; Otsuka *et al.*, 1987; Lantz *et al.*, 1993). Also some have found a requirement for metal ions (Yoshimura *et al.*, 1984; Fujimura and Nakamura, 1987; Sorsa *et al.*, 1987; Sundqvist *et al.*, 1987; Tsutsui *et al.*, 1987) but others have found the opposite (Otsuka *et al.*, 1987; Suido *et al.*, 1987). Also, the figures for pH optimum range from 6.0–8.5 (Yoshimura *et al.*, 1984; Fujimura and Nakamura, 1987; Otsuka *et al.*, 1987; Suido *et al.*, 1987; Sundqvist *et al.*, 1987; Tsutsui *et al.*, 1987), whilst estimates for molecular weight range from 18–300 kDa (Fujimura and Nakamura, 1987; Otsuka *et al.*, 1987; Smalley and Birss, 1987; Sorsa *et al.*, 1987; Tsutsui *et al.*, 1987; Lantz *et al.*, 1993).

The most likely explanation for these variations is that there is more than one trypsin-like enzyme. In this regard, one study obtained four distinct factions of trypsin-like activity all of which appeared to be cysteine proteinases (Fujimura and Nakamura, 1989). Another separated two cysteine proteinases, both of which cleaved arginine bond and one of which also cleaved lysine bonds and a third serine proteinase (Hinode *et al.*, 1991). Similar findings (Nakamura *et al.*, 1991) have been reported by other workers. In addition, many reports on trypsin-like proteinases include descriptions of collagenase activity which is almost certainly due to separate proteinases (*see below*).

Shah *et al.* (1991) separated the trypsin-like activity from *P. gingivalis* outer membrane vesicles and culture supernatant. They showed that it was a thiol-dependent cysteine proteinase which cleaved synthetic arginine substrates. They proposed the name gingivain for this enzyme. A similar and probably identical proteinase was isolated from the culture supernatant by Chen *et al.* (1992) and they gave it the name of gingipain. They showed that it had a narrow spectrum of activity against peptide bonds containing arginine, was resistant to inhibition by serine proteinase inhibitors and was activated by glycine-containing dipeptidides. They found that it had a molecular weight of 50 k Daltons (kDa) and a pH optimum of 6.0.

Pike *et al.* (1994) separated the trypsin-like activity in *P. gingivalis* culture supernatants and found that there were two separate cysteine proteinase activities, one with arginine and one with lysine specificity respectively. The arginine specific proteinase was a high molecular weight form of gingipain and proved to be 50 kDa gingipain complexed with 44 kDa binding proteins which were shown to be haemagglutinins. The lysine specific activity had a molecular weight of 60 kDa and a pH optimum of 8.0–8.5 and was also complexed with haemagglutinin binding proteins. They called this enzyme lys-gingipain. They thought that these proteinase/haemagglutinin complexes might be involved in the uptake of haemin which is a vital metabolite for *P. gingivalis*, by haemagglutination and subsequent haemolysis of erythrocytes.

Scott *et al.* (1993) also isolated and identified this lysine specific activity and called the enzyme lys-gingivain. They showed that it was capable of cleaving high molecular weight kininogens to generate bradykinin and could also degrade fibrinogen. Thus, *P. gingivalis* produces two cysteine proteinases with trypsin-like activity. One of these is arginine specific and is called either gingivain or gingipain and the other is lysine specific and is called lys-gingivain or lys-gingipain.

As well as being essential for *P. gingivalis* nutrition these trypsin-like proteinases could be involved in periodontal tissue degradation. They degrade protein substrates such as albumin (Fujimura and Nakamura, 1987; Otsuka *et al.*, 1987; Tsutsui *et al.*, 1987; Hinode *et al.*, 1992) as well as fibronectin and other cell surface glycoproteins (Smalley *et al.*, 1988a; Uitto *et al.*, 1989b; Lantz *et al.*, 1991a), immunoglobulin A (Sato *et al.*, 1987) and lysozyme (Endo *et al.*, 1989). The reports of its collagenolytic activity (Smalley *et al.*, 1988a;

Sorsa *et al.*, 1987; Tsutsui *et al.*, 1987) probably reflect contamination of the enzyme preparation with the true collagenases (Fujimura and Nakamura, 1987), (*see below*). However, there is some evidence that the breakdown of Type I collagen by *P. gingivalis* may involve the concerted action of both a collagenase and trypsin-like enzyme (McDermid *et al.*, 1988).

Collagenolytic proteinases

Collagenolytic activity has frequently been reported in *P. gingivalis* (Robertson *et al.*, 1982; Toda *et al.*, 1984; Birkedal-Hansen *et al.*, 1988). The activity is usually described as cell bound and has also been found in extracellular outer membrane vesicles (Grenier and Mayrand, 1987). Unlike mammalian collagenase it degrades collagen into multiple fragments (Robertson *et al.*, 1982; Sundqvist *et al.*, 1987; Toda *et al.*, 1984; Birkedal-Hansen *et al.*, 1988) but the initial attack is in the triple helical region, indicating that it is a true collagenase (Birkedal-Hansen *et al.*, 1988). Further breakdown probably involves other proteases. The activity is activated by sulphydryl compounds and inhibited by thiol-blocking agents and metal chelating agents (Robertson *et al.*, 1982; Sundqvist *et al.*, 1987; Toda *et al.*, 1984; Birkedal-Hansen *et al.*, 1988). Thus, it appears to be a cysteine proteinase with a requirement for metal ions and it probably has a binding specificity for arginine residues (Toda *et al.*, 1984; Birkedal-Hansen *et al.*, 1988). Type IV collagen is also degraded by *P. gingivalis* but its activity is not affected by thiol blocking agents indicating that another enzyme is involved (Uitto *et al.*, 1988).

The separate collagenolytic enzymes from *P. gingivalis* have been investigated by several workers and separate proteinase activities have been only recently isolated.

Lawson and Meyer (1992) purified the collagenolytic activities from *P. gingivalis* using electrophoretic techniques. They showed that the enzymes were present in the bacterial cell wall and were released into the culture medium. The purified enzyme was capable of cleaving basement membrane collagen Type IV and synthetic substrates for bacterial collagenases. The activity had the characteristics of a cysteine proteinase and appeared to exist as an active precursor protein of 94 kDa molecular weight which undergoes proteolytic cleavage to 75, 56 and 19 kDa forms. It appeared to function also as an adhesin permitting the bacteria to attach to collagenous tissue.

Sojar *et al.* (1993) purified the proteases from *P. gingivalis* which were capable of cleaving the bacterial collagenase substrate called the pZ-peptide. They showed that the purified enzyme activity was present in the bacterial cell wall and was also released into the culture medium. The purified enzyme was capable of hydrolysing salt-solubilized Type I collagen, kininogen and transferrin in the presence of both calcium and dithiothreitol (a reducing agent required by cysteine proteinases) and could also function as a gelatinase. However, it failed to degrade acid-soluble Type I or Type IV collagens and fibrinogen and also did not cleave either terminal arginine or lysine or glycyl-prolyl synthetic peptide substrates. It thus appeared to be a collagenolytic cysteine proteinase with no trypsin-like or dipeptidyl peptidase activities which had a calcium and salt requirement for its activity. The native enzyme had a molecular weight of 120 kDa and its range of activity suggested that it had specificity for the Pro X Gly sequence found on several proteins including collagen.

Kato *et al.* (1992) isolated a gene (prt C) from *P. gingivalis* which coded for a protein with collagenolytic activity. They cloned the gene into *Escherichia coli* and harvested the resultant protein which was purified by gel filtration and ion exchange chromatography. The purified enzyme had a molecular weight of 35 kDa and the active enzyme behaved as a dimer. It degraded soluble and reconstituted fibrillar Type I collagen, heat denatured Type I collagen but did not degrade gelatin or synthetic substrates for bacterial collagenases. Its activity was not dependent on reducing agents, was enhanced by calcium ions and inhibited by chelating agents. It was therefore not a cysteine proteinase and had some properties of a metalloproteinase.

The three collagenolytic proteinases described above all differ from each other in important respects so it appears that at least 3 distinct collagenolytic proteinases are produced by *P. gingivalis*. These enzymes are also distinct from the two trypsin-like cysteine proteinases, the dipeptidyl peptidase and probably other proteinases degrading other proteins such as fibrinogen.

Other proteases

Another protease coding gene (tpr) has been isolated from *P. gingivalis* and cloned into *E. coli*. The resultant enzyme had a molecular weight of 64 kDa and was active against general protein substrates but not collagen (Bourgeau *et al.*, 1992). In addition, two proteinases of 120 and 150 kDa which degraded fibrinogen (Lantz *et al.*, 1991b) and fibronectin (Lantz *et al.*, 1991a,b) and a 70 kDa collagenase-like neutral protease (Sorsa *et al.*, 1987) have been isolated from *P. gingivalis*. The 150 kDa fraction has been shown to be a cysteine proteinase with trypsin-like activity and to bind to both fibrinogen and fibronectin prior to degrading them (Lantz *et al.*, 1991a). It has also been shown to be located on the outer cell membrane and to mediate attachment of the bacteria to these proteins (Lantz *et al.*, 1993). Since it cleaves fibrinogen in an identical way to plasmin it may also activate pro-collagenase and degrade fibrin and glycoproteins in the extracellular matrix and basement membrane.

Finally, *P. gingivalis* produces dipeptidyl peptidase activity against glycyl-prolyl and alanyl-prolyl dipeptides (Suido *et al.*, 1986; Nakamura *et al.*, 1991; Cox *et al.*, 1993). Glycyl-prolyl arylamidase activities have also been studied by several groups (Abiko *et al.*, 1985; Grenier and McBride, 1987; Suido *et al.*, 1987; Barua *et al.*, 1989; Kay *et al.*, 1989). These are serine proteases with a pH optima of 7.5–8.5. These activities are found in bacterial cells in association with the outer membrane and are also present in extracellular outer membrane vesicles (Grenier and McBride, 1987; Kay *et al.*, 1989).

All of the collagenolytic, trypsin-like, dipeptidyl peptidases and other proteases described above (*Table 5.1*) would appear to be located in the cell wall, to be concentrated in outer membrane vesicles and to be released into the surrounding environment in extracellular vesicles. Thus, they could enter the periodontal tissues and play a role in periodontal pathology. In summary, these proteases could:

• degrade basement membrane and extracellular matrix proteins including collagen, proteoglycans and glycoproteins such as fibronectin. This would both destroy periodontal connective tissue and facilitate bacterial invasion of the host tissues.

- Interfere with tissue repair by inhibiting clot formation or lysing the fibrin matrix in periodontal lesions.
- Activate latent host tissue collagenases which would enhance host tissue enzyme-mediated tissue destruction.
- Inactivate proteins important in host defence.

Other hydrolytic enzymes

P. gingivalis also produces hyaluronidase and chondroitinase activities (Steffen and Hengtes, 1981; Tipler and Embery, 1985; Fiehn, 1986; Seddon and Shah, 1989) which could hydrolyse the glycosaminoglycan components of proteoglycans. These activities could be present in the outer membrane vesicles (Smalley *et al.*, 1988b). It also produces neuraminidase activity (Moncla *et al.*, 1990) which might attack sialoproteins in the epithelium. Finally, it produces strong acid and alkaline phosphatase activities (Slots, 1981; Laughton *et al.*, 1982b).

Prevotella intermedia

Proteolytic enzymes

P. intermedia is capable of degrading a number of tissue proteins including collagen, fibronectin, fibrin and immunoglobulins (Wikström and Lindhe, 1986; Larjava *et al.*, 1987; Smalley *et al.*, 1988a; Uitto *et al.*, 1989b; Kilian, 1981) and proteolytic activity has also been demonstrated against gelatin (Uitto *et al.*, 1989b; Seddon and Shah, 1989). However, this proteolytic activity only showed weak trypsin-like activity (Gazi *et al.*, 1994) and had no aminopeptidase, chymotrypsin- or elastase-like activity (Slots, 1981; Laughton *et al.*, 1982a; Suido *et al.*, 1988a; Seddon and Shah, 1989). On the other hand, it has been shown to have moderate dipeptidyl peptidase activity (Suido *et al.*, 1986; Cox *et al.*, 1993).

Other hydrolytic enzymes

This bacteria also produces strong acid and alkaline phosphatase (Slots, 1981; Laughton *et al.*, 1982a).

Treponema species

Proteolytic enzymes

Treponema denticola shows significant proteolytic activity against a range of host components such as collagens Types I and IV, fibronectin, keratin and fibrin (Uitto *et al.*, 1988; Wikström and Lindhe, 1986; Larjarva *et al.*, 1987; Smalley *et al.*, 1988a; Lantz *et al.*, 1991a; Mikx and De Jong, 1987). This species also hydrolyses a number of synthetic peptide substrates including those from aminopeptidase, trypsin-, chymotrypsin- and bacterial collagenase-like activities (Laughton *et al.*, 1982a; Mäkinen *et al.*, 1986; Uitto *et al.*, 1988) (*Table 5.1*). In contrast, *T. vincentii* has negligible trypsin- and chymotrypsin-like activities (Laughton *et al.*, 1982a; Mäkinen *et al.*, 1986; Uitto *et al.*, 1988), though it does possess collagenase-like and aminopeptidase activities (Mäkinen *et al.*, 1986).

The capacity of *T. denticola* to degrade proteins appears to be mostly associated with its chymotrypsin-like activity. The partially purified activity has a molecular weight of 95 kDa, a pH optimum of 7.5 and the characteristics of a cysteine proteinase (Uitto *et al.*, 1988). The enzyme has a broad range of proteolytic activity and extensively breaks down transferrin, fibrinogen and gelatin and a limited cleavage of α_1-antiproteinase inhibitor and immunoglobulins. It has also been found to attack the basement membrane components collagen Type IV, fibronectin and laminin and this ability, together with location on the outside of the cell envelope, indicates a possible role in destruction and invasion of the epithelium by *T. denticola* (Grenier *et al.*, 1990).

The gene coding for the *T. denticola* chymotrypsin-like activity has been inserted into *E. coli* and the protein product (the cloned enzyme) showed similar properties to the bacteria itself (Que and Kuramitsu, 1990).

The trypsin-like proteinases of *T. denticola* are active against BANA and BAPNA substrates and there is evidence that two different enzymes cleave each of these substrates and furthermore the activity may vary in different strains of this bacterium. The activity against BAPNA has a molecular weight in the range of 40–69 kDa and a pH optimum of about 8.5 (Ohta *et al.*, 1986). It had the characteristics of a serine proteinase but was not able to degrade protein substrates such as haemoglobin or gelatin.

Both *T. denticola* and *T. vincentii* are able to cleave synthetic substrates for bacterial collagenase activity (Mäkinen *et al.*, 1988). Cell extracts from *T. vincentii* yielded two fractions active against this substrate with molecular weight of 23 and 75 kDa and pH optima of 7.0–8.0 and 6.5–7.5 respectively (Mäkinen *et al.*, 1988). Both activities have the characteristics of metalloproteinases and the 75 kDa fraction hydrolysed gelatin at a low rate. The gene coding for the *T. denticola* collagenase-like activity has been inserted into *E. coli* and the cloned enzyme purified and characterized (Que and Kuramitsu, 1990). This has a molecular weight of 36 kDa and a pH optimum of 7.5. Like the *T. vincentii* collagenase enzyme it has the characteristics of a metalloproteinase. However, it is unable to hydrolyse collagens Type I and IV or gelatin.

T. denticola produces both an iminopeptidase and aminopeptidase. The iminopeptidase has a molecular weight of 100 kDa, a pH optimum of 7.5 and the characteristics of a cysteine protease (Mäkinen *et al.*, 1986, 1987). As collagen is rich in proline, it is possible that the enzyme acts on degradation products to provide nutrition for the organism. Some *T. denticola* strains also produce an aminopeptidase cleaving terminal aspartic acid residues (Mäkinen *et al.*, 1986). *T. vincentii* gave the highest aminopeptidase activity cleaving terminal arginine residues and this has a molecular weight of about 200 kDa and a pH optimum of 7.0–8.0 (Mäkinen *et al.*, 1988).

Other hydrolytic enzymes

Hyaluronidase and chondroitinase activities are produced by *T. denticola* (Steffen and Hengtes, 1981; Tipler and Embery, 1985; Fiehn, 1986; Seddon and Shah, 1989) and these could hydrolyse the glycosaminoglycan components of proteoglycans.

Capnocytophaga species

Proteolytic enzymes

Capnocytophaga species show low to moderate activity against host proteins and may degrade collagen Types I and IV and immunoglobulins (Seddon and Shah, 1989;

Kilian, 1981). In a recent study both smooth and rough surfaced strains were found to possess weak to moderate activity against Type I collagen, gelatin, collagen polypeptides and synthetic bacterial collagenase substrates (Söderling *et al.*, 1991). The main fraction of the separated sample which contained these activities had a molecular weight of 54 kDa. The cleavage of IgA1 by *C. gingivalis*, *C. ochracea* and *C. sputigena* protease was inhibited by metal chelators, suggesting that metalloproteinases were involved.

Weak trypsin-like activity has been shown in *C. gingivalis*, *C. ochracea* and *C. sputigena* (Slots, 1981; Laughton *et al.*, 1982a; Nakamura and Slots, 1982; Suido *et al.*, 1986; Seddon and Shah, 1989; Söderling *et al.*, 1991; Gazi *et al.*, 1994). Chymotrypsin-like activity has also been detected in various *Capnocytophaga* species (Gazi *et al.*, 1995). In addition, weak elastase activity has been found in *C. sputigena* and very weak activity in *C. gingivalis* and *C. ochracea* (Gazi *et al.*, 1995).

A number of studies have found all *Capnocytophaga* strains and species possess high aminopeptidase and dipeptidase activity (Slots, 1981; Suido *et al.*, 1986; Söderling *et al.*, 1991).

Other hydrolytic enzymes

Hyaluronidase and chondroitinase activities are produced by *C. ochracea* (Steffen and Hengtes, 1981; Tipler and Embery, 1985; Fiehn, 1986; Seddon and Shah, 1989) which could hydrolyse the glycosaminoglycan components of proteoglycans. Strong acid and alkaline phosphatase activities are also present in *Capnocytophaga* species (Slots, 1981; Laughton *et al.*, 1982b).

Actinobacillus actinomycetemcomitans

Proteolytic enzymes

Some studies have shown that *A. actinomycetemcomitans* is able to degrade native Type I collagen (Robertson *et al.*, 1982; Rozanis and Slots, 1982; Rozanis *et al.*, 1983) and a synthetic substrate for bacterial collagenases (Rozanis *et al.*, 1983). The activity is found both in the bacterial cell and the culture medium (Robertson *et al.*, 1982, Rozanis and Slots, 1982) and it produces multiple scissions in the collagen molecule (Robertson *et al.*, 1982). The activity has the characteristics of a metalloproteinase (Robertson *et al.*, 1982; Rozanis and Slots, 1982; Rozanis *et al.*, 1983). Weak gelatinase activity has also been reported. However, surveys with a variety of other substrates have shown that this bacteria produces no trypsin-, chymotrypsin-, elastase-, dipeptidyl peptidase- or aminopeptidase-like activity (Slots, 1981; Laughton *et al.*, 1982a; Suido *et al.*, 1986; Seddon and Shah, 1989).

Fusobacterium nucleatum

Proteolytic enzymes

F. nucleatum appears to have little ability to degrade proteins or synthetic substrates for trypsin-, chymotrypsin-, elastase-, dipeptidyl peptidase-, or aminopeptidase-like activity (Suido *et al.*, 1986).

Other hydrolytic enzymes

Hyaluronidase and chondroitinase activities are produced by *F. nucleatum* (Steffen and Hengtes, 1981; Tipler and Embery, 1985; Fiehn, 1986; Seddon and Shah, 1989).

Campylobacter recta

Proteolytic enzymes

C. recta produces aminopeptidases but so far no proteinases have been detected (Umemoto *et al.*, 1991).

Eikenella corrodens

Proteolytic enzymes

E. corrodens produces proteases connected with its nutritional use of protein but these have not yet been characterized.

Bacterial metabolites and toxic factors

There are many bacterial metabolites and toxic products which can damage the tissues or stimulate inflammation. They include ammonia, toxic amines, indole, organic acids, hydrogen sulphide, methylmercaptan and dimethyl disulphide (Slots and Genco, 1984).

Gram negative bacterial cell walls contain lipopolysaccharides (LPS, endotoxins) which are released when they die. Distinct LPSs are produced by individual species but they share common properties, including activating complement by the alternative pathway and stimulating bone resorption in tissue culture. Lipoteichoic acid and peptidoglycans present in Gram positive bacterial cell walls also stimulate bone resorption (Meikle *et al.*, 1986). Extracts from Gram negative bacteria isolated from periodontal pockets can cause polyclonal B-cell activation, which could contribute to periodontal pathology by inducing B lymphocytes to produce antibodies with determinants unrelated to the activating agent. They can also induce the release of lymphokines that mediate inflammation and bone resorption.

Bacterial antigens

Each bacterial species contains many antigens which can stimulate the immune system and lead to a variety of immune and hypersensitivity reactions which may contribute to both host protection and tissue damage.

Sites of periodontal infections

The sites of periodontal infection are shown in *Figure 5.1* and listed below:

1. Supragingival plaque
2. Subgingival flora which are
   (a) Attached to the root
   (b) Free within the pocket
   (c) Within cementum
   (d) On or within the soft tissue wall of the pocket.

In all stages of periodontitis bacteria are present on the root surface and free within the pocket and from here bacterial products may enter the tissues through the pocket epithelium which is often ulcerated. *Actinomyces* species may penetrate small distances into cementum and bacterial products such as LPS may contaminate the cementum. However, the degree of penetration of these products into cementum appears superficial (Moore *et al.*, 1986). Many Gram negative bacteria have the ability to attach to Gram positive bacteria and epithelial cells (Slots and Genco, 1984). This ability is an important factor in their colonization of the subgingival environment and also

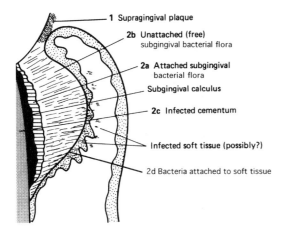

1 Supragingival plaque

2b Unattached (free) subgingival bacterial flora

2a Attached subgingival bacterial flora

Subgingival calculus

2c Infected cementum

Infected soft tissue (possibly?)

2d Bacteria attached to soft tissue

Figure 5.1 Sites of periodontal infection

allows them to colonize the surface cells of the pocket epithelium.

Bacterial invasion

It can be shown from evidence of transient bacteraemias which can follow gingival trauma that, from time to time, bacteria penetrate into the soft tissues of the pocket. However, infection of the soft tissue appears to be rare because of the ability of the immune and inflammatory systems to destroy bacteria in the tissues.

Bacterial invasion of the tissues in periodontitis has only been described occasionally in cases of advanced chronic periodontitis (Frank, 1980; Saglie *et al.*, 1982b) and juvenile periodontitis (Gillett and Johnson, 1982). Other studies of advanced chronic and juvenile periodontitis (Liakoni *et al.*, 1987) have concluded that the few bacteria in the tissues were more likely to result from passive entry in tissue processing than from active invasion. It has been suggested that bacterial invasion could be a factor in the production of an acute episode of progression in chronic periodontitis by the production of local necrosis or micro-abscesses (Allenspach-Petrzilka and Guggenheim, 1983).

Saglie *et al.* (1987) attempted to test this hypothesis by monitoring 20 patients with advanced chronic periodontitis for episodic progression. When active sites were detected

by significant attachment loss periodontal surgery was performed. Biopsies of the active sites and control inactive sites in the same patient with similar pocket depths were obtained. These tissues were examined by a number of electron microscopical and immunocytochemical techniques. They found statistically significant higher numbers of bacteria in the gingival connective tissue in active as opposed to control sites. *Porphyromonas gingivalis* and *Actinobacillus actinomycetemcomitans* were found most frequently at active sites. Several recent studies have specifically identified bacterial species in the periodontal tissues of patients with advanced chronic periodontitis or juvenile periodontitis using immunofluorescent techniques or DNA probes (Chapter 13). These are listed in *Table 5.2.*

In these studies care was taken to avoid translocation of bacteria during the surgery and tissue processing. Saglie *et al.* (1987) claimed that translocation was ruled out in their work because control biopsies did not contain bacteria, a pattern of invasion of the gingival connective tissue was seen in the intercellular spaces, bacteria were seen in the same plane as the tissue elements and bacteria were also seen within phagocytic cells.

Animal studies using normal and immuno-suppressed rats (Savani *et al.*, 1985) showed that bacterial invasion of the gingiva only occurred when virulent bacteria overcame normal host defences or when the host defences were compromised by immunosuppression.

Saglie *et al.* (1988b) have also studied the cellular infiltration associated with bacterial invasion of the gingival connective tissue. On the basis of their findings they postulated that inactive periods were associated with T-helper lymphocytes, NK-cells and macrophages and active periods with B-lymphocytes, T-cytotoxic/suppressor lymphocytes, Langerhans cells, pan lymphocytes and polymorphs. In addition, it has also been shown that bacteria in gingival connective tissue were always associated with specific antibodies and often also complement (Pekovic and Fillery, 1984). This indicates that a strong immune reaction is mounted against bacteria invading the gingiva. In most situations the local defence mechanisms will rapidly kill invading bacteria and prevent any multiplication. It would seem that

Table 5.2 Specific identification of bacteria in gingival tissue

Author	Year	Method	Bacteria	Disease
Courant and Bader	1966	Immunofluorescence	*Bacteroides melaninogenicus*	Chronic periodontitis
Takeuchi *et al.*	1974	Immunofluorescence	*Bacteroides melaninogenicus Corynebacterium*	Chronic periodontitis
Saglie *et al.*	1982a	Immunoperoxidase	*Actinobacillus actinomycetemcomitans*	Juvenile periodontitis
			Capnocytophaga sputigena	Chronic periodontitis
Pekovic and Fillery	1984	Immunofluorescence	*Actinomyces viscosus A. naeslundii Porphyromonas gingivalis Prevotella intermedia*	Chronic periodontitis
Saglie *et al.*	1988b	Immunoperoxidase	*Porphyromonas gingivalis Actinobacillus actinomycetemcomitans Capnocytophaga Fusobacterium nucleatum Bacterionema matruchotii*	Chronic and juvenile periodontitis
Saglie *et al.*	1988a	DNA Probes	*Mycoplasma pneumoniae*	Chronic and juvenile periodontitis
Christersson *et al.*	1987	Immunofluorescence	*Actinobacillus actinomycetemcomitans*	Juvenile periodontitis
Wolinsky *et al.*	1987	Immunoperoxidase	*Treponema vincentii*	Chronic periodontitis

bacteria only multiply in the gingival tissues very rarely and then only in advanced periodontitis leading to the formation of a lateral periodontal abscess.

Indirect tissue damage

Immunity

The role of the immune system in tissue degradation

Bacterial antigens penetrate the crevicular epithelium to enter the tissue and stimulate immunity. Both arms of the immune system have the potential for host protection and tissue damage. Activation of humoral immunity leads to an accumulation of plasma cells and the production of immunoglobulins, which will activate the complement cascade and lead to inflammation and generation of prostaglandins. The accumulated inflammatory cells can release tissue destructive enzymes (*see below*).

Stimulation of cellular immunity leads to the production of lymphokines from activated T lymphocytes which modulate macrophage activity. Activated macrophages (Chapter 3) release a number of cytokines and these can affect other cells leading to tissue damage. The cytokines released include interleukin-1 (IL-1), tumour necrosis factor (TNF), and gamma interferon (IFNγ) (*Table 5.3*). IL-1 can induce the release of collagenase from a variety of connective tissue cells including fibroblasts. Osteoclast activation factor (*see pp. 60–61*) has now been shown to be identical to IL-1 (Dewhirst *et al.*, 1985). Activated T-8 lymphocytes (Chapter 3) also release cytotoxic lymphokines known as perforins which disrupt cell membranes and connective tissue cells close to activated T-8 cells could be damaged.

Some clinical findings support the idea that immune responses take part in the pathogenesis of periodontal disease:

1. Patients receiving immunosuppressive drugs or who have immunodeficiency diseases have less gingival inflammation than might be expected from their oral hygiene status.
2. When drugs which enhance the immune response are given the severity of gingivitis increases.
3. Patients with a deficiency of white cells (agranulocytosis) have much more severe periodontal disease.
4. Patients with immunosuppression are prone to develop to acute ulcerative gingivitis. This can occur as a complication of HIV infections and these patients are also prone to develop an aggressive form of periodontitis (Winkler *et al.*, 1988).

Inflammation

Inflammation leads to the accumulation of PMNs, macrophages and mast cells which are very important in protecting against infection. They do, however, contain destructive enzymes within lysosomes which are capable of damaging tissue if released. Such enzymes may be released by inflammatory cells during function or when they degenerate and die. Cells and tissues in the vicinity of these cells will be damaged and this process is known as *bystander damage*. In order to understand the possible roles of these enzymes it is necessary briefly to consider collagen and proteoglycan degradation.

Collagen degradation

Collagen degradation is a multistage process. Each collagen molecule consists of two distinct regions. The larger (96% by weight) is the triple helical region which is resistant to attack by most proteinases except collagenase. The smaller terminal regions consist of peptides known as the terminal peptides, which contain the sites of intra- and intermolecular cross links. These areas can be attacked by a number of proteinases. Collagen fibrils, with intermolecular cross links are resistant to the action of collagenases and under physiological conditions a number of enzymes may act in concert (Harris and Cartwright, 1977). Mammalian collagenases

are metalloproteinases which act at neutral pH, in the presence of metal ions to cleave the triple helix into two fragments. They cannot cleave the molecule further but expose it to the action of other proteinases in the tissues or within cells. Collagenases are present in many cells and tissues as latent enzymes either as pro-enzymes or enzyme inhibitor complexes (Meikle *et al.*, 1986) and need to be activated by other proteinases. Under physiological conditions the tissues are at neutral pH and neutral proteinases are most likely involved. In inflammatory states the tissues surrounding inflammatory cells may be acidified and could also provide suitable conditions for the action of acid proteinases (Burleigh, 1977).

Proteoglycan degradation

When connective tissue is degraded in disease, the catabolism of collagen is often preceded by that of proteoglycans. Proteoglycans consist of glycosaminoglycan (GAG) molecules linked to a protein core (Bartold, 1987). Several interactions occur between individual proteoglycans and cell surfaces, basal lamina and collagen. The principal proteoglycans of gingiva and periodontal ligament are hyaluronic acid, heparin sulphate, dermatan sulphate and chondroitin sulphate 4 (Chapter 1). In bone and cementum the principal proteoglycan is chondroitin sulphate 4 with small amounts of chondroitin sulphate 6, dermatan sulphate and keratan sulphate. In proteoglycan degradation protein cleavage occurs first to release GAGs from the protein core. A number of metallo-, serine and cysteine proteinases can do this. The released GAG usually remains intact but may be further degraded. The role of the hydrolytic enzymes such as hyaluronidase, chondroitinases, aryl sulphatase and glucuronidases, in degrading proteoglycans is confusing since none of them are proteolytic. They could be involved in the subsequent degradation of the released GAGs but observations of GAGs isolated from inflamed gingiva indicate that they remain intact despite the abundance of hydrolytic enzymes in the tissues.

Proteolytic enzymes with inflammatory cells (Figure 5.2)

The proteolytic enzymes present within inflammatory cells will now be considered.

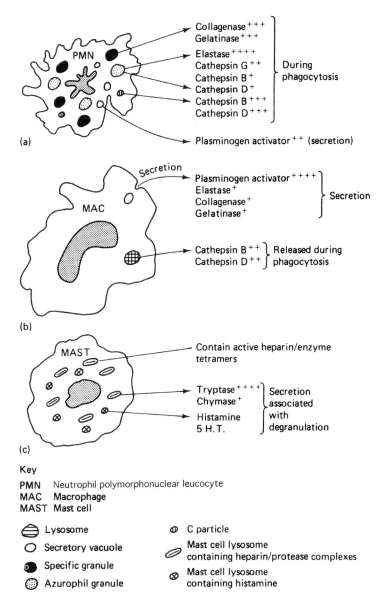

Figure 5.2 Release of proteolytic enzymes and vasoactive substances from inflammatory cells. (*a*) Neutrophil polymorphonuclear leucocyte; (*b*) macrophage; (*c*) mast cell

PMNs, macrophages and mast cells will be considered separately.

Neutrophil polymorphonuclear leucocytes (Figure 5.2a)

PMNs contain and release acid and neutral proteinases (Baggiolini *et al.*, 1980). Four distinct types of cytoplasmic body – azurophilic, specific, C-particles and secretory vacuoles – are formed during polymorph maturation.

The azurophil granules contain neutral serine proteinases, the most important of which are elastase, cathepsin G and small amounts of acid proteinases. The specific granules contain collagenase and other metalloproteinases, known as gelatinases, which can degrade collagen further once it has been cleaved by collagenase. The C granules contain the acid hydrolases cathepsins B and D. Plasminogen activator is stored in secretory vacuoles. While the granule-bound proteinases are only released during phagocytosis, plasminogen activator is secreted. Proteinases can leak from the cells into the tissues during the process of phagocytosis and are also released when cells degenerate.

Elastase can only occasionally be detected in PMNs in inflamed human gingiva using histochemical peptide substrates which only detect active enzyme (Kennett *et al.*, 1995a). In contrast elastase can be immunocytochemically detected in all gingival PMNs using a monoclonal antibody which can detect both active and inactive enzyme. This suggests that the vast majority of gingival PMNs contain inactive elastase. Using immunocytochemistry, PMNs containing elastase are found throughout the periodontal lesion and in the junctional epithelium migrating into the crevice. Numerous PMNs containing elastase can also be found in the crevice (Kennett *et al.*, 1995b). Occasional PMNs containing active elastase were only seen in a few individuals with severe periodontitis (Kennett *et al.*, 1995a) and were found in the junctional epithelium and at the active front of the lesion and could have been associated with disease activity.

Macrophages (Figure 5.2b)

Macrophages synthesize a variety of proteinases (Baggiolini *et al.*, 1980). The levels are usually low compared with those in PMNs but the amounts produced become sizeable with time. Acid and neutral proteinases are confined to different intracellular compartments. Acid proteinases (cathepsins B and D) are found in lysosymes and neutral proteinases in secretory vacuoles. The major neutral proteinase of activated inflammatory macrophages is plasminogen activator. The other neutral proteinases are present in small amounts and include the serine proteinase elastase and the metalloproteinases collagenase and gelatinase. The acid lysosomal proteinases are released during phagocytosis and although small quantities may leak out during this process they are generally confined to the cell. The neutral proteinases are all secreted. Enzyme secretion, in particular of plasminogen activator, is a characteristic property of activated macrophages.

Cathepsin B can be detected in both macrophages and fibroblasts in human gingiva either histochemically using peptide substrates detecting only active enzyme and immunocytochemically using an antibody which detects both active and inactive enzyme (Kennett *et al.*, 1994). This suggests that lysosomal cathepsin B in gingival cells is in an active form. Macrophages containing the enzyme were seen in areas of inflammatory cellular infiltration and also within the junctional epithelium migrating into the crevice. In addition, cells containing these enzymes are present in the crevice (Kennett *et al.*, 1995b).

Mast cells (Figure 5.2c)

Mast cells are important in inflammation since they release histamine and other vasoactive compounds. They also contain heparin and a number of proteinases, which are associated with heparin as active tetramers. In the absence of heparin the enzymes dissociate into inactive monomers. The principal proteolytic enzymes are tryptase and a chymotrypsin-like enzyme.

Tryptase can be histochemically detected in mast cells in the healthy and inflamed human gingiva using synthetic peptide substrates (Kennett *et al.*, 1993). Mast cells are mainly present in the lamina propria but were also found in the junctional epithelium migrating into the crevice. Greater numbers of these cells are found in inflamed as compared to healthy gingiva. Mast cells containing tryptase are also found in the gingival crevice (Kennett *et al.*, 1995b).

Control of proteolytic enzymes

Macrophages and fibroblasts and the extracellular environment contain the proteinase inhibitor alpha-1-proteinase inhibitor (α_1PI) and alpha-2-macroglobulin (α_2M) which are responsible for inactivating proteinases in the tissues (Kennett *et al.*, 1995a). Active enzyme in the tissues can only cause damage if there is an enzyme/inhibitor imbalance. This could take place in the close environment of these cells where bystander damage could occur. It might also be a local feature of episodic periodontal disease activity.

Connective tissue degradation by inflammatory cell proteinases

Proteoglycans can be degraded at neutral pH by elastase and cathepsin G (serine proteinases, SP) and at acid pH by cathepsin B (cysteine proteinase, CP) and cathepsin D (carboxylproteinase).

Collagenase (metalloproteinase, MP) can be activated at neutral pH by tryptase and plasmin (SP) and at acid pH by cathepsin B (CP).

The terminal peptide regions of collagen can be cleaved at neutral pH by elastase and at acid pH by cathepsin B.

The triple helix of collagen is specifically cleaved by collagenase and further degraded at neutral pH by gelatinases (MP) and elastase (SP) and at acid pH by cathepsin B (CP).

Tryptase (SP) can also cleave complement to generate C3a and thus increase vascular permeability; mast cell chymase (SP) can attack basal lamina, increasing epithelial permeability.

The degradation products of proteoglycans (GAGs) have been found in crevicular fluid (Embery *et al.*, 1982); collagenase, elastase, cathepsins B, D and G, tryptase, chymotrypsin and aminopeptidases have been found in gingival tissue and/or crevicular fluid (Cox and Eley, 1987, 1989a, b, c; Meikle *et al.*, 1986). The activity of a number of crevicular fluid proteases have been positively correlated with the severity of chronic periodontitis and also significantly decrease following basic periodontal treatment and periodontal surgery (Cox and Eley, 1992; Eley and Cox, 1992a, b and c). To date elastase and cathepsin B have been shown to be predictors of disease activity in longitudinal studies (Eley and Cox, 1995, 1996) (*see* also Chapter 13).

Bone resorption

The host and bacterial factors involved in bone resorption are summarized in *Table 5.3*. All understanding of how these work requires a knowledge of the physiology of bone resorption which is briefly described in this section.

Bone resorption is probably the most critical factor in periodontal attachment loss leading to eventual tooth loss. Substances produced by the subgingival bacterial flora and the tissues during inflammation and immune reactions may affect bone turnover by either

Table 5.3 Host and bacterial factors involved in bone resorption

Bacterial
  Capsular and surface associated material
  Lipopolysaccharides
  Lipoteichoic acids
  Peptidoglycan
  Muramyl dipeptide
  Lipoprotein
Host
Inflammatory mediators
  Prostaglandins e.g. PGE_2
  Leukotrienes
  12-HETEs
  Heparin
  Thrombin
  Bradykinin
Cytokines
  Interleukin-1
  Interleukin-6
  Tumour necrosis factors
  Transforming growth factor β
  Platelet derived growth factor

causing the differentiation and stimulation of osteoclasts or by inhibiting bone formation by osteoblasts.

Host and bacterial factors involved in bone resorption

The factors thought to be involved in bone resorption have been studied with tissue culture systems using embryonic bone labelled with radioactive calcium and bone loss can be detected and measured by the release of this marker. The substances which can induce resorption in periodontal disease come from two sources:

- Subgingival bacteria
- Periodontal tissues

Bacterial factors

Substances from bacteria include lipopolysaccharides (LPS) from Gram negative bacteria (Hausmann *et al.*, 1970; Hausmann, 1974), lipoteichoic acid from *Actinomyces viscosus* (Hausmann, 1974; Hausmann *et al.*, 1975), peptidoglycan (Lensgraf *et al.*, 1979), muramyl dipeptide (MDP) (Dewhirst, 1982), bacterial lipoprotein (Millar *et al.*, 1986) and capsular or surface associated material (SAM) from Gram negative bacteria (Wilson *et al.*, 1985). The potency to cause resorption *in vitro* varies with each source and LPS is 10 times more potent than lipoteichoic acid and capsular material is 1000 times more potent than the corresponding LPS (Hopps and Sisney-Durrant, 1991). Peptidoglycan, MDP and bacterial lipoprotein are all less potent than the 3 materials above. There are also differences in effect from different bacterial sources of these materials. In this regard, LPS from *P. gingivalis* is more active than those from *A. actinomycetemcomitans, C. ochracea* or *F. nucleatum*.

Capsular material or SAM stimulates the production of prostaglandin E_2 (PGE_2) and collagenase from bone cells (Harvey *et al.*, 1987). The SAMs from *P. gingivalis* and *Eikenella corrodens* appear to achieve this by first releasing IL-1 which then stimulates the release of PGE_2 and collagenase (Henderson and Blake, 1992). The SAM from *A. actinomycetemcomitans*, however, appears to mimic the action of IL-1 in its action. The main cytokine released from connective tissue and bone cells by these materials is IL-6 and it seems that this release is itself stimulated by IL-1. This is of particular relevance because IL-6 has been shown to stimulate the formation of osteoclasts (Löwick *et al.*, 1989; Löwick, 1992).

Some bacterial LPS, such as that from *E. corrodens*, also release these cytokines from these cells but most do not. LPS is however known to activate the complement cascade by the alternative pathway which generates prostaglandins.

Host factors

The main host-derived bone-resorbing factors appear to be the eicosanoids and cytokines which are generated in the gingiva and periodontium during the inflammatory and immune reactions.

Eicosanoids

Prostaglandins, hydroxyeicosatetraenoic acids (HETEs) and leukotriennes are inflammatory mediators derived from cell membrane phospholipids by the action of cyclo-oxygenase or lipoxygenases on arachadonic acid. These compounds are secreted by cells involved in inflammatory and immune reactions such as macrophages, PMNs and endothelial cells. These are also released by some cells during normal function such as fibroblasts and osteoblasts. Many of these compounds have been implicated in the pathogenesis or periodontal diseases (Seymour and Heasman, 1988).

The prostaglandins (PG) were the first mediators of local bone resorption to be discovered and may be one of the most important factors in periodontal bone loss. PGE_1, PGE_2 and prostacyclin (PGI_2) all stimulate bone resorption in tissue culture systems but PGE_2 is the most potent and stimulates increasing resorption in concentrations ranging from 1nM–10µM (Dietrich *et al.*, 1975). The levels of PGE_2 found in inflamed gingival tissue (Ohm *et al.*, 1984) and GCF from inflamed sites (Offenbacher *et al.*, 1984) fall well within the levels stimulating bone resorption *in vitro*. The GCF levels of PGE_2 also correlate with the periodontal disease status and have been claimed to predict periodontal attachment loss (Offenbacher *et al.*, 1986).

The role of prostaglandins in alveolar bone loss is supported by numerous experiments in which the effects of non-steroidal anti-inflammatory drugs (NSAIDs) on periodontal bone loss have been studied. Drugs such as indomethacin and flurbiprofen, which inhibit the synthesis of prostaglandins, markedly reduce bone loss in experimental periodontitis in animals induced by ligaments (Nyman *et al.*, 1979; Weaks-Dybvig *et al.*, 1982; Williams *et al.*, 1988) or diet (Lasfargues and Saffir, 1983).

In addition, lipo-oxygenase products of arachadonic acid also stimulate bone resorption in tissue culture experiments (Meghji *et al.*, 1988). Leukotrienes and 12-HETE are potent stimulators of bone resorption at picomolar or nanomolar concentrations. Relatively high levels of leukotrienes and HETEs are present in inflamed gingival tissue (Sighagen *et al.*, 1982; El Attar and Lin, 1982) and diseased periodontal pocket tissue (El Attar *et al.*, 1986). These experiments also showed that gingival tissue in culture metabolized arachadonic acid mainly through the lipo-oxygenase pathway and if this also occurs *in vivo* then these would be important bone resorbing factors.

Other products of inflammation

Heparin from mast cell can enhance bone resorption in tissue culture systems induced by

Table 5.4 Action of IL-1 on non-immune cells

Tissue/cell type	Prostaglandin synthesis	Proliferation	Protein synthesis	Other effects
Brain	+	–		Fever
Synovial cells	+	–	Collagenase	Proteolytic enzyme release
Bone/ osteoblasts	–	–	Collagenase	–
Cartilage/ chondrocytes	+	–	Collagenase Plasminogen activator	–
Muscle cells	+	–	–	Proteolytic enzyme release
Fibroblasts	+	+	Collagenase	–
Endothelium	+	+	Pro-coagulant activity	Boosts macrophage and PMN adhesion
Epithelium	–	–	Type IV collagen	–
Liver/ hepatocytes	–	–	Acute phase proteins	–

LPS and lipoteichoic acid, but cannot induce bone resorption on its own. Thrombin, an inflammatory mediator and end product of the blood coagulation cascade is a potent bone resorbing agent (Dziak, 1993). Another inflammatory agent, bradykinin, evokes similar effects and in both cases these effects are independent of prostaglandin production.

Cytokines

Several cytokines produced during inflammation stimulate bone resorption *in vitro* and these represent a potentially important major group of host derived bone resorbing factors which may play a role in alveolar bone loss in periodontal disease. The cytokines which have been shown to stimulate bone resorption *in vitro* include IL-1α and β (Gowen and Munday, 1986), TNFα and β (Bertolini *et al.*, 1986), transforming growth factor (TGF) (Tashjian *et al.*, 1985) and platelet derived growth factor (PDGF) (Tashjian *et al.*, 1982). In addition, IL-6 produced by fibroblasts, endothelial cells and osteoblasts may stimulate the formation of osteoclasts from precursor cells (Löwick *et al.*, 1989; Löwick, 1992). Out of all these cytokines, IL-1 and TNF are the most potent stimulators of bone resorption and are the only ones so far to be implicated in periodontal pathology (Hopps and Sisney-Durrant, 1991). IL-1 has

widespread effects on non-immune cells and these are shown in *Table 5.4.*

IL-1 is 100 times more potent than TNF and can produce resorption in picomolar concentrations. Osteoclast activation factor (OAF) has now been shown to be identical with IL-1β (Dewhirst *et al.*, 1985). IL-1β has been found in significant amounts in inflamed gingiva but has not been detected in healthy gingiva (Hönig *et al.*, 1989). Both IL-1α and β have been found in GCF from diseased sites in nanomolar concentrations which are sufficient to cause bone loss *in vitro* (Masada *et al.*, 1990). TNFα has also been detected in GCF but in low levels which are below those necessary for bone resorption *in vitro* (Rossomanda *et al.*, 1990).

The mechanism of bone resorption

The account below is based upon a wealth of experimental evidence reviewed in articles by Vaes (1988), Dziak (1993) and Meghji (1992).

Bone is continually remodelled by the combined activities of osteoblasts and osteoclasts and in pathological situations like chronic periodontitis there may be a preponderance of bone resorption over formation due to a variety of factors discussed in the previous section. The bone loss in periodontal

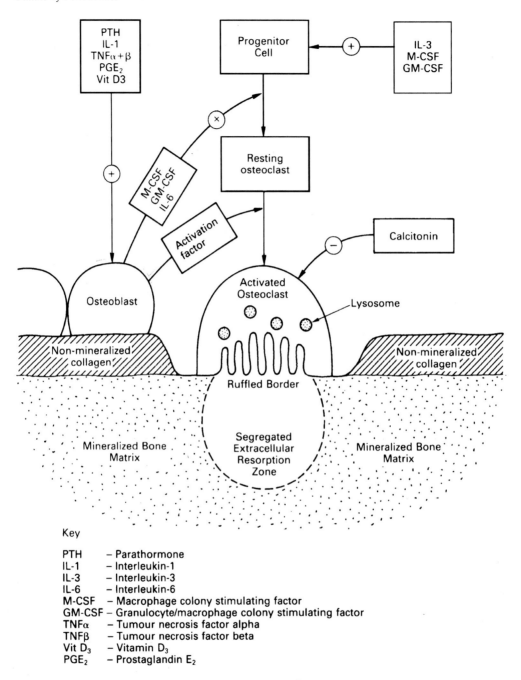

Figure 5.3 Regulation of bone resorption

disease occurs at local sites but it is regulated by both systemic and local factors.

Osteoclasts are the main effector cells in the resorptive process but it has been shown in tissue culture experiments that bone resorption cannot occur without the presence of both osteoblasts and osteoclasts. All systemic and local bone resorbing factors exert their influence by stimulating the osteoblast (*Figure 5.3*). Osteoblasts are involved in the regulation of osteoclast function at several levels. Osteoblasts have receptors for systemic

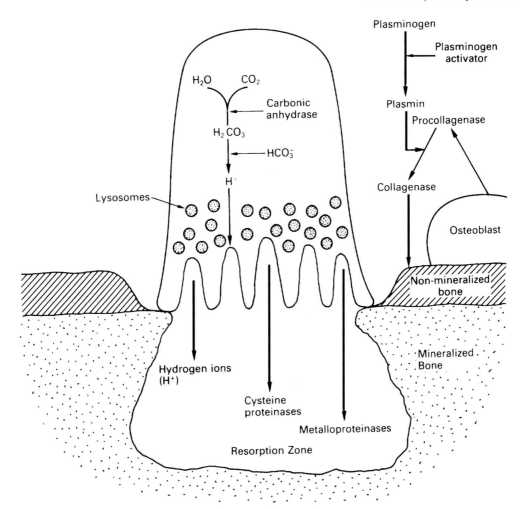

Figure 5.4 Osteoclastic function in bone resorption

factors such as parathormone (PTH) and 1,25(OH)$_2$ vitamin D$_3$ (vitamin D$_3$) which affect general remodelling, and locally produced factors such as prostaglandins, leukotrienes and cytokines which affect local changes and all exert their influence by stimulating the osteoblast in a specific way (Meikle *et al.*, 1986). In distinction, the systemic hormone, calcitonin, which favours bone deposition directly inhibits osteoclasts and causes their disaggregation into mononuclear cells. Osteoclasts have numerous receptors for calcitonin (*Figure 5.3*).

As explained in the previous section several of the locally produced factors are increased by the inflammatory and immune reactions of chronic periodontitis and some are produced by subgingival bacteria (*Table 5.3*). Osteoblasts stimulated by these factors (*Figure 5.3*) mediate their response through a series of intracellular secondary messenger systems. One pathway involves cyclic AMP and a second involves membrane phospholipids, dicycloglycerol, protein kinase C and cystolic calcium. Both of these mechanisms are stimulated by PGE$_2$ and prostocyclin (PGI$_2$) and thrombin and bradykinin. The leukotrienes and cytokines (Il-1, TNFs) do not appear to affect these intracellular mechanisms and must involve others at present unknown. In response to this stimulus osteoblasts secrete factors which both prepare the bone surface for osteoclastic resorption and stimulate the development of functional osteoclasts.

Osteoclast production involves the formation of precursor cells from stem cells in the bone marrow and the migration of these to the bone surface where they remain as pre-osteoclasts until they receive the appropriate stimulus (*Figure 5.3*). Osteoblasts stimulate osteoclast formation by the secretion of cytokines and cell to cell contact. Osteoblasts secrete growth factors, in particular granulocyte/ macrophage colony stimulating factor (GM-CSF) and macrophage colony stimulating factor (M-CSF) and IL-6. IL-6 secretion is stimulated by IL-1 attachment to its osteoblast receptor. In combination with GM-CSF and by the attachment of IL-1 to M-CSF and IL-3 it can stimulate the development of precursor cell in the marrow. IL-6 also stimulates the differentiation and maturation of these cells into osteoclasts. It cannot, however, stimulate the mature osteoclast.

Stimulated osteoblasts secrete prostaglandins and a protein made of two components (activation factor) which is responsible for activating the mature osteoclast (*Figure 5.3*). Prostaglandins also modulate osteoclast function. The pre-osteoclasts divide and fuse into multinucleated osteoclasts and spread over the bone surface prior to resorption. Stimulated osteoblasts also secrete pro-collagenase and plasminogen activator. Plasminogen activator generates plasmin from plasminogen and this activates pro-collagenase. This is then responsible for removing the non-mineralized collagenous surface layer which covers most bone surfaces in preparation for osteoclastic resorption.

Osteoclastic resorption involves firstly a solubilization of the mineral phase and secondly a dissolution of the organic matrix and these processes take place extracellularly (*Figure 5.4*). The resorption area is defined beneath the ruffled border of the osteoclast. This is a highly specialized region of cytoplasmic infolding of the plasma membrane below which is outlined a sealing or clear zone. This contains podosomes, which are specialized protrusions of the ventral membrane of the osteoclast, which adhere directly to the bone surface being broken down.

The mineral is dissolved by acid secretion which is brought about by an electrogenic hydrogen ion transporting. This is an ATPase-driven proton pump (*Figure 5.4*). Intracellular pH regulation is achieved by carbonic anhydrase, which is abundant in the osteoclast cytoplasm. Bicarbonate, generated by carbonic anhydrase appears to be secreted from the basal outer membrane via HCO_3^-/Cl^- exchange. The hydrogen ions are released into the functionally extracellular lysosomal compartment and here they solubilize the mineral and create a suitable pH for the lysomal cysteine proteinase enzyme activity which is involved in the first stage of the degradation of the demineralized bone matrix. This involves the secretion of acid cysteine proteinases including cathepsins B, L and N which have been shown to be capable of degrading collagen and proteoglycans under these conditions (*Figure 5.4*). However, recently it has been shown that the degradation of the demineralized organic matrix of bone by osteoclasts involves the production, secretion and function of both cysteine- and metallo-proteinases (Everts *et al.*, 1992; Everts, Creemers and Beertsen, 1994). Using a bone tissue culture system, they showed that when selective inhibitors of either cysteine proteinases or metalloproteinases were separately added to the system, bone demineralization occurred but there was no degradation of the remaining organic bone matrix. Therefore, degradation of the organic matrix involves both cysteine- and metalloproteinases (*Figure 5.4*). It seems likely that the cysteine proteinases are responsible for the first stage of degradation when the environment within the bone resorbing compartment below the ruffled border of the osteoclast is acid. They probably degrade the proteoglycans of the bone matrix and attack the non-helical terminal portions of the collagen molecules. In addition, they may also function to activate the metalloproteinase pro-enzymes. As the pH in this environment increases the metalloproteinase may become functional and then attack the helical portion of the collagen molecules.

References

Allenspach-Petrzilka, G.E. and Guggenheim, B. (1983) Bacterial invasion of the periodontium; an important factor in the pathogenesis of periodontitis? *Journal of Clinical Periodontology* **10**, 609–617

Abiko, Y., Hayakawa, M., Murai, S. and Takiguchi, H. (1985) Glycylprolyl dipeptidyl aminopeptidase from *Bacteroides gingivalis*. *Journal of Dental Research* **64**, 106–111

Baggiolini, M., Schnyder, J., Bretz, U. *et al.* (1980) Cellular mechanisms of proteinase release from inflammatory cells and degradation of extracellular proteins. In: Evered, D. and Whelan, J. (eds) *Protein Degradation in Health and Disease. Ciba Foundation Symposium* **75**, pp. 105–121

Bartold, P.M. (1987) Proteoglycans in the periodontium. Structure, role and function. *Journal of Periodontal Research* **22**, 431–444

Barua, P.K., Neiders, M.E., Topolnyeky, A. *et al.* (1989) Purification of an 80,000 M_r glycylprolyl peptidase from *Bacteroides gingivalis. Infection and Immunity* **57**, 2522–2528

Betolini, D.R., Nedwin, G.E., Bringman, T.S. *et al.* (1986) Stimulation of bone resorption *in vitro* by human tumour necrosis factors. *Nature* **319**, 516–519

Birkedal-Hansen, H., Taylor, R.E., Zambon, J.J. *et al.* (1988) Characterization of collagenolytic activity from strains of *Bacteroides gingivalis. Journal of Periodontal Research* **23**, 258–264

Bourgeau, G., Laponte, H., Péloquin, P. and Maryland, D. (1992) Cloning, expression and sequencing of a protease gene (*tpr*) from *Porphyromonas gingivalis* W83 in *Escherichia coli. Infection and Immunity* **60**, 3186–3192

Bulkacz, J., Newman, M.G., Socransky, S.S. *et al.* (1979) Phospholipase A activity of micro-organisms from dental plaque. *Microbiology Letters* **10**, 79–88

Bulkacz, J., Schuster, G.S., Singh, B. and Scott, D.F. (1985) Phospholipase A activity of extracellular products from *Bacteroides melaninogenicus* on epithelial tissue cultures. *Journal of Periodontal Research* **20**, 146–153

Burleigh, M.C. (1977) Degradation of collagen by non-specific proteinases. In: Barrett, A.J. (ed) *Proteinases in Mammalian Cells and Tissues.* Amsterdam: Elsevier/North-Holland Biomedical Press, pp. 185–209

Carlsson, J., Hofling, J.F. and Sundqvist, G.K. (1984) Degradation of albumin, haemopexin, heptoglobin and transferrin by black-pigmented *Bacteroides* species. *Journal of Medical Microbiology* **18**, 39–46

Carlsson, J., Hermann, B.F., Hofling, J.F. and Sundqvist, G.K. (1984) Degradation of the human proteinase inhibitors alpha-1-antitrypsin and alpha-2-macroglobulin by *Bacteroides gingivalis. Infection and Immunity* **43**, 644–648

Chen, Z., Potempa, J., Polanowski, A. *et al.* (1992) Purification and characterization of a 50-kDa cysteine proteinase (gingipain) from *Porphyromonas gingivalis. Journal of Biological Chemistry* **267**, 18896–18901

Cox, S.W. and Eley, B.M. (1987) Preliminary studies on cysteine and serine proteinase activities in inflamed human gingiva using different 7-amino-4-trifluoromethyl coumarin substrates and protease inhibitors. *Archives of Oral Biology* **32**, 599-605

Cox, S.W. and Eley, B.M. (1989a) Identification of a tryptase-like enzyme in extracts of inflamed human gingiva by effector and gel filtration studies. *Archives of Oral Biology* **34**, 219–221

Cox, S.W. and Eley, B.M. (1989b) Tryptase-like activity in crevicular fluid from gingivitis and periodontitis patients. *Journal of Periodontal Research* **24**, 41–44

Cox, S.W. and Eley, B.M. (1989c) The detection of cathepsin B and L-, elastase-, tryptase-, trypsin-, and dipeptidyl peptidase IV-like activities in crevicular fluid from gingivitis and periodontitis patients with peptidyl derivatives of 7-amino-4-trifluoromethyl coumarin. *Journal of Periodontal Research* **24**, 353–361

Cox, S.W. and Eley, B.M. (1992) Cathepsin B/L-, elastase-, tryptase-, trypsin- and dipeptidylpeptidase IV-like activities in gingival crevicular fluid: a comparison of levels before and after basic periodontal treatment. *Journal of Clnical Periodontology* **19**, 333–339

Cox, S.W., Gazi, M.I., Clark, D.T. and Eley, B.M. (1993) Host tissue and *Porphyromonas gingivalis* dipeptidyl peptidase activities in gingival crevicular fluid. *Journal of Dental Research* **72**, 705

Christersson, L.A., Wikesjö, U.M.A., Albini, B. *et al.* (1987) Tissue localisation of *Actinobacillus actinomycetemcomitans* in human periodontitis. 1. Light, immunofluorescent and electron microscopic studies. *Journal of Periodontology* **58**, 529–539

Courant, P. and Bader, H. (1966) *Bacteroides melaninogenicus* and its products in the gingiva of man. *Periodontics* **4**, 131–136

Dewhirst, F.E. (1982) N-acetyl muramyl dipeptide stimulation of bone resorption in tissue culture. *Infection and Immunity* **35**, 133–137

Dewhirst, F.E., Stashenko, P.P., Mole, J.E. and Tsurumachi, T. (1985) Purification and partial sequence of osteoclast-activation factor: identity with interleukin-1-beta. *Journal of Immunology* **135**, 2562–2568

Dietrich, F.E., Goodson, J.M. and Raisz, L.G. (1975) Stimulation of bone resorption by various prostaglandins in organ culture. *Prostaglandins* **10**, 231–240

Dziak, R. (1993) Biochemical and molecular mediators of bone metabolism. *Journal of Periodontology* **64**, 407–415

El Attar, T.M.A. and Lin, H.S. (1982) Relative conversion of arachidonic acid through lipo-oxygenase and cyclo-oxygenase pathways by homogenates of diseased periodontal tissues. *Journal of Oral Pathology* **12**, 7–10

El Attar, T.M.A., Lin, H.S., Killoy, W.J. *et al.* (1986) Hydroxy fatty acids and prostaglandins formation in diseased periodontal pocket tissue. *Journal of Periodontal Research* **21**, 169–176

Eley, B.M. and Cox, S.W. (1992a) Cathepsin B/L-, elastase-, tryptase-, trypsin- and dipeptidylpeptidase IV-like activities in gingival crevicular fluid: correlation with clinical parameters in untreated chronic periodontitis patients. *Journal of Periodóntal Research* **27**, 62–69

Eley, B.M. and Cox, S.W. (1992b) Correlation of gingival crevicular fluid proteases with clinical and radiological measurements of periodontal attachment loss. *Journal of Dentistry* **20**, 90–99

Eley, B.M. and Cox, S.W. (1992c) Cathepsin B/L-, elastase-, tryptase-, trypsin- and dipeptidylpeptidase IV-like activities in gingival crevicular fluid: a comparison before and after periodontal surgery. *Journal of Periodontology* **63**, 412–417

Eley, B.M. and Cox, S.W. (1995) A 2-year longitudinal study of elastase in gingival crevicular fluid and periodontal attachment loss. *Journal of Clinical Periodontology* (in press)

Eley, B.M. and Cox, S.W. (1996) The relationship between gingival crevicular fluid cathepsin B and periodontal attachment loss in chronic periodontitis patients. A 2-year longitudinal study. *Journal of Clinical Periodontal Research* (in press)

Embery, G., Olivier, W.M., Stanbury, J.B. and Purvis, J.A. (1982) The electrophoretic detection of acid glycosaminoglycans in human gingival sulcular fluid. *Archives of Oral Biology* **27**, 177–179

Endo, J., Otsuka, M., Ohara, E. *et al.* (1989) Cleavage action of a trypsin-like protease from *Bacteroides gingivalis* 381 on reduced egg-white lysozyme. *Archives of Oral Biology* **34**, 911–916

Everts, V., Creemers, L. and Beertsen, W. (1994) The use of selective inhibitors in the study of collagen breakdown. *Proceedings of Royal Microscopical Society* **29**, 216. Abstract 7c

Everts, V., Delaissé, J.M., Korper, W. *et al.* (1992) Degradation of collagen in the bone-resorbing compartment of the osteoclast involves both cysteine-proteinase and matrix metalloproteinases. *Journal of Cell Physiology* **150**, 221–231

Fiehn, N-E. (1986) Enzyme activities from eight small-sized oral spirochaetes. *Scandinavian Journal of Dental Research* **94**, 132–140

Frank, R.M. (1980) Bacterial penetration in the apical pocket wall of advanced human periodontitis. *Journal of Periodontal Research* **15**, 563–573

Fujimura, S. and Nakamura, T. (1987) Isolation and characterization of a protease from *Bacteroides gingivalis*. *Infection and Immunity* **55**, 716–720

Fujimura, S. and Nakamura, T. (1989) Multiple forms of proteases of *Bacteroides gingivalis* and their cellular location. *Oral Microbiology and Immunology* **4**, 227–229

Gazi, M.I., Cox, S.W., Clark, D.T. and Eley, B.M. (1994) Cathepsin B, tryptase and *Porphyromonas gingivalis* trypsin-like activities in gingival crevicular fluid. *Journal of Dental Research* **73**, 799

Gazi, M.I., Cox, S.W., Clark, D.T. and Eley, B.M. (1995) Cysteine and serine proteinases in gingival crevicular fluid: comparisons with host tissue, saliva and bacterial enzymes by analytical isoelectric focusing. *Journal of Dental Research* (in press)

Gillett, R. and Johnson, N.W. (1982) Bacterial invasion of the periodontium in a case of juvenile periodontitis. *Journal of Clinical Periodontology* **9**, 93–100

Gowen, M. and Mundy, G.R. (1986) Actions of recombinant interleukin 1, interleukin 2 and interferon γ on bone resorption *in vitro*. *Journal of Immunology* **136**, 2478–2482

Grenier, D., Chao, D. and McBride, B.C. (1989)

Characterisation of sodium dodecyl sulfate-stable *Bacteroides gingivalis* proteases by polyacrylamide gel electrophoresis. *Infection and Immunity* **57**, 95–99

Grenier, D. and McBride, B. (1987) Isolation of membrane-associated *Bacteroides gingivalis* glycylprolyl protease. *Infection and Immunity* **55**, 3131–3136

Grenier, D. and Mayrand, D. (1987) Functional characterization of extracellular vesicles produced by *Bacteroides gingivalis*. *Infection and Immunity* **55**, 111–117

Grenier, D., Mayrand, D. and McBride, B.C. (1989) Further studies on the degradation of immunoglobulins and black-pigmented *Bacteroides*. *Oral Microbiology and Immunology* **4**, 12–18

Grenier, D., Uitto, V-J. and McBride, B.C. (1990) Cellular location of a *Treponema denticola* chymotrypsin-like protease and the importance of the protease in migration through basement membrane. *Infection and Immunity* **58**, 347–351

Harris, E.D. and Cartwright, E.C. (1977) Mammalial collagenases. In: Barrett, A.J. (ed.) *Proteinases in Mammalian Cells and Tissues*. Amsterdam: Elsevier/North-Holland Biomedical Press, pp. 247–283

Harvey, W., Kamin, S., Meghji, S. and Wilson, M. (1987) Interleukin 1-like activity in capsular material from *Haemophilus actinomycetemcomitans*. *Immunology* **60**, 415–418

Hausmann, E. (1974) Potential pathways for bone resorption in human periodontal disease. *Journal of Periodontology* **45**, 338–343

Hausmann, E., Raisz, L.G. and Miller, W.A. (1970) Endotoxin: stimulation of bone resorption in tissue culture. *Science* **168**, 862–864

Hausmann, E., Ludereitz, E.O., Knox, K. and Weinfeld, N. (1975) Structural requirements for bone resorption by endotoxin and lipoteichoic acid. *Journal of Dental Research* **54**, 94–99

Henderson, B. and Blake, S. (1992) Therapeutic potential of cytokine manipulation. *Trends in Pharmacological Science* **13**, 145–152

Hinode, D., Hayashi, H. and Nakamura, R. (1991) Purification and characterization of three types of proteases from culture supernants of *Porphyromonas gingivalis*. *Infection and Immunity* **59**, 3060–3068

Hinode, D., Nagata, A., Ichimiya, S. *et al.* (1992) Generation of plasma kinin by three types of protease isolated from *Porphyromonas gingivalis* 381. *Archives of Oral Biology* **37**, 859–861

Hönig, J., Rordorf-Adam, C., Siegmund, C. *et al.* (1989) Increased interleukin-1-beta (IL-1β) concentration in gingival tissue from periodontitis patients and healthy controls. *Journal of Periodontal Research* **24**, 362–367

Hopps, R.M. and Sisney-Durrant, H.J. (1991) Mechanisms of alveolar bone loss in periodontal disease. In: Hamada, S., Holt, S.C. and McGhee, J.R. (eds) *Periodontal Disease Pathogens and Host Immune Response*. Quintessence Publishing Co. Ltd, Tokyo, pp. 307–320

Kato, T., Takahashi, N. and Kuramitsu, H. (1992)

Sequence analysis and characterization of the *Porphyromonas gingivalis ptrC* gene, which expresses a novel collagenase activity. *Journal of Bacteriology* **174**, 3889–3895

Kay, H.M., Birss, A.J. and Smalley, J.W. (1989) Glycylprolyl dipeptidase activity of *Bacteroides gingivalis* W50 and the avirulent variant W50/DE1. *FEMS Microbiology Letters* **57**, 93–96

Kennett, C.N., Cox, S.W., Eley, B.M. and Osman, I.A.R.M. (1993) Comparative histochemical and biochemical studies of mast cell tryptase in human gingiva. *Journal of Periodontology* **64**, 870–877

Kennett, C.N., Cox, S.W. and Eley, B.M. (1994) Comparative histochemical, biochemical and immunocytochemical studies of cathepsin B in human gingiva. *Journal of Periodontal Research* **29**, 870–877

Kennett, C.N., Cox, S.W. and Eley, B.M. (1995a) Localisation of active and inactive elastase, alpha-1-proteinase inhibitor and alpha-2-macroglobulin in human gingiva. *Journal of Dental Research* **74**, 667–674

Kennett, C.N., Cox, S.W. and Eley, B.M. (1995b) Investigations into the cellular contribution to host tissue protease activity in gingival crevicular fluid. *Journal of Clinical Periodontology* (in press)

Kilian, M. (1981) Degradation of immunoglobulins A1, A2 and G by suspected principal periodontal pathogens. *Infection and Immunity* **34**, 757–765

Lantz, M.S., Allen, R.D., Duck, R.D. *et al.* (1991a) *Porphyromonas gingivalis* surface components bind and degrade connective tissue proteins. *Journal of Periodontal Research* **26**, 283–285

Lantz, M.S., Allen, R.D., Vail, T.A. *et al.* (1991b) Specific cell components of *Bacteroides gingivalis* mediate binding and degradation of human fibrinogen. *Journal of Bacteriology* **173**, 495–504

Lantz, M.S., Allen, R.D., Chiorowski, P. and Holt, C.S. (1993) Purification and immunolocalisation of a cysteine protease from *Porphyromonas gingivalis*. *Journal of Periodontal Research* **28**, 467–469

Larjava, H., Uitto, V-J., Haapasalo, M. *et al.* (1987) Fibronectin fragmentation induced by dental plaque and *Bacteroides gingivalis*. *Scandinavian Journal of Dental Research* **95**, 308–314

Lasfargues, J.J. and Saffir, J.L. (1983) Effect of indomethacin on bone destruction during experimental periodontal disease on the hamster. *Journal of Periodontal Research* **18**, 110–117

Laughton, B.E., Syed, S.A. and Loesche, W.J. (1982a) API ZYM system for the identification of *Bacteroides* spp., *Capnocytophaga* spp. and spirochaetes of oral origin. *Journal of Clinical Microbiology* **15**, 97–102

Laughton, B.E., Syed, S.A. and Loesche, W.J. (1982b) The rapid identification of *Bacteroides gingivalis*. *Journal of Clinical Microbiology* **15**, 345–346

Lawson, D.A. and Meyer, T.F. (1992) Biochemical characterization of *Porphyromonas (Bacteroides) gingivalis* collagenase. *Infection and Immunity* **60**, 1524–1529

Lensgraf, E.J., Greenblatt, J.J. and Bowden, J.W. (1979) Effect of group A streptococcal peptidoglycan and

group A streptococcal cell wall on bone in tissue culture. *Archives of Oral Biology* **24**, 495–498

Liakoni, H., Barber, P. and Newman, H.N. (1987) Bacterial penetration of pocket soft tissues in chronic adult and juvenile periodontitis cases. An ultrastructural study. *Journal of Clinical Periodontology* **14**, 22–28

Loesche, W.J., Syed, S.A., Schmidt, E. and Morrison, E.C. (1985) Bacterial profiles of subgingival plaques in periodontitis. *Journal of Periodontology* **56**, 447–456

Löwick, C.W.G.M., van der Pluijm, G., Bloys, H. *et al.* (1989) Parathyroid hormone (PTH) and PTH-like protein (PLP) stimulate interleukin-6 production by osteogenic cells: a possible role of interleukin-6 in osteoclastogenesis. *Biochemical and Biophysical Research Communications* **162**, 1546–1552

McDermid, A.S., McKee, A.S. and Marsh, P.D. (1988) Effect of pH on enzyme activity and growth of *Bacteroides gingivalis* W50. *Infection and Immunity* **56**, 1096–1100

Mäkinen, K.K., Syed, S.A., Mäkinen, P-L. and Loesche, W.J. (1986) Benzlarginine peptidase and immunopeptidase profiles of *Treponema denticola* strains isolated from the human periodontal pocket. *Current Microbiology* **14**, 85–89

Mäkinen, K.K., Syed, S.A., Mäkinen, P-L. and Loesche, W.J. (1987) Dominance of immunopeptidase activity in the human oral bacterium *Treponema denticola* ATCC 35405. *Current Microbiology* **14**, 341–346

Mäkinen, K.K., Syed, S.A., Loesche, W.J. and Mäkinen, P-L. (1988) Proteolytic profile of *Treponema denticola* ATCC 35580 with special reference to collagenolytic and arginine aminopeptidase activity. *Oral Microbiology and Immunology* **3**, 121–128

Masada, M.P., Persson, R., Kenney, J.S. *et al.* (1990) Measurement of interleukin-1α and 1β in gingival crevicular fluid: implications for the pathogenesis of periodontal disease. *Journal of Periodontal Research* **25**, 156–163

Meghji, S. (1992) Bone remodelling. *British Dental Journal* **172**, 235–242

Meghji, S., Sandy, J.R., Scutt, A.M. and Harvey, W. (1988) Stimulation of bone resorption by lipo-oxygenase metabolites of arachidonic acid. *Prostaglandins* **36**, 139–149

Meikle, M.C., Heath, J.K. and Reynolds, J.J. (1986) Advances in understanding cell interactions in tissue resorption. Relevance to the pathogenesis of periodontal diseases and a new hypothesis. *Journal of Oral Pathology* **15**, 239–250

Mikx, F.H. and De Jong, M.H. (1987) Keratinolytic activity of cutaneous and oral bacteria. *Infection and Immunity* **55**, 621–625

Millar, S.J., Goldstein, E.J., Levine, M.J. and Hausmann, E. (1986) Lipoprotein: a Gram negative cell wall component that stimulates bone resorption. *Journal of Periodontal Research* **21**, 256–259

Minhas, T. and Greenman, J. (1989) Production of cell-bound and vesicle-associated trypsin-like protease, alkaline phosphatase and N-acetyl-betaglucosaminidase by *Bacteroides gingivalis* W50. *Journal of General Microbiology* **135**, 577–564

Moncla, B.L., Braham, P. and Hillier, S.L. (1990) Sialidase (neuraminidase) activity among Gram-negative anaerobic and capnophilic bacteria. *Journal of Clinical Microbiology* **28**, 422–425

Moore, J., Wilson, M. and Kieser, J.B. (1986) The distribution of bacterial lipopolysaccharide (endotoxin) in relation to periodontally involved root surfaces. *Journal of Clinical Periodontology* **13**, 748–751

Mortensen, S.B. and Kilian, M. (1984) Purification and characterization of immunoglobulin A1 protease from *Bacteroides melaninogenicus. Infection and Immunity* **45**, 550–557

Nakamura, R., Hinode, D., Terai, H. and Morioka, M. (1991) Extracellular enzymes of *Porphyromonas (Bacteroides) gingivalis* in relation to periodontal destruction. In: Hamada, S., Holt, S.C. and McGhee, J.R. (eds) *Periodontal Disease: Pathogens and Host Immune Responses*. Quintessence Publishing Co. Ltd, Tokyo, pp. 129–141

Nakamura, M. and Slots, J. (1982) Aminopeptidases of *Capnocytophaga. Journal of Periodontal Research* **17**, 597–603

Nilsson, T., Carlsson, J. and Sundqvist, G. (1985) Inactivation of key factors of the plasma proteinase cascade systems by *Bacteroides gingivalis. Infection and Immunity* **50**, 467–471

Nyman, S., Schroeder, H. and Lindhe, J. (1979) Suppression of inflammation and bone resorption by indomethacin during experimental periodontitis in dogs. *Journal of Periodontology* **50**, 450–461

Offenbacher, S., Odle, B.M., Gray, R.C. and van Dyke, T.E. (1984) Crevicular fluid prostaglandin E levels as a measure of periodontal disease status of adult and juvenile periodontitis patients. *Journal of Periodontal Research* **19**, 1–13

Offenbacher, S., Odle, B.M. and van Dyke, T.E. (1986) The use of crevicular fluid prostaglandin E_2 levels as a predictor of periodontal attachment loss. *Journal of Periodontal Research* **25**, 101–112

Ohm, K., Albers, von H.-K. and Lisboa, B.P. (1984) Measurement of 8 prostaglandins in human gingival and periodontal disease using high pressure liquid chromatography and radioimmunoassay. *Journal of Periodontal Research* **33**, 253–249

Ohta, K., Mäkinen, K. and Loesche, W.G. (1986) Purification and characterization of an enzyme produced by *Treponema denticola* capable of hydrolysing synthetic trypsin substrates. *Infection and Immunity* **53**, 213–220

Otsuka, M., Endo, J., Hinode, D. *et al.* (1987) Isolation and characterization of a protease from culture supernatant of *Bacteroides gingivalis. Journal of Periodontal Research* **22**, 491–498

Page, P.C. and Schroeder, H.E. (1976) Pathogenesis of inflammatory periodontal disease. A summary of current work. *Laboratory Investigation* **33**, 235–249

Pekovic, D.D. and Fillery, E.D. (1984) Identification of

bacteria in immunopathological mechanisms of human periodontal diseases. *Journal of Periodontal Research* **19**, 329–351

Pike, R., McGraw, W., Potempa, J. and Travis, J. (1994) Lysine- and arginine-specific proteinases from *Porphyromonas gingivalis*. Isolation, characterization and evidence for the existence of complexes with hemagglutinins. *Journal of Biological Chemistry* **269**, 406–411

Que, X-C. and Kuramitsu, H.U. (1990) Isolation and characterization of the *Treponema denticola prtA* gene coding for chymotrypsin-like protease activity and detection of a closely linked gene encoding Pz-PLGPA-hydrolysing activity. *Infection and Immunity* **58**, 4099–4105

Robertson, P.B., Lantz, P.T., Marucha, K.S. *et al.* (1982) Collagenolytic activity associated with *Bacteroides* species and *Actinobacillus actinomycetemcomitans. Journal of Periodontal Research* **17**, 275–283

Rossomando, E.F., Kennedy, J.E. and Hadjimichael, J. (1990) Tumour necrosis factor alpha in gingival crevicular fluid as a possible indicator of periodontal disease in humans. *Archives of Oral Biology* **35**, 431–434

Rozanis, J. and Slots, J. (1982) Collagenolytic activity of *Actinobacillus actinomycetemcomitans* and black-pigmented *Bacteroides. Journal of Dental Research* **61**, 275

Rozanis, J., Van Wart, H.E., Bond, M.B. and Slots, J. (1983) Further studies on collagenase of *Actinobacillus actinomycetemcomitans. Journal of Dental Research* **62**, 300

Saglie, F.R., Carranza, F.A. Jnr., Newman, M.G. *et al.* (1982a) Identification of tissue-invading bacteria in human periodontal diseases. *Journal of Periodontal Research* **17**, 452–455

Saglie, F.R., Newman, M.J., Carranza, F.A. Jnr, and Pattison, G.L. (1982b) Bacterial invasion of gingiva in advanced periodontitis in humans. *Journal of Periodontology* **53**, 217–222

Saglie, F.R., Carranza, F.A. Jnr. and Newman, M.J. (1985) The presence of bacteria within the oral epithelium of human periodontal disease. 1. A scanning and transmission electron microscopic study. *Journal of Periodontology* **56**, 618–624

Saglie, F.R., Rezende, J.H., Pertuiset, J. *et al.* (1987) Bacterial invasion during disease activity as determined by significant attachment loss. *Journal of Periodontology* **58**, 837–846

Saglie, F.R., Cheng, I. and Sadighi, R. (1988a) Detection of *Mycoplasma pneumoniae* DNA within diseased gingiva in-situ hybridization using a biotin labelled probe. *Journal of Periodontology* **59**, 121–123

Saglie, F.R., Rezende, J.H., Pertuiset, J. *et al.* (1988b) *In situ* correlative immuno-identification of mononuclear infiltrates and invasive bacteria in diseased gingiva. *Journal of Periodontology* **59**, 688–696

Sato, M., Otsuka, M., Maehara, R. *et al.* (1987) Degradation of human secretory immunoglobulin A by a protease isolated from the anaerobic periodontopathic bacteria *Bacteroides gingivalis. Archives of Oral Biology* **32**, 235–238

Savani, F., Listgarten, M.A., Boyd, F. *et al.* (1985) The colonization and establishment of invading bacteria in the periodontium of ligature-treated immunosuppressed rats. *Journal of Periodontology* **56**, 273–280

Schenkein, H.A. (1988) The effect of proteolytic *Bacteroides* species on the proteins of the human complement system. *Journal of Periodontal Research* **23**, 187–192

Schenker, B. J. (1987) Immunologic dysfunction in the pathogenesis of periodontal disease. *Journal of Clinical Periodontology* **14**, 489–498

Scott, C.F., Whitaker, E.J., Hammond, B.F. and Colman, R.W. (1993) Purification and characterization of a potent 70-kDa thiol lysyl-proteinase (Lys-gingivian) that cleaves kininogens and fibrinogen. *Journal of Biological Chemistry* **268**, 7935–7942

Seddon, S.V. and Shah, H.N. (1989) The distribution of hydrolytic enzymes among Gram-negative bacteria associated with periodontitis. *Microbial Ecology in Health and Disease* **2**, 181–190

Seymour, R.A. and Heasman, P.A. (1988) Drugs and the periodontium. *Journal of Clinical Periodontology* **15**, 1–16

Shah, H.N., Garbia, S.E., Kowlessur, D. *et al.* (1991) Gingivian; a cysteine proteinase isolated from *Porphyromonas gingivalis. Microbial Ecology in Health and Disease* **4**, 319–328

Sighagen, B., Hamberg, M. and Fredholm, B.B. (1982) Formation of 12L-hydroxyeicosatetraenoic acid (12 HETE) by gingival tissue. *Journal of Dental Research* **61**, 761–763

Slots, J. (1981) Enzymic characterization of some oral and non-oral Gram-negative bacteria with the API ZYM system. *Journal of Clinical Microbiology* **14**, 288–294

Slots, J. and Genco, R. J. (1984) Black pigmented *Bacteroides* species, *Capnocytophaga* species and *Actinobacillus actinomycetemcomitans* in human periodontal disease: virulence factors in colonisation, survival and tissue destruction. *Journal of Dental Research* **63**, 412–421

Smalley, J.W. and Birss, A.J. (1987) Trypsin-like enzyme activity of the extracellular membrane vesicles of *Bacteroides gingivalis* W50. *Journal of General Microbiology* **133**, 2883–2894

Smalley, J.W., Birss, A.J. and Suttleworth, C.A. (1988a) Degradation of type I collagen and human plasma fibrinogen by trypsin-like enzyme and extracellular membrane vesicles of *Bacteroides gingivalis* W 50. *Archives of Oral Biology* **33**, 323–329

Smalley, J.W., Birss, A.J. and Suttleworth, C.A. (1988b) Effect of the outer membrane fraction of *Bacteroides gingivalis* W50 on the glycosaminoglycan metabolism by human fibroblasts. *Archives of Oral Biology* **33**, 547–553

Söderling, E., Mäkinen, P.L., Syed, S.A. and Mäkinen, K.K. (1991) Biochemical comparison of proteolytic enzymes present in rough- and smooth-surfaced *Capnocytophaga* isolated from the subgingival plaque of periodontitis patients. *Journal of Periodontal Research* **26**, 17–23

Sojar, H.T., Lee, J-Y., Bedi, G.S. and Genco, R.J. (1993) Purification and characterization of a protease from *Porphyromonas gingivalis* capable of degrading salt-solubilized collagen. *Infection and Immunity* **61**, 2369–2376

Sorsa, T., Uitto, V.J., Suomalainen, K. *et al.* (1987) A trypsin-like protease from *Bacteroides gingivalis*. Partial purification and characterization. *Journal of Periodontal Research* **22**, 375–380

Steffan, E.K. and Hengtes, D.J. (1981) Hydrolytic enzymes of anaerobic bacteria isolated from human infections. *Journal of Clinical Microbiology* **14**, 153–156

Suido, H., Eguchi, T. and Nakamura, M. (1988a) Investigation of periodontopathic bacteria based upon their peptidase activities. *Advances in Dental Research* **2**, 304–309

Suido, H., Nakamura, M., Mashimo, P.A. *et al.* (1986) Arylaminopeptidase activities of oral bacteria. *Journal of Dental Research* **65**, 1335–1340

Suido, H., Neiders, M.E., Barua, P.K. *et al.* (1987) Characterization of the N-CBz-glycyl-glycyl-arginyl peptidase and glycyl-prolyl peptidase of *Bacteroides gingivalis. Journal of Periodontal Research* **22**, 412–418

Suido, H., Zambon, J.J., Mashimo, P.A. *et al.* (1988b) Correlations between gingival crevicular fluid enzymes and the subgingival microflora. *Journal of Dental Research* **67**, 1070–1074

Sundqvist, G., Carlsson, J. and Hänström, L. (1987) Collagenolytic activity of black-pigmented *Bacteroides* species. *Journal of Periodontal Research* **22**, 300–306

Sundqvist, G., Carlsson, J., Herrmann, B. and Tarnvik, A. (1985) Degradation of human immunoglobulins G and M and complement factors C3 and C5 by black pigmenting *Bacteroides. Journal of Medical Microbiology* **19**, 85–94

Takeuchi, H., Sumitani, M., Tsubakimoto, K. and Tsutsui, M. (1974) Oral organisms in the gingiva of individuals with periodontal disease. *Journal of Dental Research* **53**, 132–136

Tashjian, A.H., Hohmann, E.L., Antoniades, H.N. and Levine, L. (1982) Platelet derived growth factor stimulates bone resorption via a prostaglandin-mediated mechanism. *Endocrinology* **111**, 118–124

Tashjian, A.H., Voelkel, E.F., Lazzaro, M. *et al.* (1985) α and β human transforming growth factors stimulate prostaglandin production and bone resorption in cultured mouse calvaria. *Proceedings of the National Academy of Science, USA* **82**, 4535–4538

Tipler, L.S. and Embery, G. (1985) Glycosoaminoglycan depolymerising enzymes produced by anaerobic bacteria isolated from the human mouth. *Archives of Oral Biology* **30**, 391–396

Toda, K., Otsuka, M., Ishikawa, Y. *et al.* (1984) Thiol-dependent collagenolytic activity in culture media of *Bacteroides gingivalis. Journal of Periodontal Research* **19**, 372–381

Tsai, C.C., McArthur, W.P., Baehni, P.C. *et al.* (1979) Extraction and partial characterization of a leukotoxin from plaque-derived Gram-negative microorganisms. *Infection and Immunity* **25**, 427–439

Tsutsui, H., Kinouchi, T., Wakano, Y. and Ohnishi, Y. (1987) Purification and characterization of a protease from *Bacteroides gingivalis*. *Infection and Immunity* **55**, 420–427

Uitto, V-J., Chan, E.C.S. and Chin Quee, T. (1986) Initial characterization of neutral proteinases from oral spirochaetes. *Journal of Periodontal Research* **21**, 95–100

Uitto, V-J., Grenier, D., Chan, E.C.S. and McBride, B.C. (1988) Isolation of a chymotrypsin-like enzyme from *Treponema denticola*. *Infection and Immunity* **56**, 2717–2722

Uitto, V-J., Grenier, D. and McBride, B.C. (1989a) Effect of *Treponema denticola* on periodontal epithelial cells. *Journal of Dental Research* **68**, 894. Abstract 223

Uitto, V-J., Larjava, H., Heino, J. and Sorsa, T. (1989b) A protease of *Bacteroides gingivalis* degrades cell surface and matrix glycoproteins of cultured gingival fibroblasts and induces secretion of collagenase and plasminogen activator. *Infection and Immunity* **57**, 213–218

Umemoto, T., Watanabe, K., Kumada, H. and Yamaji, Y. (1991) The role of motile rods in periodontal disease. In: Hamada, S., Holt, S.C. and McGhee, J.R. (eds) *Periodontal Disease: Pathogens and Host Immune Responses*. Quintessence Publishing Co. Ltd, Tokyo, pp. 65–76

Vaes, G. (1988) Cellular biology and biochemical mechanism of bone resorption. *Clinical Orthopaedics and Related Research* **23**, 239–271

Weakes-Dybvig, M., Sanavi, F., Zander, H. and Rifkin, B.R. (1982) The effect of indomethacin on alveolar bone loss in experimental periodontitis. *Journal of Periodontal Research* **17**, 90–100

Wikström, M. and Lindhe, A. (1986) Ability of oral bacteria to degrade fibronectin. *Infection and Immunity* **51**, 707–711

Williams, R.C., Jeffcoat, M.K., Howell, T.C. *et al.* (1988) Ibuprofen: an inhibitor of alveolar bone resorption in beagles. *Journal of Periodontal Research* **23**, 225–229

Wilson, M., Kamin, S. and Harvey, W. (1985) Bone resorbing activity from purified capsular material from *Actinobacillus actinomycetemcomitans*. *Journal of Periodontal Research* **20**, 484–491

Winkler, J.R., Grassi, M. and Murray, P.A. (1988) Clinical description and aetiology of HIV-associated periodontal diseases. In: Robertson, P.B. and Greenspan, J.S. (eds) *Oral Manifestations of AIDS*. PSG Publishing Company, Littleton, MA, USA. pp. 49–70

Wolinsky, L.E., Saglie, F.R., Carranza, F.A. Jnr, and Newman, M.J. (1987) The identification of *Treponema vincentii* in the gingival tissue of humans with adult periodontitis. *Journal of Periodontology* **58**, 337

Yoshima, F., Nishikata, M., Suzuki, T. *et al.* (1984) Characterization of a trypsin-like protease from the bacterium *Bacteroides gingivalis* isolated from human dental plaque. *Archives of Oral Biology* **29**, 559–564

6

The effect of systemic factors on the periodontal tissues

The systemic conditions which can potentially affect the periodontal tissues are numerous and will be described under the following headings:

- Physiological changes
- Systemic diseases
- Infections
- Drug reactions
- Dietary and nutritional factors

Physiological changes

The sex hormones

Oestrogens and progesterone are the predominant female sex hormones and are controlled by the ovary. Oestrogens produce the physiological changes in women at puberty and progesterone prepares the female reproductive tract for fertilization. The androgen, testosterone, is the predominant male hormone which produces the male characteristics at puberty and also promotes protein synthesis. Synthetic hormones which mimic the effects of the endogenous female hormones are used as oral contraceptives.

These hormones can affect the periodontal tissues. Oestrogens can promote keratinization and increase the mucopolysaccharide content of the connective tissue. Progesterone can increase the permeability of gingival blood vessels. Changes in the periodontal tissues may become clinically apparent principally at puberty, during pregnancy and during the use of oral contraceptives when there may be an exaggerated response to plaque products.

Puberty

The increasing levels of the sex hormones in the circulation at puberty have been linked to the increased prevalence and severity of gingivitis at this time (Sutcliffe, 1972) and this is supported by the observation that gingivitis peaks earlier in girls (11–13) than boys (13–14). However, a six-year longitudinal study (Yanover and Ellen, 1986) failed to show any increase in gingivitis at puberty in 18 hormonally stable girls, and a significant increase of gingivitis was seen in girls experiencing precocious puberty.

It would appear that a small amount of plaque which at a different age might cause minimal gingival inflammation produces in puberty an obvious inflammation with gingival swelling and bleeding. When puberty is passed the inflammation tends to subside but does not disappear until adequate plaque control is achieved.

Menstruation

With pre-existing gingivitis, gingival crevicular exudate increases at the time of ovulation in the menstrual cycle owing to the increased production of oestrogens and progesterone (Lindhe and Attström, 1967). However, no such increase was seen in healthy tissues (Holm-Pedersen and Lindhe, 1967). This may explain why in a few women a deterioration of a pre-existing gingivitis may occur at this time in their menstrual cycle.

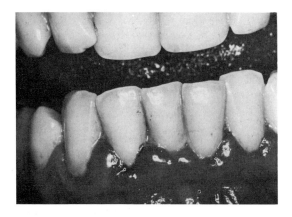

Figure 6.1 Gingival inflammation caused by poor oral hygiene, the tissue response exaggerated by hormonal changes associated with pregnancy

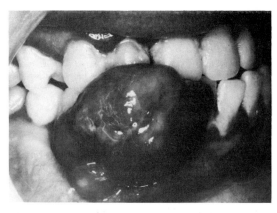

Figure 6.2 Pyogenic granuloma ('pregnancy tumour') in a pregnant patient. (Courtesy of Professor C. Scully)

Pregnancy

Folklore has always associated pregnancy with gingivitis and tooth loss but where the mouth is clean gingivitis does not occur in pregnancy. However, as in puberty an otherwise low-grade plaque-induced inflammation will become more severe in pregnancy (*Figure 6.1*).

The incidence of gingivitis in pregnancy has been reported as between 30 and 100% (Löe, 1965; Adam *et al.*, 1973). The changes usually start about the third month of gestation and the severity of the inflammation gradually increases during pregnancy, with partial or complete resolution after parturition (Löe and Silness, 1963; Silness and Löe, 1964; Hugoson, 1970; Samant *et al.*, 1976). Gingivitis has also been reported to peak at 6 months' gestation and then resolve slightly in the third trimester (Cohen *et al.*, 1971). The gingivae may become bright red, swollen, sensitive and bleed spontaneously. There is also an increase in gingival exudate and tooth mobility.

It is believed that increasing levels of progesterone produce an increase in vascularity with alterations in the walls of the gingival vessels which makes them more permeable. It has also been shown that the numbers of black-pigmented anaerobics in the subgingival flora increase as pregnancy progresses (Kornman and Loesche, 1980). This appears to be associated with raised levels of oestrogen and progesterone as the bacteria demonstrate an increased steroid uptake in pregnancy. This may relate to oestrogen becoming a substitute

for methadione which is a growth requirement for these bacteria.

To control gingivitis in the pregnant patient or in the adolescent it is important to explain the nature of the condition and the special care which she needs to take during this period. Regular scaling and instruction in home care are essential; at the same time all plaque retentive factors should be eliminated.

Pregnancy epulis (pyogenic granuloma of pregnancy)

The pregnancy epulis is a soft pedunculated granuloma which usually arises from an inflamed gingival papilla. It is usually deep red in colour and bleeds easily and may cause the patient great concern (*Figure 6.2*). It may arise from any gingival site but tends to be most prevalent on the labial aspect of the anterior part of the mouth. It may appear at any time during pregnancy but is most common about the third month. It usually grows slowly but can sometimes become quite large. It usually regresses partially or completely after parturition. It is usually associated not only with plaque deposits but also with an additional factor, such as a carious cavity, poor tooth contact or overhanging filling.

Histologically it resembles a pyogenic granuloma. It is composed of numerous, wide-spaced and thin-walled blood vessels within a delicate connective tissue stroma, which can intensify with age. A moderate to dense inflammatory infiltrate is present with numerous PMNs. The covering epithelium is thin and in areas of ulceration a thin fibrin exudate covers the surface.

An epulis should only be surgically removed in pregnancy if it is being traumatized by opposing teeth or restoration causing bleeding. The lesion can bleed profusely when excised and electrocautery of the base of the lesion may be necessary to control this. The excised lesion should be placed in formal saline and sent for histological examination to confirm the diagnosis. Any secondary irritating factor associated with the lesion should also be corrected. There is a high recurrence rate of these lesions and for this reason removal should be delayed until after parturition whenever possible. At this stage the lesion usually regresses considerably and becomes more fibrous. It is therefore easier to remove the remnant lesion at this time and the return of hormone levels to normal means that recurrence is rare.

Oral contraceptives

The hormonal oral contraceptive pill contains progestogen, often combined with an oestrogen. Many studies have shown that these produce a greater flow of gingival fluid and a higher prevalence of gingival inflammation (Chevallier, 1970). The degree of inflammation seems to be related to the length of time the woman is taking 'the pill'. As with pregnancy these changes do not affect healthy tissues in a clean mouth and the effect is to exaggerate a pre-existing gingivitis and is secondary to irritation from plaque. The exogenous hormones can also enhance the development of an anaerobic plaque in which black-pigmented anaerobic rods predominate (Jensen *et al.*, 1981).

As for the pregnant patient special care with oral hygiene should be advised and this combined with any necessary periodontal treatment brings about a resolution of the condition (Pearlman, 1974).

Systemic diseases

Endocrines

Diabetes mellitus

Diabetes mellitus is a metabolic disorder characterized by glucose intolerance. It can be classified into two major categories, Type I or insulin-dependent diabetes mellitus (IDDM) and Type II or non-insulin-dependent diabetes.

IDDM has a sudden onset and occurs usually before the age of 25. Symptoms include thirst, polyuria, hunger and weight loss and it is controlled by daily injections of insulin. It is a primary disease of the cells of the islets of Langerhans.

Type II has a gradual onset and mainly affects obese middle-aged people. It is controlled by diet and hypoglycaemic drugs.

IDDM produces atherosclerotic changes in the arterioles, capillaries and venules in a wide range of organs and renal, retinal and neural changes can occur.

The precise aetiology of IDDM is unclear but it appears to involve genetic factors relating to the HLA system and has some features of an auto-immune condition. A large number of IDDM patients have antibodies to Coxsackie 6B virus and it has been suggested that peptide sequences from viral proteins mimic those in certain protein antigens in the islet cells, such as glutamic acid dehydrogenase (GAD). T-cell immunity directed against these antigens would then damage or kill the islet cells. This would probably only occur in a group of susceptible individuals with the appropriate HLA (MHC) antigens which would present the appropriate peptide sequence from the virus (Chapter 3). Approximately 2% of the population has IDDM and the numbers are increasing.

Although scientific evidence is not clear cut, uncontrolled IDDM does appear to alter the periodontal tissues' response to plaque, especially in the longstanding and severe cases. Diabetic children have more severe gingivitis than healthy children (Bernick *et al.*, 1975). However, opinion is somewhat divided with regard to adult diabetics' susceptibility to periodontitis. The studies fall into two categories, those that investigated a mixed group of type I and II diabetics and those who just included IDDM cases. In both categories, some studies showed no relationship between diabetes and periodontal progression (Tervonen and Knuuttila, 1986; Goteiner *et al*, 1986), some showed slightly increased susceptibility (Glavind et al., 1968; Cohen et al., 1970) and some which showed a marked increase in susceptibility (Sznajder et al., 1978; Cianciola et al., 1982; Rylander et al., 1986). A full list of studies can be seen in Seymour and Heasman (1992).

The consensus from these studies would seem to be that the well controlled diabetic is at no greater risk from periodontal destruction than the normal population. However, several studies have shown that longstanding diabetics and particularly those who show systemic complications do appear to have greater rates of periodontal progression than age-matched healthy people. Diabetic patients with advanced periodontal disease also seem to suffer more frequently with complications such as lateral abscesses.

The possible reasons for their increased susceptibility could be the vascular changes and changes in polymorphonuclear leucocyte (PMN) function in IDDM.

The underlying mechanism of the vascular changes relates to the lack of heparin sulphate in basement membranes. The changes in the capillary basement membranes could have an inhibitory effect on the transport of oxygen, white blood cells, immune factors and waste products, all of which could affect the defence mechanism and tissue repair and regeneration. These vascular changes have been reported in the gingival tissues from IDDM patients (Lin *et al.*, 1975).

Impairment of PMN function is a feature of IDDM and this includes reduced phagocytosis, intracellular killing and adherence (Saadoun, 1980). Diabetic patients and their relatives also have an impaired PMN chemotactic response (Clark, 1978). In addition, impairment of the chemotactic response of PMNs from the gingival crevice has been demonstrated in diabetic patients with severe periodontitis (Manouchehr-Pour *et al.*, 1981) and in families with a history of diabetes (McMullen *et al.*, 1981). It has been suggested that the defect is at the cellular level and may involve inhibition of the glycolytic pathway, abnormal cyclic nucleotide metabolism, which disrupts the organization of microtubules and microfilaments, or a reduction in leucocyte membrane receptors (Seymour and Heasman, 1992).

Nearly all diabetic patients respond to conventional periodontal treatment and benefit from regular monitoring and maintenance. If periodontal problems are to be avoided a high standard of oral hygiene must be established and maintained. Diabetic patients are susceptible to infections and these can disturb their metabolic control. It is therefore important that periodontal infections such

as acute ulcerative necrotizing gingivitis (AUNG) or lateral periodontal abscesses should be promptly treated with the appropriate antibiotic. Also, if a diabetic requires periodontal surgery than it is advisable to carry this out under antibiotic cover.

Genetic conditions

A number of conditions of genetic origin can affect the periodontal tissues and these are listed below:

- Down's syndrome
- Hypophosphatasia
- Papillon–Lefèvre syndrome
- Ehlers–Danlos syndrome
- Hereditary gingival fibromatosis
- Mucopolysaccharidoses
- Hyperoxaluria
- Cyclic neutropenia
- Familial neutropenias
- Chediak–Higashi syndrome

Down's syndrome

Down's syndrome results from trisomy of chromosome 21 caused by non-dysjunction during oogenesis. A few cases of the syndrome have a normal number of 46 chromosomes but have a reciprocal translocation of chromosomes groups 13–15 and groups 21–22. The overall incidence of Down's syndrome is about 1 in 700 births but increases to 1:100 if the mother is 45 or over. People with the syndrome have a variable degree of mental handicap and typical mongoloid facial features.

Orally, they typically have a Class III occlusion, an anterior open bite, a large tongue and a lack of lip seal. They are prone to infections and their incidence of leukaemia is 20 times greater than the normal population. This is probably related to the presence on chromosome 21 of the genes for leucocyte development.

If living at home with their family or in a well-ordered community they usually have a very happy and trusting personality and if they receive an appropriate education they can develop reasonable skill levels.

It is now well established by a large number of epidemiological studies that Down's syndrome cases are much more prone to destructive periodontitis than either the normal

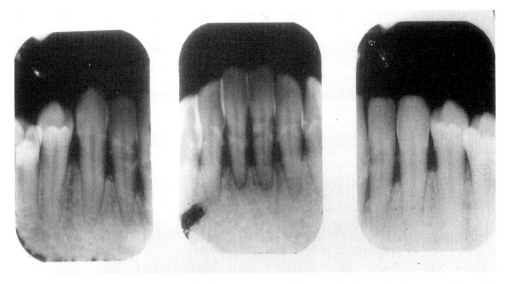

Figure 6.3 Radiograph showing advanced alveolar bone loss around the lower incisors of a 14-year-old boy with Down's syndrome

population or other mentally handicapped cases (Reuland-Bosma and van Dijk, 1986; Seymour and Heasman, 1992). The overall incidence of periodontitis is in excess of 90% but tends to be less in those living at home rather than in institutions. The distribution of disease is uneven with the lower permanent incisors most commonly involved and these teeth often have short conical roots. These are followed by the upper incisors and first molars and the deciduous molars, premolars and canines. The commonest clinical presentation is mobility of the lower incisors with radiographical evidence of advanced alveolar bone loss (*Figure 6.3*). They also have an increased susceptibility to AUNG. In this regard numerous black-pigmented anaerobic rods and spirochaetes can be frequently isolated from the subgingival flora of Down's cases (Brown, 1973).

The susceptibility to periodontitis is most likely related to systemic disorders that are a feature of the syndrome, particularly those relating to the immune system. Many abnormalities have been reported in PMN from Down's cases. Their numbers in the peripheral blood are normal but the many cells are immature possibly relating to a high rate of cell turnover (Kahn *et al.*, 1975). Impaired chemotaxis (Barkin *et al.*, 1980a), reduced phagocytosis (Rosner *et al.*, 1973) and intracellular killing (Kretschmer *et al.*, 1974) have

been reported. This last feature may be related to disturbances in the intracellular oxidative metabolism in PMNs. Monocyte function is also impaired but less so than PMNs (Barkin *et al.*, 1980b). However, monocyte sensitivity to interferon is 3 times higher than normal and this may prevent their maturation to macrophages (Epstein *et al.*, 1980). B-lymphocytes display abnormalities in the form of capping of their immunoglobulin surface receptors (Naeim and Walford, 1980). This phenomenon also occurs in old age in normal people and this suggests that there may be a premature ageing of B-lymphocytes in Down's syndrome. T-lymphocyte function is profoundly affected in Down's syndrome and the numbers of these cells in the circulation are low. There also appears to be impaired maturation of these cells, possibly due to a defect in thymic processing (Levin *et al.*, 1979). Abnormalities have been seen in the thymus gland and these include calcifications of Hassall bodies and a depletion of lymphocytes in the glands cortex. In addition, there is a reduced T-lymphocyte response to mitogenic stimulation (Nishida *et al.*, 1981) and the response decreases further with age.

There are also some vascular changes in people with Down's syndrome. They suffer from circulatory problems due to abnormally thin and narrow peripheral arterioles and capillaries (Dallapiccola *et al.*, 1971). Capillary fragility is high in comparison to normal children or children with other forms of mental retardation. This could be due either to a connective tissue disorder or diminished platelet activity. These vascular changes could lead to local tissue anoxia.

Patients with Down's syndrome need special care if dental problems are to be avoided or kept under control. They need frequent monitoring with prompt treatment of any problem. Good plaque control must be established to combat periodontal problems and scaling needs to be carried out frequently. Patient cooperation and acceptance of treatment and the support of the family and carers are of paramount importance. If the patient lacks the dexterity necessary for immaculate oral hygiene then these functions will need to be carried out by relatives or carers and they will need to be trained in this function and informed about dental disease and its control and the increased susceptibility in Down's syndrome. These functions are considerably more difficult to carry out in an institution than in the home environment.

Hypophosphatasia

Hypophosphatasia is a rare condition with an autosomal recessive mode of inheritance. There is a deficiency of the enzyme alkaline phosphatase and a urinary excretion of phosphoethanolamine. It is characterized by abnormal mineralization of bones and dental tissues. In the infantile form which appears at birth there is softening of bones, fever, anaemia, hypocalcaemia and vomiting which leads to death in infancy of more than half of the cases. The juvenile form, where the signs become apparent around 6 months of age, is less severe.

Several reports have appeared describing the dental and periodontal manifestations (Seymour and Heasman, 1992). These are fairly specific to the condition and include premature exfoliation of the deciduous teeth, absence of gingival inflammation, presence of 'shell' teeth, and loss of alveolar bone which is usually limited to the deciduous incisors and canines (Baer *et al.*, 1964). Microscopically these teeth show either complete absence of cementum or isolated areas of abnormal cementum (Bruckner *et al.*, 1962). The loss of the deciduous teeth seems to result from the

bone and cementum changes. The permanent dentition does not appear to be affected.

Papillon–Lefèvre syndrome

Papillon–Lefèvre syndrome is an autosomal recessive inherited disease characterized by a diffuse palmar-plantar keratosis and premature loss of both deciduous and permanent dentitions (Papillon and Lefèvre, 1924). Haneke (1979) reviewed 111 cases; 45 of these cases were from 22 families and consanguinity of the parents was found in about a third of the cases. Males and females are equally affected. The condition is very rare with an incidence of 1–4 per million although 2–4 persons per 1000 are heterozygous (Gorlin *et al.*, 1964).

The characteristic skin lesions are diffuse erythematous, keratotic areas on the palms of the hand and soles of the feet. Ectopic calcifications of the falx cerebri and choroid plexus have also been reported in some cases. In the review of 111 cases (Haneke, 1979), 26 cases showed an increased susceptibility to infections. The dental condition affects the primary and permanent dentitions. The primary teeth are affected from the second year and are all prematurely exfoliated by the sixth year and are lost in order of eruption (Baer and Benjamin, 1974). The tissues then heal and the permanent teeth erupt early. A similar destructive rapidly progressive periodontitis affects these teeth and results in progressive bone loss and exfoliation. The clinical signs resemble those of an advanced adult periodontitis with severe gingival inflammation. The prognosis of the teeth is very poor and most subjects are edentulous by the age of 16.

Periodontal treatment is usually unsuccessful (Haneke, 1979; Glenwright and Rock, 1990). Recently some clinicians have suggested extraction of the primary teeth at 3 years with systemic antimicrobial therapy (tetracycline 250–500 mg per day) for 10 days during the period of the eruption of permanent teeth (Preus and Gjermo, 1987; Preus, 1988). A very high standard of oral hygiene is necessary for this treatment and regular monitoring and treatment is required thereafter.

Ehlers–Danlos syndrome

Ehlers–Danlos syndrome is an inherited condition affecting the connective tissues and is a disorder in collagen molecular biology. The main effects are excessive joint mobility, skin hyperextensibility, easy bruising and peculiar scarring after skin wounds. Ten variants of this condition have been described (Seymour and Heasman, 1992) and the mode of inheritance of four types is autosomal dominant (I, II, III, VIII), three types is autosomal recessive (IV, VI, VII) and three other types is X-linked (V, IX, X). The precise nature of the defect is unknown for most types but in Type IV the defect in collagen is due to reduced lysyl hydroxylation of the molecule. Also in Type IV there is a deficiency in the synthesis, structure and secretion of Type III collagen and a deficiency of the enzyme procollagen peptidase.

The oral mucosa, gingival tissue, periodontium, teeth and temporomandibular joint are all affected. The oral mucosa is fragile and is susceptible to bruising. The gingival tissues bleed easily particularly after brushing and post-extraction haemorrhage may be a problem. The teeth are fragile and fracture easily and recurrent subluxation of the temporomandibular joint can occur.

Patients with Type VIII Ehlers–Danlos syndrome have been reported to be susceptible to a rapidly progressive periodontitis (Stewart *et al.*, 1977) but this does not appear to be a feature of other variants (Barabas and Barabas, 1967).

Conventional periodontal treatment is difficult because of the oral mucosal and gingival fragility. This can give rise to serious complications if root planning or surgery is attempted. The tissues split under the slightest provocation and are very difficult to suture. Extractions are complicated by haemorrhage. Periodontal treatment should be as atraumatic as possible and very careful, atraumatic oral hygiene techniques should be taught using a soft toothbrush.

Hereditary gingival fibromatosis

Hereditary gingival fibromatosis may occur singly or in association with other inherited syndromes. It is inherited as an autosomal dominant trait (Witkop, 1971) and has an incidence of 1:350 000. The condition does not become manifest until after the eruption of the teeth and is most commonly seen associated with the permanent teeth. The hyperplasia is due to excessive production of collagen in the

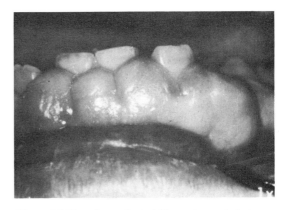

Figure 6.4 Hereditary gingival fibrous hyperplasia in a girl of 15. Regrowth of tissue has followed gingivectomy on three occasions. The fibrous overgrowth is associated with incomplete eruption of posterior teeth

gingival corium. The enlarged gingival tissues (*Figure 6.4*) appear firm and pink with exaggerated stippling (Becker *et al.*, 1967). The tissue often completely covers the crowns of the teeth and may interfere with speech and mastication. It may delay the eruption of teeth. The gingival hyperplasia may be generalized or localized and local involvement mainly affects the maxillary tuberosities and lingual surfaces of the lower molars.

Histologically, the tissues show a vast excess of collagen in an avascular corium with overlying parakeratinized epithelium.

The condition may occur with a number of other rare inherited syndromes when it may be associated with some of the following: hypertrichosis, hypopigmentation, mental deficiency, epilepsy, optic and auditory defects, cartilage and nail defects and dentigerous cysts (*see* Seymour and Heasman, 1992).

Mucopolysaccharidoses

The mucopolysaccharidoses (MPS) are a group of inherited disorders characterized by disturbances of mucopolysaccharide metabolism and this results in increased storage of these substances in various tissues. They include Hurler's syndrome (MPS I), Hunter's syndrome (MPS II), I-cell disease and MPS III, IV, V and VI. Hurler's syndrome is inherited as an autosomal recessive trait, whilst Hunter's syndrome is an X-linked recessive trait and I-cell disease probably represents the homozygous state of a recessive mutation (McKusick, 1969). Hurler's syndrome manifests in early childhood and children usually die before 10 from respiratory infection or cardiac disease consequent on deposition of mucopolysaccharides in the heart valves and intima of the coronary arteries. The main clinical features of this syndrome are mental retardation, dwarfism, hernia, deformed head, typical facies, short neck and spinal deformities (Gardiner, 1971). Hunter's syndrome is less severe and the survival rate is greater. In both syndromes there are increased levels of chondroitin sulphate B and heparitin sulphate in the urine.

The teeth in these conditions are small and widely spaced and exhibit delayed eruption (Cawson, 1962). Gingival enlargement may occur and the tissue is nodular, fibrotic, oedematous and haemorrhagic (Cawson, 1962; Gardiner, 1971). The gingival tissues often contain the characteristic Hunter cells within the lamina propria. They are probably macrophages and they contain large amounts of metachromatic material in their cytoplasm (Gardiner, 1968).

Hyperoxaluria and oxalosis

Primary hyperoxaluria is a rare autosomal recessive inherited disease of glycoxalate metabolism and is due to an enzyme deficiency. It results in the deposition of calcium oxalate in various tissues throughout the body. Its clinical features are nephrolithiasis, nephrocalcinosis, acute arthritis, heart block and peripheral neuropathy. The life expectancy is poor and death is usually due to renal failure. Secondary hyperoxaluria can also occur in chronic renal failure where oxalate deposits in the kidney possibly due to recurrent dialysis failing to remove all the calcium oxalate.

The main oral changes of oxalosis are root resorption, both external and internal, and histologically these areas show deposits of calcium oxalate crystals and granulomatous foreign body reaction (Wysocki *et al.*, 1982). Pain may arise from an inflammatory reaction in the pulp and periodontal ligament to calcium oxalate crystal deposition. These crystals may also deposit in the gingiva and periodontal ligament where they also evoke a chronic inflammatory response (Moskow,

1989). The crystals become surrounded by macrophages, multinucleated giant cells (macrophage polykaryons), lymphocytes and plasma cells. This reaction in the periodontal ligament or pulp may be the cause of root resorption (Fantasia *et al.*, 1982).

The only effective treatment of the root resorption appears to be extraction of the grossly involved teeth.

Granulomatous conditions

Crohn's disease

Crohn's disease or regional enteritis is a chronic inflammatory condition primarily of the terminal ileum and was first described by Crohn *et al.* (1932). It affects the submucosa of the gastrointestinal tract and produces stenosis, necrotic breakdown and scarring of the mucosa. All areas of the tract including the mouth can be affected but the initial lesion is in the terminal ileum. Symptoms include abdominal pain, pyrexia, intermittent diarrhoea, joint pains and generalized malaise. The overall incidence is about 15 per 100 000 but is higher in Jews and siblings of affected patients (Sandler and Golden, 1986).

The aetiology is unknown but intolerance to certain foods particularly those containing gluten may be an important factor and there is a familial tendency although no genetic pattern has been established. A gluten-free diet is recommended for these subjects.

The oral manifestations of Crohn's disease are aphthous-like ulceration and a cobblestone appearance of the oral mucosa, labial and buccal gingival swellings, mucosal tags, fissuring of the midline of the lip and angular cheilitis (Bernstein and McDonald, 1978).

The characteristic gingival lesion is diffuse, erythematous, granular enlargement of the attached gingiva. The cobblestone appearance of the oral mucosa is mainly confined to the buccal mucosa and the lesions are lobulated, oedematous and fissured and ulceration may be present. The tag-like lesions in the mucobuccal fold resemble denture granulomata (Seymour and Heasman, 1992).

Severe periodontitis has been seen in patients with this condition (Lampster *et al.*, 1978, 1982; Engel *et al.*, 1988). Patients with active bowel disease have been reported to have high levels of circulating immune complexes and metabolically active PMNs compared to healthy controls (Lampster *et al.*, 1982). It has also been found that the PMNs from these patients had elevated levels of alkaline phosphatase which is an indication of early release of these cells from the marrow (Koldjaer *et al.*, 1977). In addition, it has been found that these patients had low circulating B-lymphocyte numbers and high numbers of T-lymphocytes (Engel *et al.*, 1988). All of these factors could exacerbate an existing periodontal condition or accelerate its progress.

These patients usually respond well to conventional periodontal treatment.

Sarcoidosis

Sarcoidosis is a granulomatous condition of uncertain aetiology which may affect the lymph nodes, lungs, liver, spleen, skin, eyes, phalangeal bones and parotid glands. The worldwide prevalence is 20 per 100 000 with higher levels in blacks than whites. Its prognosis is good with most cases showing spontaneous healing which can be accelerated by the administration of corticosteroids.

Oral lesions occur rarely with swelling of the parotid glands and cervical lymph nodes as the most common and gingival involvement as least common. It may also affect the minor salivary glands. The histopathology is a collection of monocyte-derived epithelioid cells with T-lymphocytes and occasional plasma cells (Gold and Sager, 1976). Several cases of sarcoid gingivitis have been reported (*see* Seymour and Heasman, 1992). The gingivae have a hyperplastic, granulomatous appearance and may have superficial ulceration. Histologically there is an infiltration of macrophages and their polykaryons.

Scleroderma

Scleroderma or systemic sclerosis is a connective tissue disorder of uncertain aetiology. It produces inflammatory, vascular and fibrotic changes in the skin and other organs and structures. The changes may be limited to the skin or generalized and in the latter form the prognosis is poor particularly if there is involvement of the lungs, heart and kidneys.

The main change in the periodontium brought about by this condition is widening of the periodontal ligament space at the expense of alveolar bone. The changes affect the posterior teeth more than the anterior teeth. The teeth remain firm and the apical level of the junctional epithelium is unaffected. There is a proportional increase in collagen and oxytalin fibres and the fibrous tissue contains areas of degeneration with sclerosis and hyalinization (Wood and Lee, 1988).

Haematological conditions (blood diseases)

Blood diseases do not appear to cause gingivitis but they do bring about tissue changes which alter the tissue response to plaque. The dentist has a special responsibility in relation to these diseases as severe gingival bleeding is a common feature of acute leukaemia and the dentist may be the first person to examine the patient. Delay in the control of such a disease could be fatal.

Red blood cell (RBC) disorders

Anaemia

Anaemia is defined as a reduction in the concentration of haemoglobin in the blood below the normal level. This is usually accepted for males as 12.5–18.0 g/dl and for females as 12.0–16.5 g/dl. There are a large number of causes of anaemia, including haemorrhage, chemical damage and disease, but the most common form is iron-deficiency anaemia which is found in about 10% of the female population. Anaemia lowers the oxygen-carrying capacity of the blood so that the patient may feel tired and faint and may have difficulty in breathing and tingling of the fingers and toes. The skin may be pale but this is frequently not the case; pallor of the tissue beneath the finger nails and pallor of the oral mucosa, including the gingiva, is a more reliable sign but even this may only occur when the anaemia is severe. The tongue may lose its normally rough papillated surface and become smooth. There may be recurrent aphthous ulcers and angular cheilitis in some cases. If anaemia is suspected blood examination is necessary.

Aplastic anaemia

Aplastic anaemia can be caused by drugs, chemicals, radiation, infections or neoplasia. The resultant anaemia, leucopenia and thrombocytopenia produce weakness, fatigue, recurrent infections, pyrexia, epistaxis and retinal haemorrhage. The main oral effects are gingival bleeding and infections.

A rare autosomal recessive inherited form of aplastic anaemia with a poor prognosis is called Fanconi's anaemia. Orally it produces a rapidly progressive destructive periodontitis with early tooth loss (Opinya *et al.*, 1988).

Acatalasia

This is a rare inherited disease caused by the absence of the enzyme catalase in RBCs and WBCs. Catalase converts hydrogen peroxide to oxygen and water. Plaque bacteria can produce hydrogen peroxide which will oxidize haemoglobin in the deficient RBCs. This results in hypoxia and necrosis of gingival tissue. A case report of two siblings with this condition described gingival necrosis and severe destructive periodontitis (Delago and Calderon, 1979).

White blood cell (WBC) disorders

Neutrophils (PMNs) and monocytes are essential cells in the defence system of the periodontium. Reductions in their numbers or their function can have a profound effect on the periodontal tissues. The term leucopenia means an absolute reduction in numbers of WBCs and neutropenia means reduction in the number of PMNs. The leukaemias are a group of neoplastic conditions in which there is uncontrolled proliferation of the affected group of WBCs.

Neutropenia

Neutropenia may be genetic, familial, idiopathic or secondary to viral, bacterial or protozoan infections or systemic disease. All forms of neutropenia profoundly affect periodontal health. The main primary neutropenias are:

- Cyclic neutropenia
- Chronic benign neutropenia
- Familial neutropenias
- Chronic idiopathic neutropenia

Cyclic neutropenia

This is a rare autosomal dominant inherited condition. It produces a cyclical depression of PMNs in the peripheral blood at intervals varying from 15–55 days with occasional longer periods of neutropenia lasting 1–2 months (Page and Good, 1957). The main clinical manifestations are pyrexia, oral ulceration and skin infections. The condition appears to be due to periodic stem cell failure in the bone marrow related to a disorder of haemopoietic feedback control (Zucker-Franklin *et al.*, 1977).

The main oral and periodontal features of this condition are oral ulceration, severe gingivitis and rapid periodontal breakdown and alveolar bone loss. In the permanent dentition the bone loss is most obvious around the teeth that erupt first, the first molars and lower incisors (Spencer and Fleming, 1985). Patients with this condition require regular periodontal maintenance for careful supra- and subgingival scaling and meticulous oral hygiene should be encouraged. Antibiotic therapy will be necessary to control acute episodes and antiseptic mouthwashes will help when oral ulceration is present.

Chronic benign neutropenia of childhood

The onset of this condition is usually between 6 and 20 months. There is a moderate neutropenia with an absolute lymphocytosis and monocytosis. The bone marrow appears normal and the neutropenia may be due to increased peripheral destruction.

Pyogenic infections of the skin and mucous membranes are a feature of this condition. However, the increased numbers of monocytes in this condition can compensate for the neutropenia and may provide a reasonable resistance to infections (Biggar *et al.*, 1974).

Several case reports of the oral and periodontal features of this condition have appeared (Seymour and Heasman, 1992) and most of these relate to boys aged 4–12 years. There is a bright red, hyperplastic, oedematous gingivitis which affects the free and attached gingivae and the gingivae bleed easily. There appears to be premature loss of primary teeth due to bone loss. Some older children show a rapidly progressive periodontitis in the permanent dentition with generalized bone loss. In most reports attempts to control the condition with periodontal treatment have been unsuccessful and early loss of primary and permanent teeth seems difficult to prevent.

Benign familial neutropenia

Benign familial neutropenia is an autosomal dominant inherited condition. There is a moderate neutropenia and an accompanying monocytosis. The bone marrow appears normal and the condition may be due to an anomaly in the marrow release mechanism (Mintz and Sachs, 1973).

The only case report of oral and periodontal changes in a 14-year-old boy with this condition (Deasy *et al.*, 1980) described a bright red, hyperplastic, oedematous gingivitis and the tissues bled profusely. There was also marked bone loss around the first molars suggesting a rapidly progressive periodontitis. The treatment was plaque control, scaling and antiseptic mouthwashes but no long-term follow up of the patient's condition was reported.

Severe familial neutropenia

This is more severe than the benign form and is inherited as an autosomal dominant trait. There is a more marked neutropenia and some monocytosis. Children are susceptible to repeated infections. The oral and periodontal changes are similar to those described above but more severe and the prognosis is poor.

Chronic idiopathic neutropenia

Chronic idiopathic neutropenia was first described by Kyle and Linman (1968) and appears to occur mainly in females. There is a persistent neutropenia from birth which is not cyclical and there is no family history of the condition. There are persistent recurrent infections throughout the life of the sufferers. The cause of the condition is uncertain but there does appear to be a maturation abnormality of granulocytes in the bone marrow which could be related to an autoimmune disorder.

The periodontal features have been reported in two case reports (Kyle and Linman, 1970; Kalkwark and Gatz, 1981). There is a severe, oedematous, hyerplastic gingivitis with early bone loss and the condition does not respond well to treatment.

Leukaemia

Leukaemias are malignant neoplastic disease of the white blood cell forming tissues. They usually result in an increased number of leucocytes in the circulation including developing blast cells and an infiltration of leukaemic cells into other tissues, particularly lymph nodes. The condition may affect granulocytes (myeloid), monocytes (monocytic) or lymphocytes (lymphocytic) and can be either chronic or acute. In acute forms large numbers of neoplastic primitive stem and blast cells proliferate in the marrow and enter the circulation. The acute forms of leukaemia are more common in children and young adults and the chronic forms in adults over 40 years.

The clinical signs and symptoms are due to reduced numbers of other marrow cells such as red cells and megakaryocytes which are crowded out by the proliferation of neoplastic cells and from the lack of normal function from the leukaemic cells themselves. Early symptoms include tiredness, lethargy and fatigue due to anaemia, malaise, sore throat, oral ulceration and skin infections due to infection from reduced white cell function and lymph nodes, splenic and hepatic enlargement due to leukaemic infiltration. Chronic leukaemias have a slow, insidious onset with tiredness, weight loss, fatigue, pyrexia and splenic enlargement being the main features.

The oral and periodontal features may reflect both the condition and its treatment with radiotherapy and chemotherapy. They include oral ulceration, petechiae and ecchymoses, gingival enlargement, gingival bleeding and bacterial, viral and fungal infections. Oropharyngeal lesions may be the initial complaint in over 10% of acute leukaemias (Scully and Cawson, 1987). The gingival enlargement (*Figure 6.5*) is due to infiltration of leukaemic cells (Barrett, 1986) and is most common in monocytic leukaemia. Gingival bleeding is secondary to the accompanying thrombocytopenia and may present as oozing or frank bleeding. It is most marked when the platelet count drops below 10 000 per ml.

Infections may be due either to an exacerbation of an existing condition or to susceptibility to a range of bacterial, viral and fungal infections. Existing periodontitis can be exacerbated by the leukaemia or by chemotherapy. A variety of infections can occur for similar reasons and include acute necrotizing ulcerative gingivitis (ANUG), acute herpetic gingivostomatitis and fungal infections such as candidiasis (Barrett, 1984).

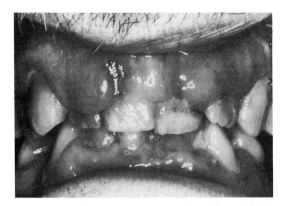

Figure 6.5 Gingival inflammation and swelling in a patient with myeloid leukaemia. (Courtesy of Professor C. Scully)

Leukaemic patients need careful hygiene care during acute episodes of the disease or during treatment with radiotherapy and chemotherapy. Regular gentle professional cleaning and swabbing with chlorhexidine can be very beneficial.

Every effort should be made to treat any periodontal condition during remission phases of the disease and during this time to encourage immaculate plaque control. Oral and periodontal infections may need to be treated with the appropriate antibiotic. The patient's physician should always be consulted before any treatment is carried out so that an appropriate regime can be discussed and agreed.

Disorders of white cell function

These conditions affect the ability of PMNs to phagocytose and destroy bacteria intracellularly. Primary functional disturbances that affect the periodontal tissues are the Chediak–Higashi syndrome and the lazy leucocyte syndrome.

Chediak–Higashi syndrome

Chediak–Higashi syndrome is a rare autosomal recessive inherited disease. Clinical features include albinism with photophobia and nystagmus and frequent pyogenic infections and ferbrile illnesses. Later a lymphoma-like condition develops with accompaning neutropenia, anaemia and thrombocytopenia. Death usually results from infection or

haemorrhage. Circulating leucocytes have large abnormal lysosomes in their cytoplasm and show defective migration and phagocytic degranulation and grossly diminished intracellular killing (Dale *et al.*, 1972).

The disease gives rise to a very severe gingivitis and periodontitis, and premature loss of the primary and permanent teeth. The condition does not appear to respond well to periodontal treatment.

Lazy leucocyte syndrome

Lazy leucocyte syndrome was first described by Miller *et al.* (1971). There is a defect in PMN chemotaxis and random mobility. A severe gingivitis has been described in two children with this condition.

Chronic granulomatous disease

Chronic granulomatous disease is an inherited condition transmitted as an autosomal recessive trait in females and as an X-linked recessive trait in males. It is characterized by the inability of phagocytes to destroy certain infective bacteria. The PMNs of subjects with this condition are unable to generate hydrogen peroxide possibly because of the absence of the enzyme NADPH oxidase. A granulomatous response occurs to inflammation and involves the lymph nodes, spleen, liver, skin and lungs. People with this condition are very prone to osteomyelitis, liver abscesses and pneumonia and their prognosis is poor.

Case reports (Allan and Straton, 1983) have described a severe and diffuse gingivitis with ulceration which spreads on to the buccal mucosa. This may respond to antibiotic therapy.

Immunological conditions

Hypogammaglobulinaemia

This can rarely occur as a X-linked recessive inherited disease. More commonly, it is secondary to chronic lymphatic leukaemia and myeloma. Patients are highly susceptible to infection, particularly of the respiratory tract. There have been some reports of severe destructive periodontitis (Roberts and Walker, 1976) but other reports have suggested that patients with primary immunodeficiencies suffer less gingivitis and caries than controls (Robertson *et al.*, 1978) but this could be associated with the extensive use of antibiotics in these cases.

Multiple myeloma

This is a multifocal malignant neoplasm of plasma cells. Deposits can occur in the mandible and maxilla. Lesions have also been reported involving the periodontium and gingiva (Petit and Ripamonti, 1990). The oral lesions described are gingival ulceration and bleeding and the condition may produce a rapidly growing, retromolar myelomatous mass with multiple foci of alveolar bone destruction.

Immunosuppressive drugs

Immunosuppressive drugs are often given to combat autoimmune disease or to prevent rejection of transplants. They include cortico-steroids, azathioprine and cyclosporin. Corticosteroids and azathioprine reduce the inflammatory response and may reduce gingivitis. Cyclosporin may produce gingival fibrous hyperplasia (*see below*).

Dermatoses

A number of skin diseases have oral manifestations which can occur on the gingivae. Some of these diseases are moderately common such as lichen planus and some are extremely rare such as pemphigus vulgaris.

Lichen planus

This disease is estimated to occur in 1% of the population. It is an inflammatory disease of doubtful aetiology which occurs in the skin and mucous membranes. It is more frequently observed in conjunction with diseases of immunity, e.g. ulcerative colitis, myasthenia gravis and hypogammaglobinaemia, and there is increasing evidence that lichen planus is immunologically mediated. Lichen planus can occur in families and there is an increasing frequency of HLA-B7 in the MHC (*see* Chapter 3). The oral lesion can occur either in the absence of skin lesions or with minimal or widespread skin lesions and there is no difference in the oral lesion with or without skin

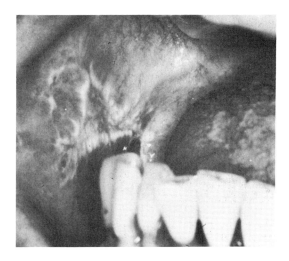

Figure 6.6 Lichen planus. Reticulated lesion in the cheek of a 50-year-old woman

involvement. The disease may be manifest in various forms (Shklar and McCarthy, 1961).

The reticulated form is the most common and consists of an interlacing network of white lines found frequently on the cheeks, vestibule and gingiva (*Figure 6.6*). In other forms, milky white patches, eroded areas or papules are present on the mucosa, especially the tongue and cheeks. Either erosive or reticular lesions can occur on the gingivae and it is the most common cause of erosive (desquamative) gingivitis. The lesion may be symptomless or painful and sore, the latter being more common with the erosive form. The lesions are sensitive to spicy and acid foods.

Some recent reports have suggested that some cases of oral lichenoid lesions in contact with amalgam restorations (contact lesions) may be caused or aggravated by an allergy to mercury from the amalgam (Eley, 1993). Mercury deposits have been found in lysosomes of fibroblasts and macrophages from contact lesions (Bolewska *et al.*, 1990). Some of these cases show remission following the replacement of amalgam restorations with alternatives restorative materials and this may support the theory that mercury allergy may be a causative or aggravating factor in certain cases of oral lichen planus.

Treatment of lichen planus is symptomatic and topical applications of triamcinolone paste (Adcortyl A in Orabase) 2–4 times per day may alleviate symptoms.

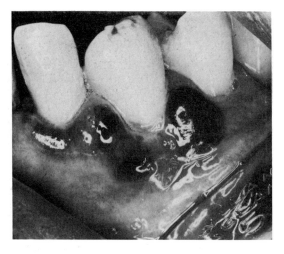

Figure 6.7 Benign mucous membrane pemphigus. Intact bullae on gingivae (Courtesy of Dr W. R. Tyldesley)

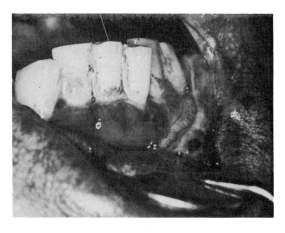

Figure 6.8 Pemphigus vulgaris (Courtesy of Dr W. R. Tyldesley)

Benign mucous membrane pemphoid

This is a disease of mucous membranes caused by an immunological disorder. Usually it occurs in older adults. The lesion is a bulla (*Figure 6.7*) which breaks down quickly to form an ulcer with an inflamed background which heals to form scarring (Shklar and McCarthy, 1959). It is most often seen in women at the menopause or after, but is not confined to women.

The disease may affect the gingivae and it is an uncommon cause of erosive gingivitis. There is a diffuse erythema of the gingivae with grey patches of desquamated epithelium. The involved areas are very sensitive and patients complain of soreness aggravated by spicy foods. The condition is chronic with periods of remission.

Treatment is symptomatic. Irritant foods or drinks or mouthwashes should be avoided. Topical applications of triamcinolone paste (Adcortyl A in Orabase) may help but Orabase alone is often just as effective. The patient needs to be reassured that the condition is benign, unless there is ocular involvement, when scarring may impair vision.

Pemphigus vulgaris

This is an autoimmune disease in which antibody and T-cells react with cells of mucous membranes thus destroying the cells. If widespread involvement occurs the disease may be fatal. The oral lesions often occur before skin lesions appear and the dentist has a special diagnostic responsibility. Most cases develop in middle age, often in patients of Jewish or Italian extraction.

The disease is characterized by the formation of bullae (large vesicles or blisters) in any part of the oral mucosa, including the gingivae (*Figure 6.8*). The bullae break down rapidly to form ragged ulcers which may heal slowly. There is pain and swelling and if the lesions involve the palate and throat, swallowing is difficult.

Sometimes it is possible to make a diagnosis by using the 'Nikolsky sign', in which sliding pressure with the finger over apparently intact mucosa dislodges the mucosa. Definitive diagnosis is made by histological examination of biopsy specimens. If pemphigus is suspected immediate referral to a physician is essential. The condition may be controlled by systemic corticosteroids.

Infections

Localized or generalized infections may involve the oral mucosa or periodontal tissues. Localized infections include acute necrotizing ulcerative gingivitis (Chapter 22) and acute lateral periodontal abscess (Chapter 19). Generalized infections include herpes simplex infections, herpes varicella/zoster infections, measles, tuberculosis, syphilis and *Candida albicans* infections (Chapter 21) and acquired immune deficiency syndrome (AIDS) (Chapter 7).

Drug reactions

In recent years it has been established that drugs which alter the haemopoietic system or the immune system, either to decrease or to enhance its activity, alter the response of the gingivae to plaque. As stated in Chapter 3 these findings support the idea of the involvement of the immune system in the pathogenesis of periodontal disease. It seems possible that in the future the influence of other drugs, e.g. antibiotics, phenacetin, sulphonamides, barbiturates, etc. which are capable of producing a hypersensitivity response with skin eruptions and oral lesions may be revealed. However, the most common response of the gingiva to drugs is gingival hyperplasia described below.

Drug-related gingival hyperplasia

The anticonvulsant drug phenytoin (Epanutin, Dilantin, DPH) given to epileptics, the immunosuppressive drug cyclosporin (Savage *et al.*, 1987) and the calcium channel blocking drug nifedipine (Barak *et al.*, 1987), given to treat cardiac angina, arrhythmias and hypertension, can produce fibrous hyperplasia of the gingiva.

Some degree of gingival enlargement occurs in a large percentage of epileptics taking phenytoin, especially those under 40 years. The condition is less common in patients on cyclosporin but when it occurs it may be very severe. Nifedipine hyperplasia is less firm than the other two and contains a higher proportion of ground substance.

The gingivae on the labial surface of the anterior teeth are usually more severely affected than the posterior teeth. The swelling is made up mainly of fibrous tissue and, unless inflammatory changes have supervened, is therefore firm, pink and lobulated (*Figure 6.9*). The swelling does not appear to be severe if oral hygiene is good but once inflammatory changes have been provoked by plaque these appear to enhance the activity of fibroblasts so that they increase in number and produce

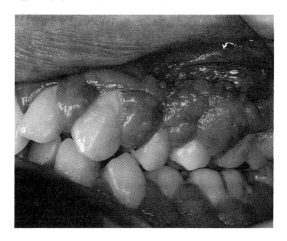

Figure 6.9 Gingival hyperplasia in an epileptic patient on Epanutin

more collagen fibres and proteoglycans appear. However, the size of the swelling does not appear to be related directly to drug dosage.

With superimposed inflammation, the gingival swelling can become soft and red and bleed when provoked. The gingival enlargement can almost cover the teeth and the condition may add to the social handicap that the epileptic patient may suffer.

Phenytoin is known to produce immunosuppression, folic acid depletion and possible suppression of adrenocortical trophic hormone (ACTH). It also produces its effect of stabilizing the neuronal cell membrane by decreasing its permeability to calcium (Seymour and Heasman, 1992). Cyclosporin also causes immunosuppression and nifedipine affects cell membrane calcium transport. All of these factors could influence fibroblast function.

Both inflammation and the effects of the drugs on androgen metabolism seem to be important in the cause of the fibrous hyperplasia (Sooryamoorthy and Gower, 1989a) Testosterone is a C19 androgenic steroid responsible for male characteristics but is also found in the tissues of both sexes. Testosterone is converted by 5α-reductase into 5α-dihydrotestosterone (DHT) which is its main biologically active metabolite. Specific cell surface receptors for DHT are present in the gingivae (Southren *et al.*, 1978) and these increase in number 2 to 3 fold in inflamed and hyperplastic gingival tissue. These DHT receptors are located on gingival epithelial cells and fibroblasts (Hernandez *et al.*, 1981) and phenytoin has been found to stimulate 5α-reductase activity in fibroblasts from inflamed gingival tissue (Sooryamoorthy and Gower, 1989b). DHT stimulates gingival fibroblasts to produce and secrete collagen and proteoglycan. Because of its sexual function there is much more testosterone available in male tissues and in healthy gingival tissue it is metabolized mainly by males. However, during inflammation gingival tissue metabolizes testosterone to the same extent in males and females (Ojanatoko *et al.*, 1980). Phenytoin stimulates the biosynthesis of DHT from testosterone in gingival fibroblasts (Sooryamoorthy *et al.*, 1988). Cyclosporin and nifedipine carry out this function also (Sooryamoorthy *et al.*, 1990).

These drugs, probably as a result of the production of DHT, may also select a subpopulation of fibroblasts which produce large amounts of collagen with the production of an inactive form of collagenase (Hassell, 1978, 1982). This would produce an imbalance between the production and removal of collagen and proteoglycan thus causing an overgrowth. This subgroup of cells may be more responsive to DHT stimulation.

Changing the drug is rarely possible with epileptics and never possible with patients taking the other two drugs. Treatment therefore must be restricted to oral hygiene instruction and supra- and subgingival scaling. Local removal of hyperplastic tissue may be carried out by gingivectomy or inverse bevel gingivectomy in some cases. Recurrence of hyperplasia is common but may be reduced if immaculate oral hygiene can be maintained.

Dietary and nutritional factors

Theoretically a deficiency of any essential nutrient might affect the status of the periodontal tissues and their resistance to plaque irritation but because of the delicately balanced interdependence of dietary elements it is extremely difficult in human beings to define the consequences of a specific deficiency. Epidemiological studies demonstrated that at any given age level there is more severe periodontal disease in African and Asian populations than in Europeans.

This could be due either to nutritional deficiency or poor oral hygiene, both of which reflect socioeconomic status. In Nigeria well-fed children have better gingival health than badly nourished children, irrespective of oral hygiene standard. Waerhaug (1967) found a correlation between the severity of periodontal destruction and the deficiency of vitamin B in a Sri Lankan population, but in general the effects of nutritional deficiency appear to be non-specific, i.e. the results of deficiency in several nutritional factors (Russell *et al.*, 1965). In severe nutritional deficiency, usually accompanied by extremely poor oral hygiene, there is rapid destruction of the periodontal tissues and early tooth loss. The prevalence of acute necrotizing ulcerative gingivitis is also increased and this may develop into a destructive and even fatal cancrum oris.

Severe periodontal destruction has long been associated with scurvy. Vitamin C is essential for collagen production and therefore normal turnover and repair, but experimental vitamin C deficiency has not produced a clear demonstration of gingival change. It seems likely that some plaque-induced inflammation is needed for gingival changes to take place in scurvy. There is no evidence to support the supplementation of a already balanced diet with extra vitamins in the treatment of periodontal disease.

References

Adam, D., Carney, J.S. and Dicks, D.A. (1973) Pregnancy gingivitis: a survey of 100 antenatal patients. *Journal of Dentistry* **2**, 106–110

Allan, D. and Straton, A.G. (1983) Chronic granulomatous disease with associated oral lesions. *British Dental Journal* **154**, 110–112

Baer, P.N. and Benjamin, S.D. (1974) In: *Periodontal Disease in Children and Adolescents*. Philadelphia: Lippincott, pp. 206–209

Baer, P.N., Brown, N.C. and Hammer, J.E. (1964) Hypophosphatasia: report of two cases with dental findings. *Periodontics* **2**, 209–215

Barabas, G.M. and Barabas, A.P. (1967) Ehlers–Danlos syndrome. A report of the oral and haematological findings in nine cases. *British Dental Journal* **123**, 473–479

Barak, S., Engelberg, I.S. and Hiss, J. (1987) Gingival hyperplasia caused by nifedipine. *Journal of Periodontology* **58**, 639–642

Barkin, R.M., Weston, W.L., Humbert, J.R. and Marie, F. (1980a) Phagocytic function in Down's syndrome. I. Chemotaxis. *Journal of Mental Deficiency Research* **24**, 243–249

Barkin, R.M., Weston, W.L., Humbert, J.R and Sunada, K. (1980b) Phagocytic function in Down's syndrome. II. Bacteriocidal activity and phagocytosis. *Journal of Mental Deficiency Research* **24**, 251–256

Barrett, A.P. (1984) Gingival lesions in leukaemia: a classification. *Journal of Periodontology* **55**, 585–588

Barrett, A.P. (1986) Leukaemic cell infiltration of the gingiva. *Journal of Periodontology* **57**, 579–581

Becker, W., Colins, C.K., Zimmerman, E.R. *et al.* (1967) Hereditary gingival fibromatosis. *Oral Surgery, Oral Medicine, Oral Pathology* **24**, 313–318

Bernstein, M.L. and McDonald, J.S. (1978) Oral lesions in Crohn's disease: report of 2 cases and update of literature. *Oral Surgery, Oral Medicine, Oral Pathology* **46**, 234–245

Bernick, S.M., Cohen, D.W., Baker, I. and Laster I. (1975) Dental diseases in children with diabetes mellitus. *Journal of Periodontology* **46**, 241–245

Biggar, W.D., Holmes, B., Page, A.R. *et al.* (1974) Metabolic and functional studies of monocytes in congenital neutropenia. *British Journal of Haematology* **28**, 233–234

Bolewska, J., Holmstrup, P., Møller-Madsen, B. *et al.* (1990) Amalgam associated accumulations in normal oral mucosa, mucosal lesions of lichen planus and contact lesions associated with amalgam. *Journal of Oral Pathology and Medicine* **19**, 39–42

Brown, R.H. (1973) Necrotising ulcerative gingivitis in mongoloid and non-mongoloid retarded and normal individuals. *Journal of Periodontal Research* **6**, 140–145

Bruckner, R.J., Rickles, N.H. and Porter, D.R. (1962) Hypophosphatasia with premature shedding of teeth and aplasia of cementum. *Oral Surgery, Oral Medicine and Oral Pathology* **15**, 1352–1369

Cawson, R.A. (1962) The oral changes in gargoylism. *Proceedings of the Royal Society of Medicine* **55**, 1066–1070

Cianciola, L.J., Park, B.H., Bruck, E. *et al.* (1982) Prevalence of periodontal disease in insulin-dependent diabetes mellitus (juvenile diabetes). *Journal of the American Dental Association* **104**, 653–660

Chevallier, M.E. (1970) Mouth manifestations and oral contraceptives. *Revue Odonto-Stomatologie du Midi de la France* **28**, 96–103

Clark, R. (1978) Disorders of granulocyte chemotaxis. In: Gallin, J. and Quie, P. (eds) *Leukocyte Chemotaxis*. New York: Raven Press, pp. 329–352

Cohen, D., Friedman, L., Shapiro, J. *et al.* (1970) Diabetes mellitus and periodontal disease: two year longitudinal observations. Part I. *Journal of Periodontology* **41**, 709–712

Cohen, D., Shapiro, J., Firedman, L. *et al.* (1971) A longitudinal investigation of the periodontal changes during pregnancy and fifteen months post partum. Part II. *Journal of Periodontology* **42**, 653–657

Crohn, B.B., Ginzburg, L. and Oppenheimer, G.D. (1932) Regional ileitis, a pathological and clinical entity. *Journal of the American Medical Aociation* **99**, 1323–1329

Dale, D.C., Clark, R.A., Root, R.K. and Kimball, H.R. (1972) The Chediak–Higashi syndrome: studies of host defences. *Annals of Internal Medicine* **76**, 293–306

Dallapiccola, B., Alboni, P. and Ballerini, G. (1971) Capillary fragility in Down's syndrome. *Coagulation* **4**, 217–220

Deasy, M.J., Vogel, R., Macedo-Sobrinho, B. *et al.* (1980) Familial benign chronic neutropenia associated with periodontal disease – a case report. *Journal of Periodontology* **51**, 206–210

Delago, W. and Calderon, R. (1979) Acatalasia in two Peruvian siblings. *Journal of Oral Pathology* **8**, 358–368

Eley, B.M. (1993) *Dental Amalgram: A Review of Safety*. London: British Dental Association. pp. 49–51

Engel, L.D., Pasquinelli, K.L., Leone, S.A. *et al.* (1988) Abnormal lymphocyte profiles and leukotriene B_4 status in a patient with Crohn's disease and severe periodontitis. *Journal of Periodontology* **59**, 841–847

Epstein, L.B., Lee, S.H.S. and Epstein, C.J. (1980) Enhanced sensitivity of trisomy 21 monocytes to the maturation-inhibiting effect of interferon. *Cellular Immunology* **50**, 191–194

Fantasia, J.E., Miller, A.S., Chen, S-Y. and Foster, W.B. (1982) Calcium oxalate deposition in the periodontium secondary to chronic renal failure. *Oral Surgery, Oral Medicine, Oral Pathology* **53**, 273–279

Gardiner, B. (1968) Metachromatic cells in the gingiva in Hurler's syndrome. *Oral Surgery, Oral Medicine, Oral Pathology* **26**, 782–789

Gardiner, D. (1971) The oral manifestations of Hurler's syndrome. *Oral Surgery, Oral Medicine, Oral Pathology* **32**, 46–57

Glavind, L., Lund, B. and Löe, H. (1968) The relationship between periodontal status and diabetes duration, insulin dosage and retinal changes. *Journal of Periodontology* **39**, 341–347

Glenwright, H.D. and Rock, W.P. (1990) Papillon–Lefèvre syndrome. A discussion of aetiology and a case report. *British Dental Journal* **168**, 27–29

Gold, R.S. and Sager, E. (1976) Oral sarcoidosis: review of the literature. *Journal of Oral Surgery* **34**, 237–244

Gorlin, R.J., Sedano, H. and Andersen, V.E. (1964) A syndrome of palmar-plantar hyperkeratosis and premature periodontal destruction of the teeth. *Journal of Paediatrics* **65**, 895–908

Goteiner, D., Vogel, R., Goteiner, C. and Deasy, M. (1986) Periodontal and caries experience in insulin-dependent diabetes mellitus. *Journal of the American Dental Association* **113**, 277–279

Haneke, E. (1979) The Papillon–Lefèvre syndrome. Keratosis palmoplantaris with periodontopathy. *Human Genetics* **51**, 1–35

Hassell, T.M. (1978) *In vivo* and *in vitro* studies of the pathogenesis of phenytoin induced connective tissue alterations in the gingiva. Dissertation, University of Washington, Seattle.

Hassell, T.M. (1982) Evidence for the production of an inactive collagenase by fibroblasts from phenytoin enlarged gingiva. *Journal of Oral Pathology* **11**, 310–317

Hernandez, M.R., Wenk, E.J., Southren, A.L. *et al.* (1981) Localization of 3H-androgens in human gingiva by radioautography. *Journal of Dental Research* **60**, 607–611

Holm-Pedersen, P. and Löe, H. (1967) Flow of gingival exudate as related to menstruation and pregnancy. *Journal of Periodontal Research* **2**, 13–20

Hugoson, A. (1970) Gingival inflammation and female sex hormones. *Journal of Periodontal Research* (Suppl.) **5**, 1–18

Jensen, J., Liljemark, W. and Bloomquist, C. (1981) The effect of female sex hormones on subgingival plaque. *Journal of Periodontology* **52**, 588–602

Kahn, A.J., Evans, H.E., Glass, L. *et al.* (1975) Defective neutrophil chemotaxis in patients with Down's syndrome. *Journal of Paediatrics* **87**, 87–89

Kalkwark, K.L. and Gatz, D.P. (1981) Periodontal changes associated with chronic idiopathic neutropenia. *Paediatric Dentistry* **3**, 189–195

Kretschmer, R.R., Lopez-Osuna, M., de la Rosa, L. and Armendares, S. (1974) Leucocyte function in Down's syndrome: Quantitative N.B.T. reduction and bactericidal capacity. *Clinical Immunology and Immunopathology* **2**, 449–455

Koldjaer, O., Klitgaard, N.A. and Schmitt, K.G. (1977) Indices of granulocyte activity in ulcerative colitis and Crohn's disease. *Danish Medical Bulletin* **24**, 72–76

Kornman, K.S. and Loesche, W.J. (1980) The subgingival microflora during pregnancy. *Journal of Periodontal Research* **15**, 111–122

Kyle, R.A. and Linman, J.W. (1968) Chronic idiopathic neutropenia: a newly recognized entity. *New England Journal of Medicine* **279**, 1015–1019

Kyle, R.A. and Linman, J.W. (1970) Gingivitis and chronic idiopathic neutropenia: a report of 2 cases. *Mayo Clinic Proceedings* **45**, 494–504

Lampster, I.B., Rodrick, M.L., Sonis, S.T. and Falchuk, Z.M. (1982) An analysis of peripheral blood and salivary polymorphonuclear leukocyte function, circulating immune complex levels and oral status in patients with inflammatory bowel disease. *Journal of Periodontology* **53**, 231–238

Lampster, I.B., Sonis, S.T., Hannigan, A. and Koldin, A. (1978) An association between Crohn's disease, periodontal disease and enhanced neutrophil function. *Journal of Periodontology* **49**, 475–479

Levin, S., Schesinger, M., Handzel, Z. *et al.* (1979) Thymic deficiency in Down's syndrome. *Pediatrics* **63**, 80–87

Lin, J., Duffy, J. and Roginsky, M. (1975) Microcirculation in diabetes mellitus: a study of gingival biopsies. *Human Pathology* **6**, 77–97

Lindhe, J. and Attström, R. (1967) Gingival exudation during the menstrual cycle. *Journal of Periodontal Research* **2**, 194–198

Löe, H. (1965) Periodontal changes in pregnancy. *Journal of Periodontology* **36**, 209–216

Löe, H. and Silness, J. (1963) Periodontal disease in pregnancy. I. Prevalence and severity. *Acta Odontologica Scandinavica* **21**, 533–551

McMullen, J.A., van Dyke, T.E., Horoszewicz, H.U. and Genco, R.J. (1981) Neutrophil chemotaxis in individuals with advanced periodontal disease and a genetic predisposition to diabetes mellitus. *Journal of Periodontology* **52**, 167–173

McKusick, V.A. (1969) The nosology of the mucopolysaccharidoses. *American Journal of Medicine* **47**, 730–747

Manouchehr-Pour, M., Spagnuolo, P.J., Rodman, H.M. and Bissada, N.F. (1981) Comparison of neutrophil chemotactic response in diabetic patients with mild and severe periodontal disease. *Journal of Periodontology* **52**, 410–415

Miller, M.E., Oski, F.A. and Harris, M.B. (1971) Lazy-leukocyte syndrome: a new disorder of leukocyte function. *Lancet* **1**, 665–669

Mintz, U. and Sachs, L. (1973) Normal granulocyte colony forming cells in the bone marrow of Yemenite Jews with genetic neutropenia. *Blood* **41**, 745–751

Moskow, E.B. (1989) Periodontal manifestations of hyperoxaluria and oxalosis. *Journal of Periodontology* **60**, 271–278

Naeim, F. and Walford, R.L. (1980) Disturbance of redistribution of surface membrane receptors on peripheral mononuclear cells of patients with Down's and aged individuals. *Journal of Gerontology* **35**, 650–655

Nishida, Y., Akaoka, I., Suzuki, T. *et al.* (1981) Serum lymphocytotoxins and lymphocyte responses to mitogens of Down's syndrome persons. *American Journal of Mental Deficiency* **85**, 596–600

Ojanatoko., Neinstedt, W. and Harri, P. (1980) Metabolism of testosterone by human healthy and inflamed gingiva (*in vitro*). *Archives of Oral Biology* **25**, 481–484

Opinya, G.N., Kaimenyi, J.T. and Meme, J.S. (1988) Oral findings in Fanconi's anaemia. *Journal of Periodontology* **33**, 266–269

Page, A.R. and Good, R.A. (1957) Studies on cyclic neutropenia. A clinical and experimental investigation. *American Journal of Diseases in Children* **94**, 623–661

Papillon, M.M. and Lefèvre, P. (1924) Deux cas de keratodermie palmaire et plantaire symmétrique familiale (maladie de Meteda) chez le frère et la soeur. Coexistence dans les deux cas d'altérations dentaire grave. *Bulletin de la Société Française de Dermatologie et de Syphilgraphie* **31**, 82–87

Pearlman, B.A. (1974) An oral contraceptive drug and gingival enlargement; the relationship between oral and systemic factors. *Journal of Periodontology* **36**, 209–216

Petit, J.C. and Ripamonti, U. (1990) Multiple myeloma of the periodontium. A case report. *Journal of Periodontology* **61**, 132–137

Preus, H. (1988) Treatment of rapidly destructive periodontitis in Papillon–Lefèvre syndrome. Laboratory and clinical observations. *Journal of Clinical Periodontology* **15**, 639–643

Preus, H. and Gjermo, P. (1987) Clinical management of

prepubertal periodontitis in 2 siblings with Papillon–Lefèvre syndrome. *Journal of Clinical Periodontology* **14**, 156–160

Reuland-Bosma, W. and van Dijk, J. (1986) Periodontal disease in Down's syndrome: a review. *Journal of Clinical Periodontology* **13**, 294–300

Roberts, W.R. and Walker, D.M. (1976) The periodontal management of a patient with a profound immunodeficiency disorder. *Journal of Clinical Periodontology* **3**, 186–192

Robertson, P.B., Wright, T.E., Mackler, B.F. *et al.* (1978) Periodontal status of patients with abnormalities of the immune system. *Journal of Periodontal Research* **13**, 37–45

Rosner, F., Kozinn, P.J. and Jervis, G.A. (1973) Leukocyte function and serum immunoglobulins in Down's syndrome. *New York State Journal of Medicine* **73**, 672–675

Russell, A.L., Leatherwood, E.C. and Consolazio, C.F. (1965) Periodontal disease and nutrition in South Vietnam. *Journal of Dental Research* **44**, 775–782

Rylander, H., Ramberg, P., Blohme, G., and Lindhe, J. (1986) Prevalence of periodontal disease in young diabetics. *Journal of Clinical Periodontology* **14**, 38–43

Saadoun, A. (1980) Diabetes and periodontal disease: a review and update. *Journal of the Western Society of Periodontology* **28**, 116–139

Sandler, R.S. and Golden, A.L. (1986) Epidemiology of Crohn's disease. *Journal of Clinical Gastroenterology* **8**, 160–165

Samant, A., Malik, C.P., Chabra, S.K. and Devi, P.K. (1976) Gingivitis and periodontal disease in pregnancy. *Journal of Periodontology* **47**, 415–418

Savage, N.W., Seymour, G.J. and Robinson, M.F. (1987) Cyclosporin-A-induced gingival enlargement – a case report. *Journal of Periodontology* **58**, 475–480

Seymour, R.A. and Heasman, P.A. (1992) In: *Drugs, Diseases and the Periodontium.*, Ch. 3. Oxford: Oxford University Press, pp. 19–54

Scully, C. and Cawson, R.A. (1987) *Medical Problems in Dentistry*, 2nd edn. Bristol: Wright, p. 119

Shklar, G. and McCarthy, P.L. (1959) Oral manifestations of benign mucous membrane pemphigus (mucous membrane pemphigoid). *Oral Surgery, Oral Medicine, Oral Pathology* **12**, 950–966

Shklar, G. and McCarthy, P.L. (1961) The oral lesions of lichen planus. *Oral Surgery, Oral Medicine, Oral Pathology* **14**, 164–171

Silness, J. and Löe, H. (1964) Periodontal disease in pregnancy. II. Correlation with oral hygiene and periodontal condition. *Acta Odontologica Scandinavica* **22**, 121–135

Sooriyamoorthy, M. and Gower, D.B. (1989a) Hormonal influence on gingival tissue: relationship to periodontal disease. *Journal of Clinical Periodontology* **16**, 201–208

Sooriyamoorthy, M. and Gower, D.B. (1989b) Phenytoin stimulation of 5α-reductase activity in inflamed gingival fibroblasts. *Medical Science Research* **17**, 989–990

Sooriyamoorthy, M., Harvey, W. and Gower, D.B. (1988) The use of human gingival fibroblasts in culture for studying the effects of phenytoin on testosterone metabolism. *Archives of Oral Biology* **33**, 353–359

Sooriyamoorthy, M., Gower, D.B. and Eley, B.M. (1990) Androgen metabolism in gingival hyperplasia induced by nifedipine and cyclosporin. *Journal of Periodontal Research* **25**, 25–30

Southren, A.L., Rappaport, S.C., Gordon, C.G. and Vittek, J. (1978) Specific 5 alpha-dihydrotestosterone receptors in human gingiva. *Journal of Clinical Endocrinology and Metabolism* **47**, 1378–1382

Spencer, P. and Fleming, J.E. (1985) Cyclic neutropenia: a literature review and report of a case. *Journal of Dentistry for Children* **52**, 108–113

Stewart, R.E., Hollister, D.W. and Rimoin, D.L. (1977) A new variant of Ehlers–Danlos syndrome: an autosomal dominant disorder of fragile skin, abnormal scarring and generalised periodontitis. *Birth Defects* **13**, 85–93

Sutcliffe, P. (1972) A longitudinal study of gingivitis and puberty. *Journal of Periodontal Research* **7**, 52–58

Sznajder, N., Carraro, J.J., Rugna, S. and Seraday, M. (1978) Periodontal findings in diabetic and non-diabetic patients. *Journal of Periodontology* **49**, 445–448

Tervonen, T. and Knuuttila, M. (1986) Relation of diabetes control to periodontal pocketing and alveolar bone level. *Oral Surgery, Oral Medicine, Oral Pathology* **61**, 346–349

Waerhaug, J. (1967). Prevalence of periodontal disease in Ceylon. Association with age, sex, oral hygiene, socio-economic factors, vitamin deficiencies, malnutrition, betel and tobacco consumption and ethnic group. Final report. *Acta Odontologica Scandinavica* **25**, 205–231

Witkop, C.J. (1971) Heterogeneity in gingival fibromatosis. *Birth Defects* **7**, 210–221

Wood, R.E. and Lee, P. (1988) Analysis of the oral manifestations of systemic sclerosis (scleroderma). *Oral Surgery, Oral Medicine, Oral Pathology* **65**, 172–178

Wysocki, G.P., Fay, W.P., Ulrichsen, R.F. and Ilan, R.A. (1982) Oral findings in primary hyperoxaluria and oxalosis. *Oral Surgery, Oral Medicine, Oral Pathology* **53**, 267–272

Yanover, L. and Ellen, R.P. (1986) A clinical and micro-biological examination of gingival disease in parapubescent females. *Journal of Periodontology* **57**, 562–567

Zucker-Franklin, L'Esperance, P. and Good, R.A. (1977) Congenital neutropenia: an intrinsic cell defect demonstrated by electron microscopy of soft agar colonies. *Blood* **49**, 425–436

7

Acquired immunodeficiency syndrome (AIDS)

The acquired immunodeficiency syndrome (AIDS) is one of the principal threats to health worldwide; the number infected with the human immunodeficiency virus (HIV) is about 19.5 million and the great majority of these will probably die of this condition.

The human immunodeficiency virus

The HIV is a retrovirus which is roughly spherical and is one ten thousandths of a millimetre across. Its outer coat or envelope consists of a double layer of lipid molecules and this is studded with proteins (*Figure 7.1*). One of these appears like a spike in electron microscope (EM) photographs and is a glyco-protein (gp). The outer part is known as gp 120 (the number stands for the mass of the protein in daltons) and the inner part embedded in the membrane as gp 41. Below this is a matrix protein (p17) which surrounds the core or capsid, made of another protein (p24), in the shape of a hollow cone. This holds the genetic material in the form of RNA of about 9200 nucleotide bases. Molecules of the enzyme reverse transcriptase, which transcribes the RNA to DNA once the virus enters the cell, lie on the surface of the strands. Also present within the capsid are integrase, protease and ribonuclease enzyme proteins.

The gp 120 protein can bind tightly to CD4 molecules present on several types of immune cells (*Figure 7.2*). When the virus binds to the cell the membranes fuse, a process governed by the gp 41 envelope protein, and the virus core and its contents are brought into the cell. The viral core then partially disintegrates releasing the RNA. The reverse transcriptase then transcribes a DNA copy with the aid of the other viral enzymes. When activated, the viral integrated DNA can code for viral RNA which leaves the nucleus, codes for structural and other proteins and buds new virus from the cell surface to infect other cells.

Pathogenesis of HIV infection and AIDS

Some CD4 bearing cells, known as dendritic cells, are present throughout the body's mucosal surfaces and it is possible that these are the first cells infected in sexual transmission. Macrophages and monocytes also carry the CD4 molecule and are similarly vulnerable. They may carry HIV to other parts of the body including the lymphoid organs and brain. The principal targets of the HIV virus are CD4 bearing T-helper lymphocytes which help to activate other parts of the immune system including the T4-effector cells, the T8-killer cells and the B-cells.

An infected person first mounts a vigorous defence when first infected. As a result of this B-cells produce antibodies to neutralize virus and killer T-cells multiply and destroy the virus infected cells. Although it is possible that the immune system may successfully fight off HIV at a very early stage by the time antibod-

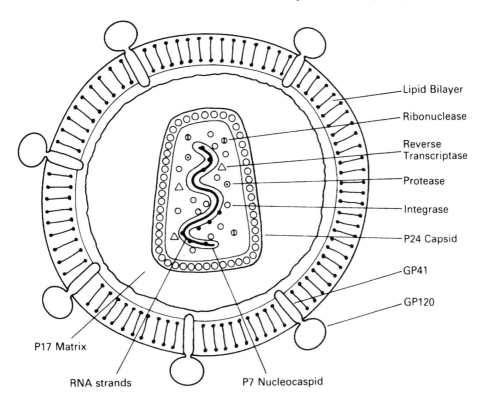

Lipid Bilayer

Ribonuclease

Reverse Transcriptase

Protease

Integrase

P24 Capsid

GP41

GP120

P17 Matrix

RNA strands

P7 Nucleocaspid

Figure 7.1 A diagram of HIV

ies to the virus have appeared in the blood the infection is generally permanent. The clinical picture is firstly a mild flu-like illness with fever and muscle aches lasting no more than a few weeks and throughout this stage large amounts of virus are present in the blood-stream and transmission is easy. The immune system mounts its response and begins to eliminate infected cells and circulating virus. However, a proportion of infected cells remain by eluding these defences and the virus contin-ues to replicate in low numbers for as long as a decade and for most of this period of chronic infection the patient is quite well. It is only after several years when the virus has signifi-cantly damaged the immune system that opportunist infections and malignancies begin to appear.

At first it was thought that the damage to the immune system was due to the progressive decline in the numbers of T4 cells in the blood as a result of the killing of these cells by the virus. In support of this is evidence that the numbers of these cells decline from 1000 per mm³ to 100 or less per mm³ during the long

subclinical phase of the illness. However, even in the late stages of the disease when there are very low numbers of T4 cells in the blood, the proportion of these cells producing virus is only 1 in 40 cells. In fact, in the early stages of the disease only about 1 in 1000 T4 cells in the blood produce virus. One reason for the decline in T4 cells could be that the unaffected T8 killer cells could progressively destroy infected cells. Another possibility is that antibodies recognizing the viral gp 120 and gp 41 proteins on the viral envelope might also interfere with the MHC on healthy cells. A further theory supported by experimental evidence is that HIV might precipitate a widespread apoptosis (programmed death) of healthy immune cells.

Recent experimental evidence suggests that the most likely reason is that HIV infection gradually and progressively destroys the lymphoid organs, particularly the lymph nodes. There is evidence that in the long chronic asymptomatic phase HIV replicates mainly in the lymph nodes and this gradually increases the body burden of infected cells in

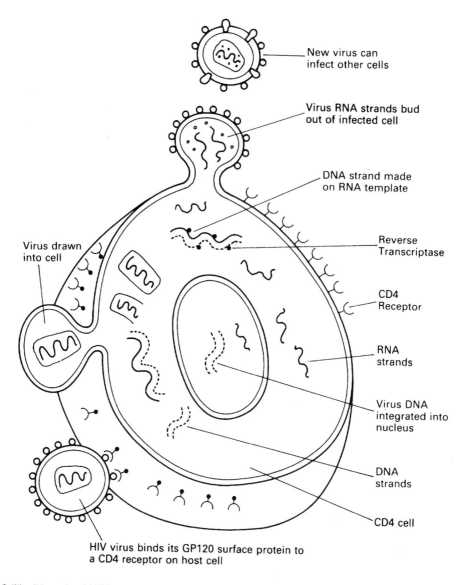

New virus can infect other cells

Virus RNA strands bud out of infected cell

DNA strand made on RNA template

Reverse Transcriptase

CD4 Receptor

Virus drawn into cell

RNA strands

Virus DNA integrated into nucleus

DNA strands

CD4 cell

HIV virus binds its GP120 surface protein to a CD4 receptor on host cell

Figure 7.2 The life cycle of HIV

these organs. Thus, it seems that in the lymph nodes the viral burden is substantial and increases steadily throughout the chronic phase. The abrupt rise in the blood levels of the virus in the late stages of the disease is most likely due to the burning out of the lymph nodes. Loss of follicular dendritic, T4 helper and memory cells probably leads to a rapid loss of immune function and the virus spills out into the blood. The patient, now with a paralysed immune system dies, from recurrent opportunistic infections and neoplasms.

Clinical features of AIDS

General

The main clinical features of AIDS are lymphadenopathy, weight loss, unexplained diarrhoea, candidiasis, pneumocystis pneumonia and Kaposi's sarcoma.

Oral

AIDS has a variety of oral manifestations and these have been classified by Pindborg (1989).

The commonest of these are candidiasis, hairy leukoplakia, Kaposi's sarcomata and periodontal infections.

Periodontal

The main periodontal infections associated with AIDS are ANUG and rapidly progressive atypical periodontitis. Two types of periodontal disease, HIV gingivitis (HIV-G) and HIV periodontitis (HIV-P) have been described in HIV patients by Winkler and Murray (1987). HIV-G manifests as a distinct erythema of the free and attached gingiva and sometimes the alveolar mucosa. It bleeds easily and may fail to respond to treatment. HIV-P involves extensive soft tissue necrosis and marked loss of periodontal attachment. Soft tissue destruction can be rapid and is often accompanied by interdental necrosis and ulceration which can expose bone. Unlike chronic periodontitis, there is no deep pocket formation but rather marked recession, ulceration and exposure and sometimes sequestration of bone. Localized pain is a feature of this condition (Winkler *et al.*, 1988). The microbiology of HIV-G and HIV-P are the same as that associated with chronic periodontitis. It is probably the disruption of immune function by HIV infection that increases the pathogenicity of these bacteria.

Other HIV associated lesions may occur on the gingiva and these include herpetic gingivostomatitis, candidiasis, human papillomavirus (HPV) causing multiple condylomas of the gingival margin and gingival ulceration due to infection with *Mycobacterium avium intracellulare* (Volpe *et al.*, 1985). Kaposi's sarcoma is the commonest oral tumour (Lozada *et al.*, 1983) and it can involve the gingival margin. Non-Hodgkin's lymphoma has been found in AIDS patients and may appear as a diffuse gingival swelling, epulis or nodule (Phelan *et al.*, 1987).

Treatment of HIV-G and HIV-P

Very careful cross infection control must be used with all these patients as all periodontal procedures produce blood in the mouth. Patients are normally treated by conventional periodontal therapy, i.e. plaque control, scaling and root planing. This may be supplemented by the use of chlorhexidine mouthwashes or local irrigation. The treatment is usually very successful in HIV infection but not in AIDS. Ulceration in HIV-P or ANUG may respond to antimicrobials such as metronidazole and amoxycillin.

References

Greene, W.C. (1993) AIDS and the Immune System. *Scientific American* (Sept.) pp. 67–73

Lozada, F., Silverman, S., Migliorati, C.A. *et al.* (1983) Oral manifestations of tumour and opportunistic infections in the acquired immunodeficiency syndrome (AIDS): finding in 53 homosexual men with Kaposi's sarcoma. *Oral Surgery, Oral Medicine, Oral Pathology* **56**, 491–494

Phelan, J.S., Saltzman, B.R., Friedland, G.H. and Klein, R.S. (1987) Oral findings in patients with acquired immunodeficiency syndrome. *Oral Surgery, Oral Medicine, Oral Pathology* **64**, 50–56

Pindborg, J.J. (1989) Classification of oral lesions associated with HIV infection. *Oral Surgery, Oral Medicine, Oral Pathology* **67**, 292–295

Volpe, F., Schwimmer, A. and Barr, C. (1985) Oral manifestations of disseminated *Mycobacterium avium intracellulare* in a patient with AIDS. *Oral Surgery, Oral Medicine, Oral Pathology* **60**, 567–570

Winkler, J.R., Grassi, M. and Murray, P.A. (1988) Clinical description and aetiology of HIV-associated periodontal diseases. In: Robertson, P.B. and Greenspan, J.S. (eds) *Oral Manifestations of AIDS* Littleton, MA, USA: PSG Publishing Company. pp. 49–70

Winkler, J.R. and Murray, P.A. (1987) Periodontal disease – a potential intra-oral expression of AIDS may be rapidly progressive periodontitis. *Journal of the Californian Dental Association* **15**, 20–24

8

The natural history of periodontal disease

In health the gingivae are firm, pink, knife-edged and do not bleed on probing. There is a shallow gingival crevice or sulcus and the junctional epithelium is attached to the enamel. The gingival fibre system is well organized. A few PMNs are present in the junctional epithelium as they pass through from the gingival vessels into the gingival crevice and into the mouth. In the subjacent connective tissue isolated inflammatory cells, mainly lymphocytes with the occasional plasma cell and macrophage, may also be seen. The picture manifests the quiet but dynamic balance of health.

Gingivitis

Because plaque accumulation is greatest in the sheltered interdental region gingival inflammation tends to start in the interdental papilla and spread from there around the neck of the tooth.

The histopathology of chronic gingivitis has been described chronologically by Page and Schroeder (1976) in a number of stages: the initial lesion at 2–4 days followed by an early gingivitis which at 2–3 weeks becomes an established gingivitis. These changes were described by examining biopsies of experimental gingivitis lesions at different time intervals.

The initial lesion

The first observed change occurs around the small gingival blood vessels apical to the junctional epithelium. These vessels begin to leak and perivascular collagen disappears to be replaced by a few inflammatory cells, plasma cells and lymphocytes – mainly T lymphocytes – tissue fluid and serum protein. There is increased migration of leucocytes through the junctional epithelium and exudation of tissue fluid from the gingival crevice. Other than the increased flow of fluid exudate and PMNs there may be no clinical signs of tissue change at this stage.

Early gingivitis

If plaque deposition persists, the initial inflammatory changes continue with an increased flow of gingival fluid and migration of PMNs. Changes occur in both the junctional and crevicular epithelia where there are signs of cell separation and some proliferation of basal cells. Fibroblasts begin to degenerate and the collagen bundles of the dentogingival fibre groups break up so that the seal of the marginal cuff of gingiva is weakened. There is a small increase in the number of inflammatory cells, 75% of which are lymphocytes. There are also a few plasma cells and macrophages. The clinical signs at this stage are few and the gingivae often appear clinically healthy. This is because the lesion, which has become more 'chronic' in nature, occupies a very small area of the gingiva. Also the signs of acute inflammation reduce as the lesion becomes chronic. This stage is probably classed as gingival health in clinical dentistry.

Established gingivitis

If satisfactory oral hygiene is not re-established, clinically obvious gingivitis becomes established within 7–14 days. Clinical signs of inflammation

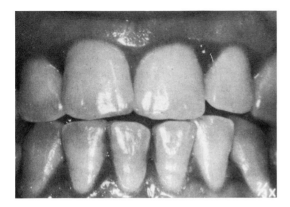

Figure 8.1 The first clinical signs of gingival inflammation: swelling of interdental papilla and involvement of gingival margin

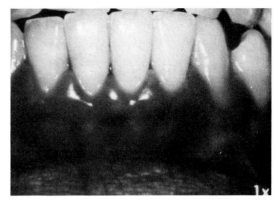

Figure 8.2 Established gingival inflammation with papillary swelling

appear and the interdental papillae may become swollen and bleed on probing (Figure 8.1). The number of lymphocytes increase and B-lymphocytes become more dominant. Many of these cells mature and develop into plasma cells which manufacture specific antibodies to the many plaque antigens. Some macrophages appear but there is a secondary stimulation of acute inflammation produced by complement activation. This results in the emigration of PMNs from blood vessels, and many of these also migrate through the junctional epithelium into the gingival crevice. The flow of gingival crevicular fluid (GCF), an inflammatory exudate, increases. Immunoglobulins, mainly IgG, are found in the gingival connective tissue and GCF. Mast cells are also found in the gingival connective tissue and junctional epithelium. These changes result in clinical gingival inflammation and the gingivae are red, swollen and bleed easily (*Figure 8.2*). The lesion increases in size and occupies a larger volume within the gingival connective tissue.

With the increased destruction of collagen and inflammatory swelling the gingival margin can be separated easily from the tooth surface giving rise to 'gingival' or 'false' pocketing (*Figure 8.3b*). If there is considerable inflammatory oedema and gingival swelling the gingival pocket can be quite deep. There is now degeneration of the cells of the junctional epithelium and some proliferation of its basal layers into the underlying connective tissue but at this stage there is no significant migration of epithelial cells on to the root surface.

As the inflammation spreads along the trans-septal fibres there may be some resorption of the alveolar crest. This is reversible on resolution of the inflammation.

One interesting feature of the disease is that no bacteria are found either in the epithelium or in the connective tissue.

As fibrous tissue is destroyed within the site of active inflammation, at more distant sites there is some proliferation of fibrous tissue and formation of new blood vessels. This productive or repair activity is a very important characteristic of the chronic lesion and where the irritation and inflammation are longstanding the fibrous tissue element can become the predominant component of the tissue change.

Thus destruction and repair continue side by side and the proportion of each affects the colour and shape of the gingivae. If the inflammation dominates, the tissues are red, soft and bleed easily; if fibrous tissue production dominates, the gingivae can be firm and pink, although swollen, and there may be little or no bleeding.

The systemic factors which determine the tissue response to plaque irritation are discussed in Chapter 6.

Effective treatment of gingivitis will remove the cause of irritation and the condition will resolve and turn back into a small lesion resembling the 'early' lesion with a small number of lymphocytes occupying a small area of gingival connective tissue subjacent to the junctional epithelium. The gingiva then appears clinically healthy.

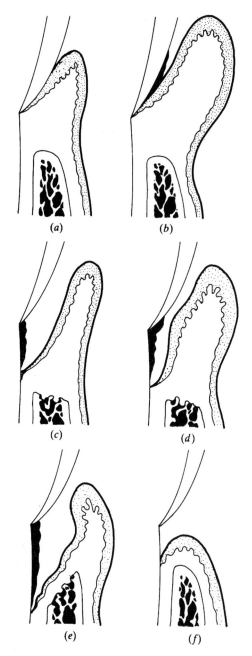

Figure 8.3 Diagram to show the various forms of periodontal pathology: (*a*) gingival health and shallow gingival crevice; (*b*) gingival swelling with production of a 'false' or gingival pocket; (*c*) 'true' or periodontal pocket with apical migration of crevicular epithelium and associated resorption of alveolar crest to form a 'suprabony' pocket; (*d*) a suprabony pocket plus gingival hyperplasia producing a deep pocket but little bone loss; (*e*) an 'infrabony' pocket where the epithelial attachment is apical to the alveolar crest; (*f*) gingival recession, i.e. equal apical movement of gingival margin and alveolar crest (is this pathological?)

The lesions described so far have been described as 'contained' because they are limited to the gingiva and are largely reversible on removal of the plaque. They may remain contained for many years; on the other hand, an established gingivitis lesion may spread into the deeper tissues to become a destructive chronic periodontitis. This progression is not inevitable, and some longitudinal studies indicate that the incidence of conversion to periodontitis is very low (Albander *et al.*, 1986; Listgarten, 1988). There is considerable debate as to whether this progression is determined by the nature of the bacterial plaque or by host factors or by both. Plasma cells appear to be related to more aggressive lesions and it is possible that the proliferation of plasma cells may be provoked by particular plaque constituents.

Chronic periodontitis

With continuing plaque irritation and inflammation the integrity of the junctional epithelium is increasingly damaged. The epithelial cells degenerate and separate and the attachment to the tooth completely breaks down. At the same time the junctional epithelium proliferates into the connective tissue and *down the root surface* as the dentogingival fibres and alveolar crest fibres are destroyed. Apical migration of the junctional epithelium continues and as this epithelium separates from the root surface a 'periodontal' or 'true' pocket is formed (*Figure 8.3c*). This seems to be an irreversible change.

Once a true pocket is formed plaque is in contact with the cementum. The connective tissue is oedematous; vessels are dilated and thrombosed; vessel walls break down with haemorrhage into the surrounding tissues. There is a massive inflammatory infiltrate of plasma cells, lymphocytes and macrophages. IgG is the predominant immunoglobulin but some IgM and IgA are present. The epithelium of the pocket wall may be intact or ulcerated. This appears to make no difference as plaque products diffuse through the epithelium. The flow of GCF and migration of PMNs continue and it is likely that the fluid flow helps to promote the deposition of subgingival calculus.

Extension of the inflammation into the alveolar crest is marked by the infiltration of some inflammatory cells into trabecular spaces, and these may increase in size. Bone resorption tends to be compensated for by deposition further away from the inflammatory zone so that the bone is remodelled but shows a net loss. Bone resorption usually starts interproximally so that where the table of interproximal bone is broad, as it is between molars, an interdental crater is formed and then as the resorption process spreads laterally the entire alveolar crest is resorbed.

The periodontal lesion also appears to be 'contained' because as it advances and connective tissue is destroyed the trans-septal fibres are continually reformed and seem to separate the main inflammatory infiltrate from the underlying bone.

The progression of the lesion is not continuous, periods of advance and remission take place, and fibrosis is a constant feature, especially in the latter phase.

With destruction of periodontal ligament and alveolar crest resorption the pocket deepens. At a later stage in the disease there may be varying degrees of suppuration and abscess formation. Finally, the teeth become loose, migrate and are lost.

Disease progression

At one time it was believed that periodontitis, once established, progresses continuously and inevitably, with a simple straight-line age correlation. This led to the notion that tooth-loss was part of the ageing process. So strong was this belief that many dentists recommended full extractions in middle age when the patient was still 'adaptable' to dentures, rather than waiting to a time when the elderly person, having lost most or all teeth, would find such adaptation difficult or impossible.

This belief about the pattern of disease progression was supported by clinical studies which reduced measurements of pocket depth or alveolar bone loss to average values for a given mouth, thus eliminating intra-oral variation and obscuring both sites of little or no disease, and sites of worst disease. Epidemiological studies on various populations also used average values for age groups, and these findings also supported the belief in a straightforward age-correlated linear progression. In this way ideas about longitudinal change were derived from the compilation of misleading findings from cross-sectional studies.

However, detailed measurement of loss of attachment at specific sites over time, i.e. valid longitudinal study, contradicts the idea of continuous and inevitable disease progression, and indicates that:

1. As stated above, gingivitis, even when persistent and untreated, does not inevitably progress to periodontitis.
2. Even when established periodontal destruction is not continuous but progresses in an episodic manner with 'bursts' of destructive activity alternating with periods of quiescence, and possibly repair.
3. There is great individual variation in the pattern of destruction, which also varies over time in the same individual.

Some research workers believe that the bursts of activity occur at random (Goodson *et al.*, 1982; Socransky, 1984), and that a past history of persistent and severe gingivitis or of periodontal destruction does not indicate future destructive activity. Thus, progress is unpredictable. Other workers find that progress is not random, and that there is a correlation between the initial degree of bone loss and the subsequent rate of bone loss (Papapanou *et al.*, 1989; Albander, 1990). Thus, progression is to some extent predictable. Others have suggested that prognosis is affected by the site of disease, i.e. whether related to incisors, molars or distributed generally.

Many studies show that, once initiated the average rate of bone loss is very slow, 0.05–0.1 mm per year (Suomi *et al.*, 1971; Sheiham *et al.*, 1986; Albander, 1990). However, this is not always the case; in some people rapid bone loss occurs early in life, and in others rapid bone loss may follow years of little or very slow tissue destruction.

It must be recognised that the amount of probing attachment loss (PAL) that can be reliably measured depends upon the threshold for the probing method used (see Chapter 12). Most of the clinical longitudinal studies which led to the development of the 'burst' theory of periodontal progression (Goodson *et al.*, 1982; Lindhe, Haffajee and Socransky, 1983; Haffajee and Socransky, 1986) used manual probing which cannot reliably measure changes in PAL of less than 2.5–3 mm. They

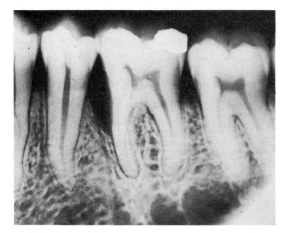

Figure 8.4 Radiographic appearance of bone defect associated with infrabony pocket mesial ⌐6. The bone defect is frequently described as an 'intrabony' defect. Note early alveolar crest resorption in other areas which are related to suprabony pockets

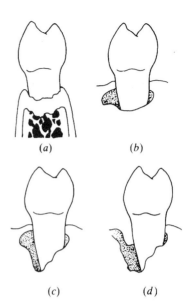

Figure 8.5 Diagram to show some forms of bone defect: (*a*) interdental crater; (*b*) three-walled defect; (*c*) two-walled defect; (*d*) one-walled defect or hemisepta

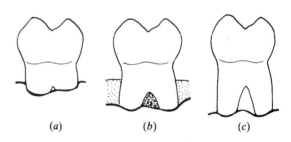

Figure 8.6 Diagram to show furcation defects: (*a*) Class 1; (*b*) Class 2; (*c*) Class 3

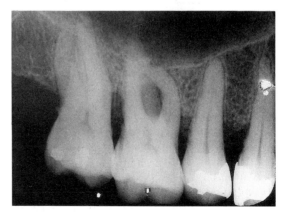

Figure 8.7 Radiographic appearance of trifurcation Class 3 defect

would therefore only detect rapidly progressive attachment loss (RAL) losing this amount or more and would not detect gradual attachment loss (GAL) losing much smaller amounts possibly over a longer time period. They therefore lead to the notion that all periodontal progression occurs in bursts of activity over short time periods.

More recently electronic probes have been developed which will measure PAL more reliably and accurately and have thresholds of 0.3–0.8 mm (see Chapter 12). Using an electronic probe which detects and measures from the cement-enamel junction (CEJ) with a threshold of 0.25 mm, Jeffcoat *et al.* (1991) monitored 30 patients with moderate-advanced chronic periodontitis for 6 months. Using a threshold of 0.4 mm they found 29% of sites with attachment loss (AL) and using one of 2.4 mm they found AL at only 2% of sites. This latter figure is similar to the percentage in the studies above which used manual probing. This indicated that using large thresholds only RAL will be detected whilst using smaller thresholds will detect both RAL and GAL with a higher proportion of GAL sites. Thus it appears that both RAL, progressing by 'bursts', and GAL occur during the progression of chronic periodontitis. GAL could either result small 'mini-bursts' of activity producing AL of less than 0.5 mm or from slow progressive AL or both. It is likely that patients susceptible to periodontal disease will tend to progress more by bursts of RAL whilst those with lesser susceptibilities would progress more slowly and gradually.

It has also been shown that in patients with moderate chronic periodontitis that further attachment loss mostly occurred at sites with previous probing depths greater than 5 mm (Gribic and Lamster, 1991, 1992).

At present we are handicapped in making precise diagnoses and prognoses by two important limitations:

1. We have no reliable markers for present disease activity (see Chapter 13).
2. We have no reliable criteria for identifying the 'at-risk' individual.

Bone defects

The pattern of alveolar resorption can vary from one tooth to the next and on different aspects of the same tooth.

It is believed that inflammation spreads from the gingiva into the deeper tissues along three pathways: through the alveolar bone, the attached gingiva and the periodontal ligament. The primary pathway appears to be through the alveolar bone in which inflammation tracks via perivascular and perineural channels into trabecular spaces. It may then travel laterally from bone into periodontal ligament and attached gingiva. If resorption of the alveolar crest is even, the base of the pocket remains coronal to the crest of the bone and a simple 'suprabony' pocket is formed, i.e. a pocket entirely surrounded by soft tissue (*Figure 8.3c*). If resorption of the alveolar crest proceeds more rapidly in one part than another at the base of the pocket becomes apical to the crest of the bone. This is known as an 'infrabony' pocket (*Figures 8.3e* and *8.4*).

As cancellous bone is more vascular and less dense than cortical bone it is likely that, as stated above, the central cancellous part of a broad alveolar septum will resorb more rapidly than the lateral parts made up of cortical bone so that an infrabony pocket is formed in relation to an interdental 'crater'.

The variety of bone defects is infinite, but for purposes of description they have been classified according to their morphology as marginal defects, intra-alveolar defects, perforation and furcation defects. These are very rough groupings with considerable overlap. In chronic inflammation the formative bone response may more than compensate for the bone resorption so that a thickened or bulbous alveolar margin is formed. Intra-alveolar defects, i.e. defects within the alveolar process, are commonly classified according to the number of bone walls, that is, one- two- or three-walled (*Figure 8.5*). This group also includes interdental craters and hemisepta.

Furcation defects have been classified according to the degree of bone loss in the furcation measured in a horizontal plane (*Figure 8.6*). An early or Class 1 defect is one which penetrates less than 2 mm into the furcation; a Class 2 defect is one where the bone loss is greater than 2 mm into the interradicular area but does not go completely through the furcation so that one aspect of the bone is intact; in a Class 3 defect so much inter-radicular bone has been lost that a probe can be passed between the roots from one side to the other (*Figure 8.7*).

There has been much speculation about the factors which might determine the pattern of bone resorption. Two factors appear to play an important role: the original morphology of the bone, and excessive occlusal stress. Variations in original bone morphology must influence the type of bone defects in disease. A thin alveolar plate of bone is more likely to be completely resorbed than a thick plate of bone; a thin interdental septum between incisors may be completely destroyed while an interdental crater will form in the septum between molars. A split or dehiscence may be formed where bone coronal to a developmental defect, a perforation or fenestration is resorbed by progressive inflammation.

Occlusal trauma

Considerable debate has centred on the role of occlusal forces in the development and progress of periodontal disease, as well as on the influence of these forces on the rate and form of alveolar bone destruction. Functional stresses on all parts of the skeleton tend to strengthen, while lack of function tends to weaken the tissues. Experimental rats fed on a coarse diet have thicker and heavier jaws than those fed on a soft diet, and the periodontal ligament is composed of more and thicker collagen bundles in the former group than in the latter.

Many experiments have been carried out on animals to determine the results of overloading teeth. A basic problem in such studies is to distinguish the effects of plaque-induced inflammation from those produced by occlusal stresses, and great care must be taken to maintain a high standard of oral hygiene in the experimental animals. A number of experiments demonstrate the kind of tissue changes produced in the tooth-supporting tissues when overloaded, e.g. when pressures are applied to teeth by different types of appliance or when a high restoration is placed so that it interferes with the occlusion.

The pattern of changes in the periodontium depends on whether the forces applied to the teeth are uni- or multidirectional. The reactions of the tissues to both of these are described below:

Orthodontic type trauma

This is brought about by single directional forces applied to a normal periodontium such as occurs in orthodontic tooth movement. This type of trauma has been investigated in animal studies by histological examination of blocks of teeth and periodontium after varying time periods (Reitan, 1951; Mühlemann and Herzog, 1961; Ewan and Stahl, 1962; Warhaug and Hansen, 1966; Karing *et al.*, 1982). The crown of the tooth is tilted in the direction of the force and the tooth moves about its fulcrum at the apical third of the root producing pressure and tension zones within the marginal and apical parts of the periodontium. On the pressure side the tissues become crushed and this produces disruption and disorganisation of the periodontal fibres leading to hyaline degeneration and necrosis of connective tissues. The blood vessels are damaged and haemorrhage and thrombosis is present. If the magnitude of the forces is within certain limits, the periodontal ligament cells remain vital and osteoclasts appear on the adjacent bone surface leading to bone resorption. This is known as direct bone resorption. However, if the force is greater then damage to the ligament cells prevents this from occurring. In this situation osteoclasts develop in the marrow spaces below the bone surface and this leads to undermining or indirect bone resorption. This bone is resorbed until it reaches the hyalinised periodontium when the tooth is able to move away from the

pressure force. Macrophages and osteoclasts remove the damaged tissues after which they become revascularised allowing new periodontal tissues to form. Bone deposition then occurs in the tension zones to compensate for the increased width of the periodontium in this area. Once the tooth has moved the pressure is nullified and the full healing of the periodontal tissues takes place in both the pressure and tension zones.

Bodily movement of the teeth with fixed orthodontic appliances produce the same changes except that the pressure and tension zones are more extended in the apical-coronal direction. If excessive forces are used root cementum and dentine may also be resorbed.

These changes affect only the intra alveolar periodontal ligament and do not involve the supra alveolar connective tissues and therefore cannot affect the marginal periodontal tissues.

Jiggling-type trauma

The kind of stress that is transmitted to the tooth in occlusal trauma is not unidirectional but rather multidirectional. Cuspal interference imposes intermittent loading on opposing teeth and this is usually resisted by soft tissues forces or secondary cuspal contacts. This produces alternating or 'jiggling' forces on the teeth. These have been investigated by a number of animal studies which have sought to reproduce these 'jiggling' forces (Wentz *et al.*, 1958; Glickman and Smulow, 1968; Svanberg and Lindhe, 1973; Meitner, 1975; Ericsson and Lindhe, 1982). These forces produce alternating pressure and tension zones within the intra-alveolar periodontium and these exhibit the same changes described above for the pressure zones in unidirectional forces. The direct or indirect bone resorption associated with this process leads to a generalised widening of the periodontal ligament space and as a result of this the tooth or teeth involved display progressive increasing mobility. When the effect of the forces is compensated by the increased width of the ligament space, the damaged tissues are removed and the widened periodontium heals. The tooth remains mobile within this widened periodontium.

As with unidirectional forces, these changes affect only the intra alveolar periodontal ligament and do not involve the supra alveolar connective tissues. Therefore, they cannot affect the marginal periodontal tissues.

Jiggling-type trauma applied to a reduced periodontium

The effects of these forces on a reduced but healthy periodontium has been studied in dogs by Ericsson and Lindhe (1977). The same changes as have been described above were produced around the whole intra-alveolar periodontium which increased in width. The affected teeth became progressively mobile over several weeks after which the enlarged space compensated for the for the forces. The bone resorption then ceased and the periodontal tissues in the enlarged space healed. The teeth remained hypermobile but were surrounded by periodontal tissues which had adapted to the increased functional forces. The supra-alveolar connective tissues and marginal periodontium were again unaffected by the changes.

Jiggling-type trauma superimposed on inflammatory chronic periodontitis

Older studies

The relation between occlusal trauma and inflammatory periodontal disease has often been discussed in connection with human case reports and autopsy material. On the basis of this Glickman (1964, 1965, 1967, 1971) claimed that the path along which the plaque-associated inflammatory lesion spread was affected by the presence of occlusal trauma. In this connection it was suggested that occlusal trauma changed the vascular pattern so that the inflammatory lesion passed into the periodontal ligament space rather than into the alveolar crest (Macapanpan and Weinmann, 1954). Glickman and Smulow (1962, 1965, 1968) claimed from the results of human autopsy and animal experiments that occlusal trauma imposed on inflammatory periodontitis produced angular bone resorption and infrabony pocketing. However, Warhaug (1979) examined human autopsy material and reported that angular bony defects and infrabony pockets usually occurred in areas unaffected by occlusal trauma. His findings supported the observations of Prichard (1965) and Manson (1976) which showed that the pattern of alveolar bone loss resulted from an interplay between the form of the alveolar bone and the apical extension of the subgingival plaque on the root surface. Furthermore, these findings did not support the concept of Glickman (1964, 1971) which described a zone

of co-destruction within the periodontium which could be affected by the combined effects of marginal inflammation and occlusal trauma. These matters have now been largely resolved by the later studies described below.

Later studies

Experiments on humans and other animals described in the previous sections have shown that trauma from occlusion cannot induce changes in the supra alveolar marginal tissues. The effect of jiggling trauma superimposed on progressive destructive periodontitis have been studied by a number of research groups (Lindhe and Svanberg, 1974; Meitner, 1975; Nyman *et al.*, 1978; Ericsson and Lindhe, 1982). In these experiments destructuve periodontitis was first initiated in dogs or monkeys and then the teeth were subject to jiggling trauma. The periodontal tissues in the combined pressure/tension zones were damaged as described before. The intra-alveolar periodontium showed signs of inflammation with hyperaemia, exudation, thrombosis and migration of inflammatory cells. Numerous osteoclasts differentiated on the adjacent bone surface and bone was resorbed. This process gradually increased the width of the periodontal ligament space and as a result the teeth became increasingly mobile. Angular bone resorption could be seen on radiographs of the affected area. The forces became nullified by the increased width of the periodontal ligament space and at this point the bone resorption ceased. The periodontium regenerated its normal tissues and within this increased space the tooth mobility stopped increasing. The angular bone resorption persisted but histological examination revealed that no further apical migration of the junctional epithelium had resulted from the imposition of occlusal trauma. This indicates that occlusal forces which allow adaptive alterations within the ligament will not aggravate inflammatory periodontal disease.

However, if this jiggling occlusal trauma generated greater forces and these were maintained for long time periods so that the periodontium could not become adapted, then the injury persisted and in some cases became permanent (Lindhe and Svanberg, 1974). In these cases the pressure/tension zones displayed continuing inflammation and damage over several months. The osteoclasts residing in the alveolar wall persisted producing continuing bone resorption and the angular bone defects remained. These changes produced gradual progressive widening of the periodontal ligament space and progressively increased tooth mobility. Under these circumstances the marginal inflammatory lesion merged with the 'trauma' lesion in the periodontium. The junctional epithelium proliferated apically and the destructive periodontal disease was aggravated.

In another set of experiments in the dog (Ericsson and Lindhe, 1982) prolonged jiggling forces for 10 months were applied to some teeth with established chronic periodontitis and these were compared with other control teeth also with established chronic periodontitis in the same dog which were not jiggled. The traumatised teeth showed an increased rate of progression compared with control teeth.

Conclusion

Unidirectional or jiggling forces applied to the healthy periodontium will not result in loss of attachment as trauma from occlusion cannot affect the marginal tissues. It does, however, produce tooth mobility within an adapted, widened periodontium. All of these changes are reversible on the removal of the trauma.

However, in teeth with established chronic periodontitis, superimposed prolonged and severe jiggling trauma may cause persistent damage within the periodontium such that adaptive changes are prevented from developing. Under these circumstances the marginal periodontal and intra alveolar 'trauma' lesions may merge and this can enhance the rate of periodontal disease progression.

The causes of excessive occlusal stress are discussed in Chapter 24. Loads can become excessive in two situations: (i) where this is an actual alteration in occlusal load, and (ii) where there is a reduced capacity of the tooth-supporting tissues to absorb stress. Tissue damage caused by applying excessive occlusal loads to a previously healthy periodontium has been called *primary occlusal trauma*. Damage caused by normal functional stress applied to an impaired periodontium has been called *secondary occlusal trauma*. The division into primary and secondary trauma is rather artificial as, more often than not, excessive loads are applied to an already impaired periodontium. However, it remains a useful conceptual distinction as primary trauma is completely

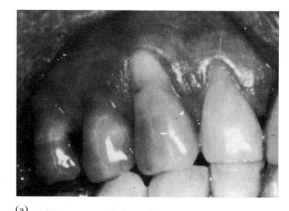

(a)

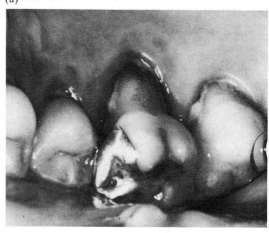

(b)

Figure 8.8 Gingival recession associated with (*a*) traumatic toothbrushing technique which has also produced tooth abrasion (note associated area of gingival irritation over the premolars) and (*b*) a divergent palatal root

reversible (as in orthodontic treatment) while the tissue changes associated with secondary trauma may be only partly reversible.

Gingival recession (*Figure 8.8*)

Gingival atrophy results in apical movement of the gingival margin to produce gingival recession and exposure of the root of the tooth. Recession involves some destruction of the periodontal tissues and it may accompany chronic periodontitis, but it is not necessarily a feature of that disease. Gingival recession is one of those tissue changes which are usually caused by the wear and tear of use and which lie between health and active pathology. Like tooth attrition gingival recession represents a departure from normal anatomy, which is not necessarily a sign of disease. It is extremely common and frequently the cause of patient concern.

A number of factors acting singly or in combination produce or affect gingival recession.

1. Physical abuse

Both healthy gingiva and the gingival wall of a periodontal pocket can atrophy under the stress of toothbrush friction, especially when an overzealous horizontal brushing technique is used. The sheltered interdental gingiva may escape this treatment so that the recession is restricted to labial tooth surfaces which may also suffer abrasion. The maxillary canines and first premolars which form the corner of the arch receive the brunt of this form of aggression and usually display the worst recession. The interdental gingiva may not escape the enthusiastic use of various interdental oral hygiene aids; some patients use woodsticks and floss like a hacksaw, and although gingiva and the underlying bone are remarkably resilient they will atrophy in the face of determined attack.

Physical damage can also result from a variety of dental procedures – the carelessly applied matrix band or temporary crown, uncontrolled condensation of an interproximal or cervical restoration, pressure from a badly designed denture clasp or denture ('gum stripping') – or from strange habits, such as pressing a pencil into the gum!

Another physical factor is that associated with deep overbite where the incisal edge of an upper incisor impinges on the lower labial gingiva or where a lower incisor strikes the palatal tissue.

2. Alveolar defects

The presence of an underlying alveolar margin defect, e.g. dehiscence, means that the overlying gingiva is unsupported and less able to withstand irritation. The Northern European skull is often dolicocephalic, i.e. long-headed, the jaws narrow and overcrowded and alveolar plates thin; developmental defects, dehiscence and fenestration are common, especially on the labial surface of canines, lower incisors and first molars. Defects of alveolar plates are frequently related to tooth position and root morphology.

3. Tooth position

The position of the tooth in the arch is a determinant of the thickness of bone overlying the root. A displaced tooth may be accompanied by some compensating thickness of overlying bone but there is a limit to such accommodation and where teeth are placed in, say, a labial position the labial alveolar margin is displaced apically or is deficient (dehiscence).

Furthermore, teeth can be moved through alveolar bone by uncontrolled orthodontic forces and excessive occlusal stress, with resultant bone perforation and gingival recession.

4. Root morphology

Where roots diverge, as they do especially on first upper molars or where the root is markedly convex as it may be on both upper and lower canines, the overlying bone may be very thin or deficient. This may not manifest in health but where some tissue destruction has taken place a divergent palatal root of an upper first molar can be related to gross recession (*Figure 8.8b*).

5. Soft-tissue attachment

The presence of a frenum or muscle attachment does not influence healthy gingiva but, in the presence of inflammation and pocketing, tension from these anatomical structures may result in retraction of the gingiva and recession. This is often the case where the zone of attached gingiva is narrow or absent. However, the mere presence of a frenum never justifies surgical intervention; only when an anatomical feature is obviously related to progressive pathology is surgical modification indicated.

6. Disease

Acute necrotising ulcerative gingivitis (*see* Chapter 22) can destroy gingival tissue which may not be reformed when the disease has resolved.

If sufficient tissue is destroyed recession results. In addition, the gingival wall of a periodontal pocket may move apically as the disease progresses or as inflammation subsides, to produce root exposure.

Recession follows surgery for the treatment of chronic periodontitis.

References

Albander, J.M., Rise, J., Gjermo, P. and Johansen, R.J. (1986) Radiographic quantification of alveolar bone level changes. *Journal of Clinical Periodontology* **13**, 195–200

Albander, J.M. (1990) A 6-year study on the pattern of periodontal disease progression. *Journal of Periodontology* **17**, 467–471

Ericsson, I. and Lindhe, J. (1977) Lack of effect of trauma from occlusion on the recurrence of experimental periodontitis. *Journal of Clinical Periodontology* **4**, 115–127

Ericsson, I. and Lindhe, J. (1982) The effect of longstanding jiggling on experimental marginal periodontitis in the beagle dog. *Journal of Clinical Periodontology* **9**, 497–503

Ewan, S.J. and Stahl, S.S. (1962) The response of the periodontium to chronic gingival irritation and long-term tilting forces in adult dogs. *Oral Surgery, Oral Medicine and Oral Pathology* **15**, 1426–1433

Glickman, I. (1964) Trauma from occlusion in the etiology of periodontal disease. In *Clinical Periodontology*, Third edition. Philadelphia, W.B. Saunders, pp. 286–299

Glickman, I. (1965) Clinical significance of trauma from occlusion. *Journal of American Dental Association* **70**, 607–618

Glickman, I. (1967) Occlusion and the periodontium. *Journal of Dental Research* **49** (Suppl. 1), 53

Glickman, I. and Smulow, J.B. (1962) Alterations in the pathway of gingival inflammation into the underlying tissues induced by excessive occlusal forces. *Journal of Periodontology* **33**, 7–13

Glickman, I. and Smulow, J.B. (1965) Effects of excessive occlusal forces upon the pathway of gingival inflammation in humans. *Journal of Periodontology* **36**, 141–147

Glickman, I. and Smulow, J.B. (1968) Adaptive alteration in the periodontium of the Rhesus monkey in chronic trauma from occlusion. *Journal of Periodontology* **39**, 101–105

Glickman, I. (1971) Role of occlusion in the etiology and treatment in periodontal disease. *Journal of Dental Research* **50**, 199–204

Goodson, J.M., Tanner, A.C.R., Haffajee, A.D., Sornberger, G.C. and Socransky, S.S. (1982) Patterns of progression and regression of advanced destructive periodontal disease. *Journal of Clinical Periodontology* **9**, 472–481

Gribic, J.T. and Lamster, I.B. (1991) Risk indicators for future clinical attachment loss in adult periodontitis. Patient variables. *Journal of Periodontology* **62**, 322–329

Gribic, J.T. and Lamster, I.B. (1992) Risk indicators for future clinical attachment loss in adult periodontitis. Tooth and site variables. *Journal of Periodontology* **63**, 262–269

Haffajee, A.D. and Socransky, S.S. (1986) Attachment level changes in destructive periodontal disease. *Journal of Clinical Periodontology* **13**, 461–472

Jeffcoat, M.K. and Reddy, M.S. (1991) Progression of probing attachment loss in adult periodontitis. *Journal of Periodontology* **62**, 185–189

Karing, T., Nyman, S., Thilander, B. and Magnusson, I. (1982) Bone regeneration in orthodontically produced alveolar bone dehiscences. *Journal of Periodontal Research* **17**, 309–315

Lindhe, J. and Svanberg, G. (1974) Influence of trauma from occlusion on progression of experimental periodontitis in the beagle dog. *Journal of Clinical Periodontology* **1**, 3–14

Lindhe, J., Haffajee, A.D. and Socransky, S.S. (1983) Progression of periodontal disease in adult subjects in the absence of periodontal therapy. *Journal of Clinical Periodontology* **10**, 433–442

Listgarten, M.A. (1988) Why do epidemiological data have no diagnostic value? In: *Periodontology Today*, ed B. Guggenheim, Basel, S. Karger, pp. 59–67

Macapanpan, L.C. and Weinmann. J.P. (1954) The influence of injury to the periodontal membrane on the spread of gingival inflammation. *Journal of Dental Research* **33**, 263–272

Manson, J.D. (1976) Bone morphology and bone loss in periodontal disease. *Journal of Clinical Periodontology* **3**, 14–22

Meitner, S.W. (1975) *Co-destructive Factors of Marginal Periodontitis and Repetitive Mechanical Injury*. Thesis, Rochester, USA: Eastman Dental Center and The University of Rochester

Mühlemann, H.R. and Herzog, H. (1961) Tooth mobility and microscopic tissue changes produced by experimental occlusal trauma. *Helvetica Odontologica Acta* **5**, 33–39

Nyman, S., Lindhe, J. and Ericsson, I. (1978) The effect of progressive tooth mobility on destructive periodontitis in the dog. *Journal of Clinical Periodontology* **7**, 351–360

Page, R.C. and Schroeder, H.E. (1989) Pathogenesis of inflammatory periodontal disease. A summary of current work. *Laboratory Investigation* **3**, 235–249

Papapanou, P.N., Wennstrom, J.L. and Grondahl, K. (1989) A 10-year study of periodontal disease progression. *Journal of Clinical Periodontology* **16**, 403–411

Prichard, J.F. (1965) *Advances in Periodontal Disease*. Philadelphia, W.B. Saunders

Reitan, K. (1951) The initial tissue reaction incident to orthodontic tooth movement as related to the influence of function. *Acta Odontologica Scandanavica* **10** (Suppl.)

Sheiham, A., Smales, F.C., Cushing, A.M. and Cowell, C.R. (1986) Changes in periodontal health in a cohort of British workers over a 14-year period. *British Dental Journal* **160**, 125–127

Socransky, S.S., Haffajee, A.D., Goodson, J.M. and Lindhe, J. (1984) New concepts of destructive periodontal disease. *Journal of Clinical Periodontology* **11**, 21–32

Suomi, J.D., Greene, J.C., Vermillion, J.R. *et al.* (1971) The effect of controlled oral hygiene procedures on the progression of periodontal disease in adults: results after third and final year. *Journal of Periodontology* **42**, 152–160

Svanberg, G. and Lindhe, J. (1973) Experimental tooth hypermobility in the dog. A methodological study. *Odontologisk Revy* **24**, 269–282

Warhaug, J. (1979) The infrabony pocket and its relationship to trauma from occlusion and subgingival plaque. *Journal of Periodontology* **50**, 355–365

Warhaug, J. and Hansen, E.R. (1966) Periodontal changes incident to prolonged occlusal overload in monkeys. *Acta Odontologica Scandanavica* **24**, 91–105

Wentz, F.M., Jarabak, J. and Orban, B. (1958) Experimental occlusal trauma imitating cuspal interferences. *Journal of Periodontology* **29**, 117–127

9

Epidemiology of periodontal disease (the size of the problem)

In the past few years, as described in Chapter 8, there has been a radical change in our ideas about the natural history of periodontal diseases. There has also been a parallel re-appraisal of their prevalence and the methods by which they are studied. Until recently periodontal disease was regarded as the main cause of tooth loss, and a WHO report of 1978 stated that 'almost all the adult population has experienced gingivitis, periodontitis or both.' These ideas are out-of-date and now seen as the result of invalid methods of data collection and interpretation.

There has been a reduction in disease prevalence, and the reasons for the improvement in periodontal health which has taken place in the industrialized countries are probably related to better personal and oral hygiene, improved standards of living, reduction in cigarette smoking, decrease in the use and dosage of oral contraceptives, plus the effects of fluoride, fewer proximal restorations and overhanging margins (Sheiham, 1990).

In order to measure the prevalence of the disease, its severity, and its relationship to other factors, such as age, oral hygiene status, nutrition and so on, special indices have been devised which attempt to provide an objective measure or score to specific identifiable features so that reliable comparisons can be made. Using these indices and applying the appropriate statistical tests should allow the interested observer to make a valid comparison of, for example, the periodontal condition of young adults in the USA with the periodon-tal condition of individuals of any age anywhere in the world. Also, if successful public health measures are to be implemented, and personnel trained and recruited, the character and size of the problems to be tackled need to be defined.

Indices

All indices should be appropriate to the nature of the investigation, and the circumstances under which this is being undertaken. Thus, the assessment of the gingival condition and oral hygiene status of 10–12-year-old children in an inner city area in Britain will require a very different approach from a study of the periodontal status of an East African nomadic cattle-breeding tribe, such as the Masai or Dinka! The application of any particular index needs to meet several criteria:

1. It must be practical and acceptable to the subject. The method of examination must not be painful or more uncomfortable than the individual can reasonably tolerate, e.g. taking six pocket measurements on every tooth in a child's mouth is impractical. Any examination in the absence of adequate illumination or sterilization facilities is not acceptable.
2. It must reflect the reality of the situation, thus pocket measurement on the buccal aspects of teeth may be irrelevant and misleading when the main site of periodon-tal destruction is interproximal. Also,

pocket depth is an indicator of past pathology, and cannot validly be used as an indicator of current disease activity.
3. It should be sufficiently standardized and reliable to allow comparison between different examiners, and between examinations at different times as in longitudinal studies.
4. It should allow numerical quantification and therefore statistical analysis. Assessment of gingival inflammation by degree of redness is subjective and quantifiable only in the grossest terms.
5. It should be sufficiently sensitive to detect small changes. Thus bleeding on probing the pocket may or may not indicate the presence of active disease and does not tell us about the strength of that activity; biochemical assessment of crevicular fluid might be sufficiently sensitive for that purpose.

Indices of the gingival condition use colour, change of contour, readiness to bleed on gentle probing, bleeding time, measurement of gingival fluid exudate, counts of white cells in gingival fluid and gingival histology. Indices of periodontal destruction depend largely on probing depth and probing attachment level measurements. Some of the tests require special equipment and special skills and are used therefore only in sophisticated laboratory studies. Conditions in the field usually do not permit other than the most simple tests to be used, especially where large numbers of individuals are inspected. The most commonly used index of gingival inflammation is the Gingival Index (Löe and Silness, 1963). The three periodontal indices to be described, the Periodontal Index (Russell, 1956), the Periodontal Disease Index (Ramfjord, 1959) and the Community Periodontal Index of Treatment Needs (CPITN; Ainamo *et al.*, 1983), score both gingival inflammation and periodontal destruction.

Gingival Index (GI)

The severity of the condition is indicated on a scale of 0 to 3:

0. Normal gingivae
1. Mild inflammation, slight change in colour, slight oedema. No bleeding on probing
2. Moderate inflammation, redness, oedema and glazing. Bleeding on probing

3. Severe inflammation, marked redness and oedema, ulceration. Tendency to spontaneous bleeding.

The mesial, buccal, distal and lingual gingival units are scored separately. This index is particularly sensitive in the early stages of gingivitis.

The gingival index is reversible as its values return to zero with the disappearance of the disease. By contrast, indices of chronic periodontitis measure the amount of periodontal destruction which is irreversible. Furthermore, as the progress of chronic periodontitis tends to be phasic, a periodontal index does not measure active disease.

Periodontal destruction indices

1. Periodontal Index (PI) (Russell, 1956)

All teeth are examined; the scores used in this index are as follows:

0. Negative: there is neither overt inflammation in the investing tissues nor loss of function due to destruction of supporting tissues
1. Mild gingivitis: there is an overt area of inflammation in the free gingivae, but this area does not circumscribe the tooth
2. Gingivitis: inflammation completely circumscribes the tooth, but there is no apparent break in the gingival attachment
6. Gingivitis with pocket formation: the epithelial attachment has been broken and there is a pocket (not merely a deepened crevice due to swelling in the free gingivae). There is no interference with normal masticatory function; the tooth is firm in its socket, and has not drifted
8. Advanced destruction with loss of masticatory function: the tooth may be loose, may have drifted, may sound dull on percussion with metallic instrument, may be depressible in its socket.

Rule: When in doubt, assign the lesser score.

This index has been applied with success to large population groups. Its limitation is that its score for periodontal destruction is so heavily weighted that it is not possible to distinguish the early stages of a chronic periodontitis.

2. *Periodontal Disease Index (PDI)* *(Ramfjord, 1959)*

The periodontal disease index introduced by Ramfjord is a development of the Russell index. The Ramfjord index is particularly designed for assessing the extent of pocket deepening below the cemento-enamel junction. Scoring is as follows:

0. Health
1. Mild to moderate inflammatory change not extending all around tooth
2. Mild to moderate inflammatory change extending all around tooth
3. Severe gingivitis, characterized by marked redness, tendency to bleed, ulceration
4. 3 mm apical extension of pocket base from enamel–cement junction
5. 3–6 mm extension
6. Over 6 mm extension.

Another feature of the PDI is that only six teeth, 6|14, 41|6 are selected for examination and measurement. The data from these teeth have been found to be representative of the dentition as a whole, and their average score is the score of the patient.

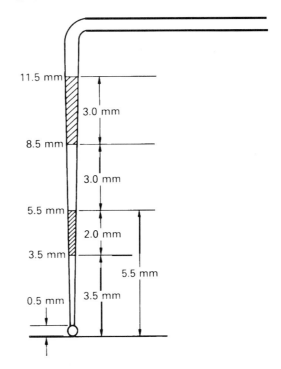

Figure 9.1 The CPITN probe

Community Periodontal Index of Treatment Needs (CPITN)

If an attempt is made to provide an adequate dental service for a particular community, it is necessary to assess its treatment need. The CPITN (Ainamo *et al.*, 1983) has become the most widely employed system for this purpose and uses the following method:

1. A specially banded probe with a ball head (*Figure 9.1*) has been designed for use with the index. It is to be used as an extension of the examiner's fingers in the gentle manipulation of the gingivae. The sensing force should correspond to about 20 g or less, and pain during probing indicates that too much pressure is being applied. A pressure guided probe has been designed to produce a standard force but it is difficult to see the relevance of such sensitive instrumentation in the context of CPITN.
2. The dentition is divided into six segments or sextants (four posterior and two anterior) in which there are two or more teeth present and not indicated for extraction. When only one tooth remains in a sextant, it is included in the adjacent sextant.
3. The scoring system is:
   Code 0 Health: no pocketing or gingival bleeding on probing
   Code 1 Gingival bleeding on probing
   Code 2 The presence of calculus or other plaque-retentive factors such as overhanging margins of restorations that can be seen or felt on probing
   Code 3 Pocketing of 4–5 mm, that is, when the gingival margin is on the black area of the probe
   Code 4 Pocketing of 6 mm or more, i.e. when the black area of the special probe is no longer visible
   Code X When only one tooth or no teeth are present in a sextant. Third molars are excluded unless they function in the place of second molars.
4. When used for epidemiological purposes (alternative 1), ten specific teeth are examined, these are 761|67, 76|167 and the worst of the two molar scores is recorded,

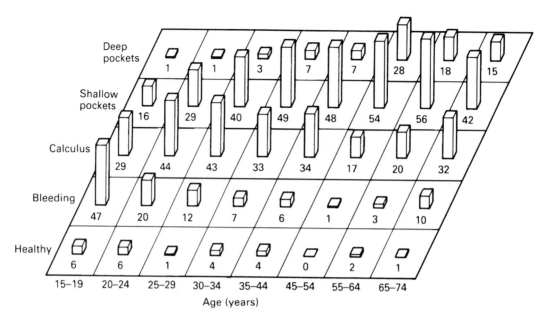

Figure 9.2 CPITN scores in Dutch National Survey. (Reproduced from *Guidelines for Community Periodontal Care,* by kind permission of FDI World Dental Press Ltd)

thus making six scores. When used for treatment purposes (alternative 2), for children and adolescents six index teeth $\left(\frac{6|1|6}{6|16}\right)$, are examined, while for adults (20 years and older) all teeth are examined.

5. It is suggested that an appropriate treatment plan can be worked out on the following basis:

    Code 0 requires no treatment

    Code 1 requires improvement in home care

    Codes 2 and 3 require supra and subgingival scaling and improvement in home care

    Code 4 requires more complicated treatment, i.e. supra and subgingival scaling and root planing, improvement in home care and surgery.

The CPITN has proved to be a very useful broad screening tool, and as such has been usefully employed in very many WHO surveys throughout the world. A good example of its use is illustrated in *Figure 9.2.* This shows on a three-dimensional bar diagram the mean number of sextants according to CPITN scores of 2784 people in a 1986 Dutch National Dental Survey (reported in

the FDI *Guidelines for Community Periodontal Care,* 1992). In a comparison of the Periodontal Index (PI) and CPITN Cuttress *et al.* (1986) demonstrated that although a partial recording index CPITN is more sensitive than PI.

However the CPITN is too insensitive to be used to produce a detailed diagnosis, prognosis and treatment plan for the individual patient in practice, or to monitor the individual patient on a regular basis.

Limitation of indices

All periodontal indices have the following limitations:

1. The criteria are subjective to some degree, and there is considerable variation in examiner assessment of degrees of inflammation and pocket depth or loss of attachment.

2. The scoring systems are arbitrary. Thus a lesion scoring Russell PI 6 is not actually three times as severe as a lesion scoring PI 2; indeed gingivitis and periodontitis cannot be compared numerically in this way.

3. Although a gingivitis score measures present inflammation, pocket measurement is a reflection of past disease. If we accept the well-established idea that periodontal breakdown is episodic, pocket depth gives us no indication of disease activity at the time of measurement. The production of bleeding on careful probing of the pocket with a blunt probe has been regarded as an indicator of disease activity, but as Nevins *et al.* (1989) point out, 'At best, bleeding on probing has a predictive value of 30%'. In this regard, the absence of bleeding on probing appears to be a good indicator of periodontal stability, whereas bleeding on probing is a very poor indicator of disease activity (Lang *et al.*, 1990). It also seems more likely that the provocation of bleeding on probing is a factor of the enthusiasm or clumsiness of the examiner than of current disease activity. However, as the mechanisms involved in tissue destruction are clarified, parameters of current disease activity are being defined. Also, some indicators of those individuals at risk from advanced periodontal disease, e.g. juvenile periodontitis, are being unravelled (*see* Chapter 20).

Oral hygiene

The most commonly used indices of oral hygiene status are the oral hygiene index (Greene and Vermillion, 1960) and the plaque index (Silness and Löe, 1964).

Oral hygiene index

This is a composite index which scores debris and calculus deposition either on all or on selected tooth surfaces.

Oral debris is any soft foreign matter which is attached to the tooth. Oral debris and calculus are scored separately. The oral debris scoring is as follows:

0. No debris or stain present
1. Soft debris covering not more than one-third of the tooth surface.
2. Soft debris covering more than one-third but not more than two-thirds of the tooth surface.
3. Soft debris covering more than two-thirds of the tooth surface.

The calculus scores are assigned according to the same criteria with the addition that individual flecks of subgingival calculus are given score 2 and a continuous heavy band of subgingival calculus is scored 3.

The debris and calculus scores are added and divided by the number of surfaces examined to give the oral hygiene score.

Plaque Index (PI)

Criteria for scoring are:

0. No plaque.
1. Film of plaque visible only by removal on probe or by disclosing
2. Moderate accumulation of plaque which can be seen by the naked eye
3. Heavy accumulation of soft material filling the niche between the gingival margin and the tooth surface. The interdental region is filled with debris.

This index has been used with the gingival index to provide precise evidence of the causal relationship between plaque and gingival inflammation. Variations of these indices measure the amount of calculus and plaque retention factors such as overhanging margins of fillings.

Prevalence of gingivitis

The prevalence of gingival inflammation varies significantly with age.

The deciduous dentition

The gingivae around deciduous teeth appear to be remarkably resistant to plaque-induced inflammation. Even when toothbrushing is withdrawn for 3 weeks there is a significant difference in tissue response to that in the adult. Early studies of American and English children under 5 years old recorded little or no gingival inflammation, but using more rigid criteria Poulsen and Moller (1972) found a 25% prevalence in Danish 3 year olds. In a study of 128 5–6-year-old Australian children, Spencer *et al.* (1983) found a high prevalence of mild inflammation around the deciduous teeth, little severe inflammation, and little correlation between the oral hygiene status and the severity of inflammation. It seems likely that this finding reflects a difference in the intensity of the immunological response in the young child, or in the microflora of the gingival crevice. The prevalence of spirochaetes and of *Bacteroides melaninogenicus* is lower at 3–7 years old than in the adult (de Araujo and MacDonald, 1964).

The transitional period

This period covers the mixed dentition from about the age of 5 or 6, through to puberty. It is marked by tooth irregularity and hormonal changes. Chronic gingivitis has been found in 80% of children under 12 years and approaches 100% by the age of 14 years (WHO, 1978). This high prevalence was also found in a UK study of 1015 11–12 year-old children, in which Addy *et al.* (1986) recorded that all the children had some inflammation as demonstrated by bleeding on probing, at one or more sites, with a good correlation between plaque and gingivitis scores.

In older studies the prevalence of inflammation, i.e. the number of individuals in whose mouth some inflammation was present, was recorded, but not the fact that this was restricted to few teeth. Therefore the figures greatly exaggerated the size of the problem.

After about 14 years there is a decrease in the severity of inflammation; a sexual difference also appears. Before 14 the severity of inflammation for girls is higher than for boys, the girls' scores peaking at about 12 years old; boys' scores peaked at 14 and were found to be higher than those for girls. This could be related to changing patterns in oral hygiene habits but in fact, in a study of the gingival status at puberty, Sutcliffe (1972) found that the increased severity of inflammation was not related to an increase in plaque deposition. One must conclude that in puberty the tissues react more vigorously to any given amount of plaque; after puberty the severity of inflammation does diminish.

The adult

After the post-puberty decline in inflammation its prevalence appears to increase and has been recorded as high as 100% of young men of 17–22. But as indicated above, such figures need to be interpreted with caution. A study of 15–19 year olds in New Zealand (Cuttress *et al.*, 1983) showed that although 79% of mouths had some gingival inflammation, only 34% of tooth sites were inflamed, and in this group only 1% showed some periodontal breakdown. In a detailed analysis of data obtained in 1981 from the examination of 7078 people aged 19 years and older in 48 states of the USA (therefore regarded as representative of 147 million Americans), Brown, Oliver and Löe (1989) found that 15% were free of any kind of periodontal disease, and that gingivitis without periodontitis occurred in 50% of the remaining people. The prevalence of gingivitis declined from 54% in the group aged 19–44 years to 44% at 45–64 years, and to 36% in people of 65 years. In most people the gingivitis was restricted to a few teeth.

There is evidence that the transition from chronic gingivitis to chronic periodontitis takes place at an earlier age in Asiatic people than in Europeans or people of European origin. Although it is possible that genetic factors influence tissue vulnerability to plaque products (as appears to be the case in juvenile periodontitis), it is more likely that this difference may be explained by differences in oral hygiene habits which relate to educational and income levels. The role of nutrition in the gingival condition is uncertain, but it is likely that in the well-nourished people of developed countries nutritional factors play little or no part (Chapter 6).

Acute ulcerative gingivitis has a very low prevalence in rich countries and a higher one in poorer countries often affecting malnourished children (Chapter 22).

Prevalence of periodontitis

There is considerable palaeontological evidence of periodontal disease in early Man, and past epidemiological studies have emphasized the general prevalence of the disease. Hence the widespread belief that all adults would at some time during their lifetime experience deterioration of the periodontal tissues, and that a large proportion of edentulousness was due to periodontal disease. Indeed, many regarded periodontal breakdown as inevitable and part of the ageing process. The influential study by Marshall-Day *et al.* (1955) was representative in demonstrating that by the age of 40 90% of adults had some periodontal disease. Such findings set the tone of attitudes to the conservation of the dentition. The question, why go to all this trouble if

I am going to lose my teeth?, reflected many people's attitudes to restorative dentistry. As stated earlier in the text, such notions were based on imperfect methods of data collection and interpretation. As Pilot (1992) points out, 'we have been brain-washed by averages; reports on mean attachment loss per year do not show those sites that are breaking down at a much faster rate than average, nor are persons indicated who have many of those sites and are in fact ,in the high risk category of losing their teeth at an early stage. Persons and sites with no attachment loss at all are also obscured in mean figures' and, 'in the early epidemiological surveys on periodontal conditions, any deviation from the ideal was recorded and implicitly considered as disease.'

More recent studies have demonstrated that periodontitis is not as prevalent, extensive or as severe as was previously believed. Even so, figures from the WHO Global Oral Dental Bank show that at 1 August 1990 in over 50 countries, 5–20% of people were affected by a serious irreversible condition at the age of 40, which is a high percentage compared with almost every other disease that afflicts mankind (Miyazaki *et al.*, 1991b).

The onset of periodontal destruction appears to take place most commonly in the young adult, and then both prevalence and severity increase with age becoming clinically significant in the fourth decade of life. However, for the large majority of most of the observed populations the progress of periodontal diseases seems to be compatible with the retention of the natural dentition into older age.

Periodontal breakdown in children is often associated with some fault in host response, as in Down's syndrome, hypophosphatasia, juvenile diabetes, etc. (*see* Chapter 6), but early destructive periodontal disease, i.e. juvenile periodontitis, has been reported by Cogen *et al.* (1992) in healthy Alabama children. This radiographic study of 4757 children, 3172 black and 1585 white, under the age of 15 revealed a prevalence of juvenile periodontitis of 1.5% in black children and 0.3% of white children. Amongst the black children the male:female ratio with JP was almost equal while among the white children it was 1:4. A further finding was that in 71.4% of the black children with JP, radiographs revealed bone loss around deciduous teeth.

The result of more than 100 WHO surveys in over 60 countries of adolescents, i.e. 15–19 years, using the CPITN have been reported by Miyazaki *et al.* (1991a). The most frequently observed condition was score 2 (calculus with or without gingival bleeding), which was much more prevalent in non-industrialized countries than in industrialized countries. Some shallow pocketing of 4–5 mm was present in two-thirds of all populations observed, but it usually affected only a minority in the sample, and then only in one or two sextants. However, a few surveys, e.g. in the West Indies, showed a relatively high prevalence of pocketing.

WHO surveys using the CPITN have been carried out in many countries on adults in the age group 35–44 years and 45–74 years. In the 35–44 years group, Miyazaki *et al.* (1991b) report that calculus and shallow pocketing were the most frequently observed conditions. They found that with a few exceptions, the percentages of persons and the mean number of sextants per person with deep pockets were small to very small. The assumed differences between industrialized and non-industrialized countries with regard to the prevalence and severity of periodontal diseases were not reflected in the survey data examined. Marked differences between the two groups of countries were only seen for the estimated national levels of edentulousness, which was very low for the non-industrialized countries (perhaps a reflection of a smaller dentist:population ratio?).

Severe periodontal destruction seemed to be a limited problem, seldom leading to tooth loss before the age of 50. For most of the population the progress of periodontal destruction seemed to be compatible with the retention of the natural dentition into older age. This finding was confirmed by the results of the CPITN studies of older people. The figures for the 45–74 years group were subdivided into three age groups, 45–54, 55–64, 65–74. Once again the assumed differences between industrialized and non-industrialized countries were not confirmed. Also, the expected increase in periodontal destruction with increasing age was not reflected in values for pocketing or deep pocketing in the successive age groups. However, on average, at age 50, almost one sextant was excluded because of missing teeth; at age 60 1.5 sextants were excluded, and almost 2.5 sextants at age 70.

From these data it appears that the progress of periodontal disease with age is not shown by an increase in CPITN scores but by an increasing number of missing teeth, which could be the result of factors other than periodontal disease. In the age group 65–74 years, this results, on average, in almost half of all sextants being excluded. Of the remaining sextants, approximately half had both shallow and deep pockets.

A similar pattern of prevalence was found in the large American survey reported by Brown *et al.* (1989) and cited above. The prevalence of periodontitis increased with age from 29% at age 19–44 years up to about 50% in people 45 years and older. Moderate periodontitis, i.e. at least one pocket of 4–6 mm deep occurred in 28% of all people, while only 8% had advanced disease, that is at least one pocket greater than 6 mm, and only 10% had 6 or more teeth with pocketing 4–6 mm. Pocketing over 6 mm deep was found in only one in twelve people, and then only around one or two teeth. The need for extraction was found in only 4%, while less than 20% of all missing teeth were listed as missing due to periodontal disease.

Douglass *et al.* (1983) compared data on periodontal disease from the US National Center for Health Statistics for the years 1960–62 and 1971–74, and found a definite downward trend in the prevalence of both gingivitis and periodontitis in younger adults.

All studies show that poor oral hygiene is the most important factor affecting both the prevalence and severity of periodontal destruction. Other factors already discussed in relation to gingivitis have, as one would expect, a similar relationship to chronic periodontitis. The severity of destruction in any given age appears to be less in women than in men, probably due to better oral hygiene habits.

Socioeconomic factors, in particular educational level and economic status, bear a significant relationship to prevalence and severity. This could well explain observed ethnic differences which were once ascribed to genetic variation. If one compares equal age groups in Asian and European populations (Löe *et al.*, 1978) the transition from gingivitis to periodontitis appears to be earlier and the severity of destruction greater in the Asian group than in the European group. Both oral hygiene habits and nutritional status were better in the latter group, and this probably reflected educational and income levels. If one compares different ethnic groups with equivalent income and educational levels the disease profile is very similar.

Summary

Worldwide epidemiological studies have shown that gingival inflammation is present in most populations, but that the more severe stages of periodontal disease, whilst not as prevalent as previously believed, are still of significant magnitude, affecting up to 15–20% of most populations over the age of 35. Although gingivitis is very common it does not inevitably progress to periodontitis. Oral hygiene and therefore periodontal health is improving in industrialized countries.

References

Addy, M., Dummer, P.M.H., Griffiths, G. *et al.* (1986) Prevalence of plaque, gingivitis and caries in 11–12-year-old children in South Wales. *Community Dentistry and Oral Epidemiology* **14**, 115–118

Ainamo, J. (1983) Assessment of periodontal treatment needs. Adaptation of the WHO Community Periodontal Index of Treatment Needs (CPITN) to European conditions. In: Frandsen, A. (ed.) *Public Health Aspects of Periodontal Disease in Europe*. Berlin: Quintessence Verlag

Brown, L.J., Oliver, R.C. and Loe, H. (1989) Periodontal diseases in the US in 1981: Prevalence, severity, extent and role in tooth mortality. *Journal of Periodontology* **60**, 363–380

Cogen, R.B., Wright, T. and Tate, A.L. (1992) Destructive periodontal disease in healthy children. *Journal of Periodontology* **63**, 761–765

Cuttress, T.W., Hunter, P.B.V. and Hoskins, D.I.H. (1983) Adult oral health in New Zealand 1976–1982. Dental Research Unit, Medical Research Council of New Zealand, Wellington, N.Z.

Cuttress, T.W., Hunter, P.B.V. and Hoskins, D.I.H. (1986) Comparison of the Periodontal Index (PI) and Community Periodontal Index of Treatment Needs (CPITN). *Community Dentistry and Oral Epidemiology* **14**, 39–42

de Araujo, W.C. and MacDonald, J.B. (1964) Gingival crevice microbiota of pre-school children. *Archives of Oral Biology* **9**, 227–228

Douglass, C., Gillings, D., Solecito, W. and Gammon, M. (1983) The potential for increase in the periodontal needs of the aged population. *Journal of Periodontology* **54**, 721–730

Greene, J.C. and Vermillion, J.R. (1960) The oral hygiene index. A method for classifying oral hygiene status. *Journal of the American Dental Association* **61**, 172–179

Johnson, E.S., Kelly, J.E. and Van Kirk, L.E. (1965) Selected dental findings in adults by age, race and sex. United States 1960–62. U.S. Dept Health Education and Welfare, National Center for Health Statistics. Series 11, No. 7, 1

Lang, N.P., Alder, R., Joss, A. and Nyman, S. (1990) Absence of bleeding on probing. An indicator of periodontal stability. *Journal of Clinical Periodontology* **17**, 714–721

Lembariti, B.S. (1983) *Periodontal Diseases in Urban and Rural Populations in Tanzania*. Tanzania: Dar es Salaam University Press

Löe, H., Anerud. A., Boysen, H. and Smith, M. (1978) The natural history of periodontal disease in man. The rate of periodontal destruction before 40 years of age. *Journal of Periodontology* **49**, 607–620

Löe, H. and Silness, J. (1963) Periodontal disease in pregnancy. I. Prevalence and severity. *Acta Odontologica Scandinavica* **21**, 532–551

Marshall-Day, C.D., Stephens, R.G. and Quigley, L.F. (1955) Periodontal disease: Prevalence and incidence. *Journal of Periodontology* **26**, 185–191

Miyazaki, H., Pilot, T., Leclercq, M-H. and Barmes, D.E. (1991a) Profiles of periodontal conditions in adolescents measured by CPITN. *International Dental Journal* **41**, 67–73

Miyazaki, H., Pilot, T., Leclercq, M-H. and Barmes, D.E. (1991b) Profiles of periodontal conditions in adults measured by CPITN. *International Dental Journal* **41**, 74–80

Nevins, M., Becker, W. and Korman, K. (1989) Proceedings of the World Workshop in Clinical Periodontics, pp. 1–24, Princeton, New Jersey: American Academy of Periodontology.

Pilot, T. (1992) Implications of the high risk strategy and of improved diagnostic methods for health screening and public health planning in periodontal diseases. In Johnson, N.W. (ed.) *Risk Makers for Oral Diseases Vol. 3. Periodontal Diseases* Cambridge, Cambridge University Press, pp. 441–453

Poulsen, S. and Moller, I.J. (1972) The prevalence of dental caries, plaque and gingivitis in 3-year-old Danish children. *Scandinavian Journal of Dental Research* **80**, 94–103

Ramfjord, S.P. (1959) Indices for prevalence and incidence of periodontal disease. *Journal of Periodontology* **30**, 51–59

Russell, A.L. (1956) A system of classification and scoring for prevalence surveys of periodontal disease. *Journal of Dental Research* **35**, 350–359

Schour, I. and Massler, M. (1948) Prevalence of gingivitis in young adults. *Journal of Dental Research* **27**, 733–738

Sheiham, A. (1990) Public Health Approaches to the Promotion of Periodontal Health, p. 2. In Monograph Series No. 3. Joint Department of Community Dental Health and Dental Practice. University College London.

Sheiham, A. and Hobdell, M.H. (1969) Decayed, missing and filled teeth in a British adult population. *British Dental Journal* **126**, 401–404

Silness, J. and Löe, H. (1964) Periodontal disease in pregnancy. II. Correlation between oral hygiene and periodontal condition. *Acta Odontologica Scandinavica* **22**, 121–135

Socransky, S.S., Haffajec, A.D., Goodson, J.M. and Lindhe, J. (1984) New concepts of destructive periodontal disease. *Journal of Clinical Periodontology* **11**, 21–32

Spencer, A.J., Beighton, D. and Higgins, T.J. (1983) Periodontal disease in five and six-year-old children. *Journal of Periodontology* **54**, 19–22

Sutcliffe, P. (1972) A longitudinal study of gingivitis and puberty. *Journal of Periodontal Research* **7**, 52–58

WHO (1978) *Epidemiology, Etiology and Prevention of Periodontal Diseases*. Technical Report Series No. 621. Geneva: World Health Organization

10

Prevention of periodontal disease

The essential requirement for the prevention of a disease is an understanding of its cause. Chapter 4 describes the cause of chronic periodontal disease but the prevalence of the disease bears sad witness to our inability to apply that knowledge to the full. Many factors, social and economic, are beyond the influence of the dental profession but the profession has certain undeniable obligations. These are to educate the patient in good oral hygiene habits, to attempt to motivate the patient to apply advice given, to provide a regular service for professional cleaning, to apply fluoride to young teeth, and if disease occurs to practise sound dentistry which does not potentiate disease.

These ideas are also discussed in the treatment of chronic gingivitis (see Chapter 14), but patients without disease represent a different starting point from the patient with established disease. Both the patient and the practitioner are faced with a slightly different psychological situation and unfortunately it is one with which few dentists by training or experience are properly equipped to deal. Conversion to the philosophy of prevention involves nothing less than a revolutionary reorientation of thoughts and attitudes of every dentist.

Patient education and motivation cannot be a once for all process but must involve a continuing commitment to the patient. Such a commitment can be fulfilled only when dental personnel are organized to that end. A preventive service can be provided in a general dental practice which is largely devoted to treatment, but it is possible that better results are obtained when both therapist and patient are freed from the constraints of the conventional dental surgery situation. In a therapeutic situation the patient adopts a passive attitude in the face of professional authority. In providing a preventive service the patient's active participation is essential; indeed, even the word 'patient' seems inappropriate in this situation – perhaps 'pupil' would be better.

In situations where the patient has to take responsibility for their own welfare, as in the control of diabetes or periodontal disease, the patient is accountable for both the success, and of great importance, the failure of what he or she does. In the latter case people used to being passive and putting the burden on to the professional person, now have only themselves to blame.

At the same time the professional person may find him or herself in an ambiguous situation. There is a conflict between the professional as expert and authority, which reflects the traditional patient–professional relationship, and the professional person as teacher and counsellor. In the preventive situation the professional sets out to help the patient help himself, and he or she needs to recognize from the outset that the professional is separated from the patient in a number of respects, the most important of which are knowledge, values and language.

Many professional people, not just doctors and dentists but lawyers, accountants and so on, seem to overlook the fact that they possess special knowledge, particular attitudes to the problems of their patients or clients, and an exclusive vocabulary that they have learned and take for granted. These factors create a gap which must be bridged by the professional person so that a creative dialogue can be pursued. The values and attitudes of the dentist do not necessarily coincide with those of the patient; the latter wants to eat in comfort and look nice, while the dentist wants a plaque score of zero and a balanced occlusion. These different levels of aspiration need to be approximated, and two factors become essential. The first is the provision of information in language the patient can understand, and secondly, the generation of motivation, i.e. an explanation of the real advantages that will result from taking the professional advice, as well as the disadvantages of ignoring it.

Unfortunately, many dentists do not feel they can give the time to this, or are ill-equipped to deal with these challenges, and become impatient and even patronizing. The problem can be solved by having someone in an ancillary capacity, the practice nurse or hygienist, who has the time, the training and the personal motivation to take on the responsibility of undertaking the preventive programme.

The provision of information and instruction in home care can take place inside or outside the dental surgery: it may be applied to an individual or a group; it can be carried out by an informed patient or schoolteacher as well as by dental personnel. Information can be given through a variety of media, films, slides, lectures, printed material. The one-to-one relationship between therapist and patient is likely to be the most effective system but where this is not possible group instruction is better than no instruction at all. Ancillary personnel, in particular the dental hygienist, have an extremely valuable role to play in prevention. Hygienist training includes a much greater emphasis on prevention than does the conventional dental undergraduate course, and in the patient's mind she is often associated with this aspect of dentistry.

Certain groups are more receptive to information and instruction than others: adolescents with a developing awareness of self and interest in their general appearance and well-being; expectant and nursing mothers; young couples whose sense of responsibility is sharp-ened by new parenthood. This is not to imply that the older person is beyond reach; the message that teeth can and should last for life is a powerful incentive to a mature person who has knowledge of the problems suffered by less fortunate members of his or her peer group.

Regular guidance and encouragement are essential and for the young patients the application of topical fluorides can be included in the periodic checks. The long-term studies in Sweden by Axelsson and Lindhe provide overwhelming evidence of the benefits of an organized programme of regular professional care.

Prior to instituting a preventive programme one must establish that disease is not already present. One cannot take it for granted in any individual that periodontal disease is not present; careful examination of every mouth is essential. Health is the starting point of a preventive programme, the aim of which is the maintenance of that state by the control of plaque deposition. By far the major part in plaque control must be played by the individual. The responsibilities of professional personnel are:

1. To provide information about dental health
2. To provide information and guidance about the techniques of plaque control
3. To attempt to change the individual's evaluation of dental health; in jargon terms, to motivate the patient.

Providing information

Providing a patient with the necessary information takes time and some insight into the limitations of the patient's understanding. It also requires the ability to express oneself in simple language. As stated, too often dentists do not have the time to provide patients with sufficient information, and sometimes patients do not appreciate the value of time spent in giving advice. Too frequently adequate knowledge is taken for granted and when a description is provided it is expressed in technical terms quite incomprehensible to the patient. It is useless to tell a patient that 'bacterial plaque in proximity to the dentogingival junction provokes gingival inflammation'. The patient may not know what plaque or the

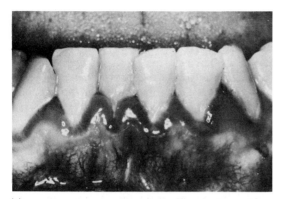

(a)

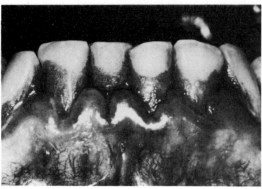

(b)

Figure 10.1 Deposits of bacterial plaque (*a*) before and (*b*) after staining with a disclosing agent which makes the presence of plaque obvious to the patient

dentogingival junction is, may not know that the mouth is full of bacteria or that gingiva means gum!

In addition, information provided in abstract may be only partly understood and quickly forgotten. Information needs to be given by demonstration in the patient's own mouth, and before any treatment is carried out. It is useful to give the patient a hand-mirror so that he or she can follow some of the examination; plaque and calculus are pointed out and the relationship to disease explained. At this time it is demonstrated that the principal cause of disease, the bacterial plaque, is almost invisible but can be revealed by using a disclosing agent. This is a completely harmless dye, e.g. 4% Erythrosin, usually pink or blue, which is absorbed by the bacterial plaque (*Figure 10.1*). To emphasize the harmful nature of the plaque a little of the stained deposit can be

scraped off the tooth with a probe and shown to the patient with some remark about its bacterial content.

The patient is then given a toothbrush (if he has brought his own so much the better) and told to attempt to remove all the stained plaque. At this stage no attempt should be made to instruct the patient in any particular brushing technique. The difficulties of the operation become apparent to the patient right away and he is thus more receptive to advice and instruction. Once the patient is aware of the problems in removing all the plaque he may be allowed to develop his own technique, but initially it is a good idea to demonstrate a formal technique as a basis for developing the necessary skill.

In starting treatment it is very important to avoid confusing the patient with too much detail about toothbrushes and other oral hygiene aids, or to make the whole exercise seem too difficult or time consuming. Over-enthusiasm at this stage can be counterproductive but it must be made quite clear that the job of cleaning the mouth needs to be carried out methodically section by section and that frantic activity with the toothbrush is likely to do more harm to the gingiva than good.

Mechanical methods of plaque removal

Toothbrushing techniques

A large number of toothbrushing techniques have been advised but the requirements of a satisfactory method of toothbrushing are few:

1. The technique should clean all tooth surfaces, in particular the area of the gingival crevice and the interdental region. A scrubbing technique will clean the tooth convexities well and yet leave plaque in more sheltered places.
2. The movement of the brush should not injure the soft or hard tissues. Vertical and horizontal scrubbing methods can produce gingival recession and tooth abrasion.
3. The technique should be simple and easy to learn. A technique which one person finds easy to use may be difficult for someone else; therefore each person needs individual guidance.

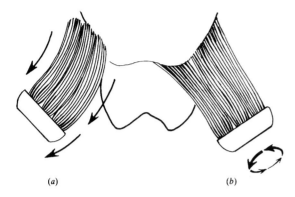

(a)   (b)

Figure 10.2 Toothbrushing techniques: (a) the roll method; (b) the Bass technique

4. The method must be well organized so that each part of the dentition is brushed in turn and no area overlooked. The mouth can be divided into a number of sections depending on the size of the dental arch and the size of the toothbrush.

Toothbrushing techniques can be demonstrated both on a model and in the patient's mouth.

The roll technique (Figure 10.2a)

This is a relatively gentle technique which is useful when the gingivae are sensitive. The side of the toothbrush is placed against the side of the tooth with the bristles pointing apically and parallel to the axis of the tooth; the back of the brush is at the level of the occlusal surface of the teeth. The brush is then rotated deliberately down in the upper jaw and up in the lower jaw so that bristles sweep across the gum and tooth. About ten strokes are given to each section and the brush is moved in turn from one section to the next. If the arch in anterior segments is narrow the brush can be used vertically. When all buccal and lingual surfaces have been brushed the biting surfaces can be brushed with a rotary movement.

The Bass technique (Figure 10.2b)

This brushing technique aims to clean the gingival crevice and to this end the brush is held so that the bristles are about 45° to the axis of the teeth, the end of the bristle pointing into the gingival crevice. The brush is pressed towards the gingiva and moved with a small circular motion so that the bristles go into the crevice and are also forced between the teeth. This may be painful if the tissues are inflamed and sensitive. When the gingivae are healthy the Bass technique is the method of choice; it has been shown to be a most effective method for the removal of plaque.

Interdental cleaning

As the interdental region is the most common site of plaque retention and the most inaccessible to the toothbrush special methods of cleaning are needed. These include the use of floss, tape, dental woodsticks, the interspace brush and the miniature interproximal brush. Once again it needs to be stated that during the first stages of instruction in home care the technique advised must be fairly easy for the patient to carry out. If it is not easy discouragement will soon set in. The point of the exercise is the removal of plaque without injuring the soft tissues and the use of woodsticks or floss where inappropriate may be harmful.

A further word of caution needs to be given about supplying the patient with too many gadgets; two implements at the most, e.g. a toothbrush and floss or a woodstick, will suffice to get the patient off the mark.

Requirements of a satisfactory toothbrush

There are now on the market a large number of toothbrushes of different sizes and shapes with bristles of various materials, textures, length and density. Overwhelmed by available choices the man in the street is as likely to choose a brush that matches his bathroom tiles as one that he thinks will work well.

A great many studies have been carried out on the specifications of a satisfactory toothbrush (*see* Fransden, 1972) with contradictory results on almost every characteristic examined.

However, certain basic requirements need to be met:

1. The brush head should be small enough to be manipulated effectively everywhere in the mouth, yet not be so small that it has to be used with extreme care in order to obtain complete coverage of the dentition.

A length of about 2.5 cm is satisfactory for an adult; about 1.5 cm is suitable for a child.

2. The bristles should be of even length so that they function simultaneously. A convex or concave brush with bristles of different lengths will not clean a flat surface without undue pressure on some bristles. Short bristles will fail to reach interdental sites and may also be so rigid that they injure the tissues.

3. The texture should allow effective use without causing damage to either soft or hard tissues. Stiffness depends on the diameter and length of the filament and its elasticity. It also depends on whether the brush is used wet or dry, and on the temperature of the water. Soft bristle may not remove plaque effectively; medium stiffness is the usual recommendation. A typical toothbrush has 1600 filaments, 11 mm long and 0.008mm diameter, arranged in about 40 tufts in 3 or 4 rows.

4. The brush should be easy to keep clean. Densely packed tufts tend to retain debris and toothpaste at the base of the bristle. Nylon bristle is said to be more hygienic than natural bristle.

5. The toothbrush handle must rest comfortably and securely in the hand. It should be broad and thick enough to allow a firm grip and good control.

Interproximal brush

The interproximal brush is an important device for cleaning between molar teeth and furca, particularly after surgery. The proximal furrow in the root is not adequately cleaned by floss or woodsticks but will accommodate an interproximal brush well.

Dental floss

Dental floss either waxed or unwaxed can be very effective in removing interproximal plaque. To be effective the floss should be pulled around the tooth curvature so that close contact with the tooth surface is made. It needs to be used with control so that the gingiva is not cut (*Figure 10.3*); many people find it difficult to use in posterior segments. A floss-threader is necessary to clean bridge abutments. As with all oral hygiene aids the use of floss must be demonstrated in the

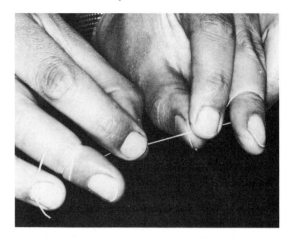

Figure 10.3 Handling dental floss so that it can be used with control when being placed against an interproximal tooth surface. Note that the floss is wound round the fingers to prevent slipping

patient's mouth, after which the patient repeats the performance under supervision. Floss-holders may make the task easier and quicker for some people.

The dental woodstick

Once upon a time it was believed that bacterial invasion was better resisted by well-keratinized gingivae, and therefore that regular gingival massage was beneficial. The definition of the junctional epithelium as the portal of entry of bacterial products has undermined the rationale for this kind of exercise. The woodstick is used not to keratinize the gingivae but to clean the interdental dentogingival junction. There must be an adequate interdental space to use a woodstick effectively and without damaging the tissues. If a woodstick is rubbed on inflamed gingiva it is more likely to stimulate the inflammation than aid its resolution.

The interspace brush

This is a single-tuft brush designed for cleaning areas difficult of access with a normal toothbrush, such as around irregular teeth, in a space where a tooth is missing and around bridge abutments and pontics. The automatic rotating brush has proved to be very effective in these situations, as well as for general interproximal cleaning.

The automatic toothbrush

The automatic toothbrush is now a well-accepted part of the home care armamentarium. There are a number of designs available with different forms of movement: arcuating, vibrating and reciprocating.

There have been many studies comparing the effectiveness of the hand and automatic brush and the results indicate that the subject is more important than the appliance. Properly used the manual brush and automatic brush can both remove plaque effectively. As many people do not use the conventional brush properly the automatic brush may be beneficial in their hands. For the uninstructed patient the automatic brush is as effective if not more effective than the manual brush. The small head allows access to difficult areas and many people find the sensation of the moving brush very pleasant.

The automatic brush is especially useful to the handicapped person; indeed it may be the only oral hygiene aid which can be used with a fair degree of success either by the individual, parent, careworker or a nurse.

Irrigating devices (Water–Pik)

An irrigating device can be a useful supplement to the toothbrush, particularly where there is fixed bridgework; however, it needs to be made clear to the patient that irrigation can remove food debris but it cannot remove plaque. In the immediate postoperative phase after periodontal surgery, irrigation with warm or even a fairly hot and weak saline solution can be very soothing. It is unlikely that the addition of antiseptics, e.g. chlorhexidine, to the irrigating fluid is of much benefit because the solution will be too dilute to affect the oral flora. On the other hand, if the taste is pleasant it might encourage the patient to use the device frequently and therefore help to make the home care process more enjoyable and less of a chore. Using the device on full strength may be hazardous. It is possible for the impact of the fluid to drive pocket bacteria into the tissues and produce a periodontal abscess.

Frequency of brushing

Theoretically one could clean the teeth once every other day and prevent plaque from accumulating to the point where it would provoke some gingival inflammation. However, few people clean their teeth so well at one time that all the plaque is removed; therefore more frequent brushing is essential. In addition, the presence of food debris or plaque build-up on the teeth is unpleasant, especially to people who are sensitive to the state of their mouth.

It has become the convention to clean teeth morning and night and certainly the establishment of regular oral hygiene habits is essential; however, the rush to start the day or the fatigue of day's end do not provide the best climate for effective home care. In advising patients about the pattern of home care it seems wise to take into account the kind of life they lead. Many people do have both the time and energy as well as access to a wash-basin to spend time on cleaning their teeth in the middle of the day. These days so many people work where good toilet facilities exist and the habit of keeping a toothbrush at the place of work is one to encourage.

The essential requirement is the acquisition of an awareness of the state of the mouth. Once an individual knows what a clean mouth feels like a dirty mouth becomes intolerable and the need to use a toothbrush is encouraged. Splaying of the bristles is the most obvious sign of toothbrush wear. This is influenced more by the quality, i.e. resilience of the bristle than by small differences in toothbrush design. Renewal of a toothbrush is usually recommended after three months' use. Market research indicates that women change their brush more frequently than men.

Toothpaste

Essentially toothpastes contain mild abrasives, which enhance the efficiency of the toothbrush in removing plaque deposits, as well as anti-bacterial agents which help retard the regrowth of plaque deposits (De La Rosa *et al.*, 1979). Many contain fluoride to retard enamel demineralization and promote remineralization, and thus help prevent and reduce caries. Some also contain chemicals to help desensitize exposed and sensitive dentine.

There is a large variety of toothpaste formulations which can be very complicated. Typical constituents are as follows:

Abrasives: Calcium carbonate, calcium pyro-
phosphate, aluminium silicate, diatomacious
earth, etc.

Anti-bacterial agents: Sodium lauryl sulphate,
zinc citrate trihydrate, triclosan, metal ions, etc.

Anti-caries agents: Sodium monofluorophosphate, sodium fluoride, stannous fluoride.

Desensitizing agents: Strontium salts, sodium
fluoride, formalin, etc.

Fillers and thickeners, e.g. Sodium carboxy-
methyl cellulose.

Humectants to keep the paste moist, e.g.
glycerine. *sorbitol, polyethylene glycol.*

Detergents e.g. sodium-lauryl sulphate.

Flavouring agents, often mint.

Colouring agents.

Sweeteners, e.g. Sodium saccharin.

In the De La Rosa study (*ibid*), after
prophylaxis, subjects brushed their teeth for
two minutes with and without toothpaste over
a 28-day period. Plaque levels were measured
immediately after brushing and then after 24
hours. After each brushing about 40% of the
plaque was removed leaving 60% to promote
plaque regrowth. The regrowth rate for the
group brushing with toothpaste was 27% lower
than that for the group brushing without
toothpaste. In subsequent studies Rustogi *et al.*
(1984) compared the effects of brushing with
tap water for one minute with that of brushing
with various abrasives, including silicon
dioxide and sodium bicarbonate, and found
that brushing with the abrasives removed
59–69% of 48-hours-old plaque compared with
only 27–33% after brushing with tap water.

Other chemotherapeutic agents are
discussed in Chapter 15.

Chemical control of plaque deposition

Mechanical methods of plaque removal
require time and manual dexterity, and therefore a high level of patient motivation. These
problems have stimulated the research for a
chemical cleaner to supplement or replace
mechanical cleaning. The central difficulty has
been to find a substance that is both effective
and harmless to the tissue.

Chemical control may be achieved in a
number of ways:

1. Suppression of the oral flora

2. Inhibition of bacterial colonization of the
tooth surface

3. Inhibition of plaque forming factors, e.g.
binding carbohydrates such as dextran

4. Dissolution of established plaque

5. Prevention of mineralization of plaque

These are discussed more fully in Chapter 15.

Mouthwashes

Mouthwashes have been used for a number of
purposes, clearing the mouth of food debris, as
carriers of anti-bacterial agents to prevent or
reduce plaque accumulation, containing anti-
caries fluorides, and to reduce the activity of
odour-producing micro-organisms.

The simplest and most frequently used
mouth rinse has been a dilute saline solution,
and when warm is especially useful in postoperative care, but much more complicated
formulations are now available to achieve the
above objectives.

Mouthwashes are commonly mixtures of:

An anti-bacterial agent; 0.2% chlorhexidine
gluconate appears to be the most effective,
but its powerful taste and tendency to stain
teeth are disadvantages. Quaternary
ammonium salts, e.g. cetylpyridinium
chloride, are frequently used.

Alcohol to enhance antibacterial activity
and taste, and to help keep flavouring agents
in solution.

A humectant, e.g. sorbitol, to prevent
drying-out.

A surfactant to help keep ingredients in
solution.

Flavourings, colouring agents, preservatives,
and water as the vehicle.

There is evidence that the activity of the
anti-bacterial agent is prolonged by absorption
to the hydroxyapatite of tooth enamel (Jensen,
1978).

It is usually recommended that the mouthwash is used for about 30 seconds twice a day,
before or after toothbrushing, or indepen-
dently of brushing. However, the evidence of
many studies (Lobene *et al.*, 1979; Ashley *et
al.*, 1984) supports the use of mouthwashes in
conjunction with regular toothbrushing.
Binney *et al.* (1993) tested five commercial
mouthwashes as pre-brushing rinses, and
found that they were of no greater use than

water, nor did they enhance the efficiency of subsequent toothbrushing; but the benefits of their use as adjuncts to normal hygiene procedures has been demonstrated.

Problems to be overcome

Satisfactory plaque control is not easy. If the practitioner is to guide the patient towards this goal he must be aware of all the problems that the patient might encounter.

Manual dexterity

By training and experience dentists achieve a high level of manual skill and it may be difficult for them to understand that many individuals are not so well endowed. Manual dexterity does not necessarily go with intellect and some of the brightest patients prove to be extremely clumsy. The extent of the patient's difficulty can be recognized by witnessing the patient's performance and directing his efforts with patience and tact. It is necessary to find out which technique the patient can best perform. It is useless to insist on a technique which the patient finds difficult. The scrubbing technique is probably the easiest to perform and if it is the only technique the patient can command, so be it, at least initially, but some effective form of interdental cleaning must also be taught. Given time and persistence, skills do come to most people, even the least dextrous. Positive encouragement is essential: criticism can be counterproductive.

Oral perception

Visual, oral and olfactory faculties vary from one person to another, and there is also considerable variation in tactile sensibility in the mouth. Just as some people are tone deaf or cannot smell the difference between curry and garlic, so some people can have a very dirty mouth without being aware of the condition while others are sensitive to the presence of the smallest foreign body in the mouth. However, sensibility can be developed although in some people it can be a slow process. The tongue is the most powerful instrument of oral tactile sensation and the patient can be instructed to run the tongue over the teeth before and after brushing and to recognize the glass-like feeling of clean teeth.

Tooth position

Malalignment is one of the most common causes of difficulty. Where teeth have been extracted and neighbouring teeth have tilted, a triangular space forms which can be difficult to clean. Areas of crowding can produce special problems as any form of interdental cleaning, even with floss, may be difficult and even harmful. Areas of special difficulty should be defined and techniques devised for those areas.

The form of tooth contact

The contact point or area takes many forms depending on tooth shapes and relationships. The smaller the area of contact the easier it is to clean. As attrition and interdental wear take place the contact area increases in size. If the teeth are rectangular in shape the contact area can be extremely wide. If the related embrasure space is filled by healthy gingiva, interdental cleaning may not be necessary but if inflammation is present interdental cleaning is essential and floss or tape may be the only effective aid.

Restorative and prosthetic dentistry

As emphasized in the text, badly executed restorative dentistry is an extremely common cause of plaque retention. The overhanging margin of the interproximal restoration creates a zone of plaque retention which is totally inaccessible to the patient's best efforts, and if possible should be removed before subgingival scaling is undertaken. Badly designed contact areas, overcontoured crowns, subgingival crown margins, badly designed bridge pontics, especially the ridge-lap pontic, extracoronal precision attachments placed too close to the gingiva, etc., create problems of plaque control which can be extremely difficult to correct. It is in these latter cases that chemical cleaning can be beneficial in the short term.

It is obviously much more satisfactory to avoid creating these problems in the first place, and all restorative and prosthetic work must be undertaken with its effect on the periodontium in mind.

Diet

Few health topics exercise people's concern as much as their diet. More myths and more neuroses attend the subject of nutrition than most other topics, and its relation to dental health is no exception. 'How does diet affect my gums?' is a constant question and a satisfactory answer should cover two aspects of this subject:

1. Nutritional deficiencies do not cause gum disease. However, if plaque-induced disease is already present nutritional deficiency might affect its development; therefore a balanced diet is necessary.
2. Both the chemical composition and the physical character of food are important. Although some tooth surfaces can be cleaned by using hard and fibrous foods it has been clearly demonstrated that such foods as apples, carrots, celery, etc. have no effect on plaque deposits in the sheltered gingival crevice, especially in the interdental regions. On the other hand, hard fibrous foods do not encourage the deposition of plaque and are therefore beneficial as *substitutes* for soft, sticky foods which do encourage plaque deposition. The consumption of sugar in any form is to be discouraged particularly between meals.

For the concerned person a simple 5-day diet analysis can be extremely revealing. All food and drinks, including between-meals snacks, are recorded, and in going through the list with the patient all refined carbohydrate is underlined. Even a superficial analysis of this sort can shed light on the idiosyncrasies and limitations of the individual's diet, and seeing their total consumption in black and white can be a salutary experience. In dealing with young people the cooperation of the parents is essential and even the help of teachers is useful.

Unfortunately there are pressures from all sides to promote the consumption of refined carbohydrate and sugar. The weight of convention and the pressure of advertising tend to limit the effectiveness of diet control advice and basic changes should not be anticipated or aimed for in the short term. Control over between-meals snacks can be achieved and can effect significant benefits.

Such an exercise must be an uphill task but in one regard dental personnel should be successful and that is in setting an example by their own performance and their own dental health.

Patient motivation

In motivating a patient to good home care one has to bring about change – change in knowledge and understanding, change in attitude and thus change in habit.

In the provision of any form of treatment some explanation of the patient's problem is essential, and this is especially the case in the control of periodontal disease where the patient must take on the responsibility for his or her own well-being. In this respect the periodontal patient is similar to the diabetic patient – both must look after themselves if the disease is to be controlled, and that control is likely to be effective if the patient has a clear understanding of the rationale behind the discipline.

In providing an explanation of the patient's problem, as already stated certain rules must be followed:

1. Do not take any prior knowledge for granted; assume that the patient knows very little about dental matters and what information he or she may have garnered is likely to be a compound of gossip, old wives' tales and pseudo-science. For example, few patients realize that teeth are held in bone and that the gum is simply a cover for the bone; many people believe that plaque is degraded food.
2. Give information in simple everyday language and avoid jargon. To say 'You have a plaque-induced gingival infection exacerbated by iatrogenic retention factors' will be meaningless to most patients. Thus, use the word 'bacteria' not 'microorganism', 'gum' instead of 'gingiva', 'stick' instead of 'adhere', 'swollen' not 'hyperplastic', etc.
3. Do not give too much information at one time, and repeat everything that you have said. When the light dawns it may dawn very slowly.

Change in attitude to dental health

Periodontal health is important: teeth are worth keeping for life. The patients must believe this; otherwise any change in habit as an immediate response to the dentist's admonitions will be short lived.

Several arguments may be employed and the experienced practitioner can tailor these to the patient's perceived needs. Adolescents and adults may respond to different arguments:

1. *Impaired function.* No appliance can function as efficiently as the natural and healthy dentition: full dentures may be an extremely poor substitute for the patient's own teeth.
2. *Personal hygiene.* These days most people are concerned about personal cleanliness and yet there may be a marked contrast between the patient's general appearance and the state of his mouth. This usually represents a lack of awareness of oral hygiene and when the true state of affairs is demonstrated the individual who is truly concerned about personal hygiene will be ready to change his habits. The patient is given a hand-mirror to witness the examination of the mouth, and deposits of plaque and calculus can be pointed out. The use of a disclosing agent is valuable.
3. *Social handicap.* Periodontal disease produces halitosis; dirty teeth and inflamed gums are unsightly. The idea of possessing offensive breath or an ugly smile is often sufficient incentive for patients to improve their home care. Today's television and screen heroes and heroines usually provide a good example to be cited if the dentist feels this is appropriate.
4. *General health.* Although there is little evidence that gingival disease can have an adverse effect on general health it is possible that where other pathology exists, e.g. gastric ulcer, oral sepsis can aggravate the condition. A healthy mouth in a healthy body could be a good maxim.

As stated earlier, the dentist and his staff should set an example and be seen to practise what they preach.

Preventive programmes

Prevention in children

Studies by Axelsson and Lindhe (1974) and Axelsson *et al.* (1976) have shown the effect of regular plaque control on periodontal disease in children. Their programmes included fortnightly attendances for dental health education and instruction in oral hygiene (IOH). The test participants were given information and IOH. At each of the fortnightly visits these children received mechanical tooth cleaning, including approximal plaque removal using dental floss and special polishing tips, combined with topical application of monofluorophosphate. Control group children brushed their teeth at school under supervision each month using 0.2% sodium fluoride solution but received no instruction or professional prophylaxis. During the first 2 years of study, the test regime resulted in reduction of disease to almost negligible levels with regard to plaque, gingivitis and caries, whereas the control group showed continuing or more severe levels of disease during this period. Similar results have been reported by Hamp *et al.* (1978).

The preventive programmes reported by other workers, e.g. Ashley and Sainsbury (1981), have achieved less success in comparison with the above studies, perhaps because the Scandinavian group were more highly motivated and disciplined. This appears to be confirmed by a more recent Swedish study by Wennstrom *et al.* (1993), in which 225 patients aged 18–65 were monitored over 12 years in a community clinic. Between 1978 and 1990 all patients received regular care, and it was found that there were fewer tooth sites with inflammation in 1990 (4%) than in 1978 (15%). The mean attachment loss over the 12 years was 0.5 mm, and radiographs showed only 0.2–0.4 mm alveolar loss. Over this period patients of 30–53 years showed a definite improvement in periodontal health, while older patients demonstrated stability rather than improvement.

Prevention in adults

Several studies have investigated the effectiveness of plaque control regimes on adult subjects. Lovdal *et al.* (1961) carried out a 5 year study on 1428 subjects who received IOH and scaling every 6 months. They found that plaque levels were reduced most in those subjects with initially good oral hygiene. Subjects with poor oral hygiene initially demonstrated minor reductions in deposits.

Lightner *et al.* (1971) investigated the influence of the frequency of IOH on the response of the patient. The study lasted 46 months and involved 470 subjects. They found that the subjects who received IOH showed decreased plaque and inflammation. They also showed the least loss of attachment.

A 3 year study by Suomi *et al.* (1972) involved 326 subjects, who were divided into a group who received scaling and IOH at 2–4 monthly intervals, and a control group who received no treatment. At the end of the study the oral hygiene score was more than four times greater in the control group than for the experimental subjects. Gingival inflammation scores were greater in the control group; there was also 3½ times greater loss of epithelial attachment and greater loss (by 0.18 mm) of alveolar bone.

These studies have been reinforced by the work of Axelsson and Lindhe (1978,1981). In a 3 year study, subsequently extended to 6 years, involving 375 test and 180 control subjects, the test group received scaling and IOH every 2–3 months. This stimulated individuals to adopt effective oral hygiene habits, with resulting resolution of inflammation, and prevented further clinical attachment loss (CAL) and caries. In contrast, the control patients showed plaque retention, gingivitis, CAL and caries.

The variation in the degree of success achieved by these studies emphasizes the need to design preventive programmes based on established educational methods and planned for the special needs of the individual. Techniques which have attempted to motivate individuals by arousing fear of tooth loss, to persuade them to participate in preventive procedures, have met with limited success; it has been found that better results have been achieved by methods using persuasion and encouragement.

Self-assessment

As previously stated, awareness of the nature of the problem is central to any preventive programme, and methods of self-assessment can form a powerful tool to self-awareness. Most methods of self-assessment of oral hygiene improvement and motivation have been directed to plaque control but in recent

years checks on gingival colour and gingival bleeding have been used as methods of monitoring their gingival status and oral hygiene regime (Glavind and Attstrom, 1979).

In a US study of about 500 14–15 year olds with gingivitis, one group received instruction in oral hygiene techniques, and a second group received in addition instruction in the self-assessment of gingival bleeding. After two years both groups demonstrated very positive benefits with indications of additional benefit in the children assessing their gingival bleeding. A similar finding was demonstrated in a study of Finnish army conscripts (Kallio *et al.*, 1990).

References

Ashley, F.P. and Sainsbury, R.H. (1981) The effect of a school-based plaque control programme on caries and gingivitis. A 3 year study in 11 to 14 year old girls. *British Dental Journal* **150**, 41–45

Ashley, F.P., Skinner, A., Jackson, P. *et al.* (1984) The effect of a 0.1% cetylpyridinium chloride mouthrinse on plaque and gingivitis in adult subjects. *British Dental Journal* **157**, 191–196

Axelsson, P. and Lindhe, J. (1974) The effect of a preventive programme on dental plaque, gingivitis and caries in schoolchildren. Results after one and two years. *Journal of Clinical Periodontology* **1**, 126–138

Axelsson, P. and Lindhe, J. (1978) The effect of controlled oral hygiene procedures on caries and periodontal disease in adults. *Journal of Clinical Periodontology* **5**, 133–151

Axelsson, P. and Lindhe, J. (1981) The significance of maintenance care in the treatment of periodontal disease. *Journal of Clinical Periodontology* **8**, 281–295

Axelsson, P. and Lindhe, J. (1986) The effect of controlled oral hygiene procedures on caries and periodontal diseases in adults. Results after 6 years. *Journal of Clinical Periodontology* **8**, 239–248

Axelsson, P., Lindhe, J. and Waseby, J. (1976) The effect of various plaque control measures on gingivitis and caries in schoolchildren. *Community Dentistry and Oral Epidemiology* **4**, 232–239

Binney, A., Addy, M. and Newcombe, R.G. (1993) The plaque removal effects of single rinsings and brushings. *Journal of Periodontology* **64**, 181–185

De La Rosa, M., Guerra, J.Z., Johnston, D.A. and Radike, A.W. (1979) Plaque regrowth and removal with daily toothbrushing. *Journal of Periodontology* **50**, 661–664

Frandsen, A. (ed.) (1972) *Oral Hygiene*. Report of a symposium held at Malmo, Sweden, May 1971. Copenhagen, Munksgaard

Glavind, L. and Attstrom, R. (1979) Periodontal self examination, a motivational tool in periodontics. *Journal of Clinical Periodontology* **6**, 238–251

Hamp, S.E., Lindhe, J. and Fornell, J. (1978) Effect of a field program based on systematic plaque control on caries and gingivitis in schoolchildren after 3 years. *Community Dentistry and Oral Epidemiology* **6**, 17–23

Jensen, J.E. (1978) Binding of dyes to hydroxyapatite treated with cetylpyridinium chloride or cetrimonium bromide. *Scandinavian Journal of Dental Research* **86**, 87–92

Kallio, P., Ainamo, J. and Dusadeepan, A. (1990) Self-assessment of gingival bleeding. *International Dental Journal* **40**, 231–236

Lightner, L.M., O'Leary, T.J., Drake, R.B. *et al.* (1971) Preventive periodontic treatment procedures: results after 46 months. *Journal of Periodontology* **42**, 555–561

Lobene, R.R., Kashket, S., Spoarkar, P.M. *et al.* (1979) The effect of cetylpyridinium chloride on human plaque bacteria and gingivitis. *Pharmacology and Therapeutics in Dentistry* **4**, 33–47

Lovdal, A., Arno, A., Schei, O. and Waerhaug, J. (1961) Combined effect of subgingival scaling and controlled oral hygiene on the incidence of gingivitis. *Acta Odontologica Scandinavica* **19**, 537–555

Rustogi, K.N., Volpe, A.R., Fishman, S. *et al.* (1984) Removal of 48-hour plaque by either brushing with dentifrices or water. *Journal of Dental Research* **63**, 312. Abstract, 1273

Sims, W. (1968) Preventive dentistry for the dental practitioner. *Dental Practitioner* **18**, 309–314

Suomi, J.D., Smith, L.W., Chang, J.J. and Barbano, J.P. (1973) Study on the effect of different prophylaxis frequencies on the periodontium of young adults. *Journal of Periodontology* **44**, 406–410

Wenstrom, J.L., Serino, G., Lindhe, J. *et al.* (1993) Periodontal conditions of adult regular care attendants. A 12 year longitudinal study. *Journal of Clinical Periodontology* **20**, 714–722

11

Clinical features of chronic periodontal disease

Chronic gingivitis

The manifestations of gingival inflammation vary considerably between individuals and from one part of the mouth to another. This variation reflects the aetiological factors at work and the tissue response to these factors. This response is essentially a mixture of inflammation and fibrous tissue repair. When the former predominates, signs and symptoms are more obvious; when the fibrous tissue component predominates, clinical manifestations can be much more subtle and recognized only by careful examination.

In making a diagnosis it is important to keep in mind the appearance of health, departures from which may indicate disease. Clinical features are:

1. Altered gingival appearance
2. Gingival bleeding
3. Discomfort and pain
4. Unpleasant taste
5. Halitosis.

Altered gingival appearance

Changes in appearance are usually described according to colour, shape, size, consistency and surface characteristics.

Healthy gingivae are pale pink and the margin is knife edged and scalloped; a stream-lined papilla is often grooved by a sluice-way and the attached gingiva is stippled.

Because the interdental embrasure is the site of greatest plaque stagnation gingival inflammation usually starts in the interdental papilla and spreads around the margin. As the blood vessels dilate the tissue becomes red and swollen with inflammatory exudate. The knife-edged margin becomes rounded, the interdental sluice-way is lost and the surface of the gingiva becomes smooth and glossy (*Figure 11.1*). As the gingival fibre bundles are broken up by the inflammatory process the gingival cuff loses tone and comes away from the tooth surface so that a shallow pocket is formed. If the inflammation becomes more diffuse and spreads into the attached gingiva the stippling disappears. If inflammation is severe it can spread across the attached gingiva to the

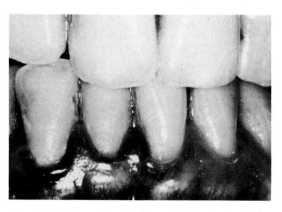

Figure 11.1 Signs of a relatively early chronic gingivitis. Gingival papillae and margins are swollen and red and bleed on probing

alveolar mucosa and so obliterate the normally well-defined mucogingival junction.

Usually the most pronounced inflammatory swelling is seen in adolescents and young adults so that 'false pocketing' is formed. It is called false as opposed to real or periodontal pocketing which is formed by apical migration of the crevicular epithelium as the periodontal ligament is destroyed by inflammation. Where several aetiological factors combine, e.g. plaque deposition plus lack of lip-seal plus the endocrinal changes of puberty, gingival swelling, especially papillary swelling, can be pronounced.

If plaque irritation is longstanding and low grade, the main tissue reaction will be fibrous tissue production so that the gingiva may remain firm and pink but become thickened and lose its streamlined shape.

Gingival bleeding

Gingival bleeding is probably the most frequent patient complaint. Unfortunately gingival bleeding is so common that people may not take it seriously and even believe it to be normal; however, unless bleeding obviously follows an episode of acute trauma, bleeding is always a sign of pathology. It occurs most frequently on toothbrushing. Bleeding may be provoked by eating hard food, apples, toast, etc. as well as by probing the gingival crevice or pocket on periodontal examination. 'Bleeding on probing' has been used as a sign of disease activity, but as stated earlier, this is an unreliable indicator of disease activity, and may be the result of injudicious examination. When gingivae are extremely soft and spongy, bleeding can occur spontaneously.

Blood may be tasted by the patient and may be smelt on the patient's breath.

If the tissue response is fibrous overgrowth, there is no bleeding even with vigorous tooth-brushing.

Discomfort and pain

These are uncommon features of chronic gingivitis and this is probably the main reason for the disease being overlooked. The gingivae may feel sore when the patient brushes his teeth and because of this he brushes more lightly and less frequently so that plaque accumulates and the condition is perpetuated.

This relative absence of pain is one of the symptoms which differentiates a chronic gingivitis from an acute ulcerative gingivitis.

Unpleasant taste

Patients may notice the taste of blood, particularly if they suck at an interdental space. Unfortunately the senses are quickly blunted and a disagreeable taste is a relatively infrequent complaint.

Halitosis

'Bad breath' frequently accompanies gingival disease and is a common cause of a visit to the dentist. The smell derives from blood and poor oral hygiene and must be distinguished from smells from different sources.

Halitosis has a number of causes, both intra-oral and extra-oral. Oral disease and residual food deposits, especially those of a volatile nature such as peppermint, garlic, curry, etc., represent the most common cause of halitosis. Pathology of the respiratory tract, nose, sinuses, tonsils and lungs can cause an embarrassing smell, as can diseases of the digestive tract. Some items of diet, e.g. garlic, are absorbed by the intestines, taken into the intestinal bloodstream and finally exhaled by the lungs so that they can be smelt a long time after they have been eaten. Mouth odour is common on waking and between meals, when it is associated with food stagnation and reduced salivary flow. Metabolic diseases, diabetes and uraemia give characteristic smells to the breath. Halitosis can increase with age.

Chronic periodontitis

The clinical features of chronic periodontitis are:

1. Gingival inflammation and bleeding
2. Pocketing
3. Gingival recession
4. Tooth mobility
5. Tooth migration
6. Discomfort
7. Alveolar bone loss
8. Halitosis and offensive taste.

Of these only pocketing and alveolar bone loss are essential features of chronic periodontitis.

Gingival inflammation and bleeding

Although gingival inflammation is a necessary precursor to periodontitis, obvious manifestations of inflammation become less apparent with the progress of periodontitis. Frequently the gingivae are pink and firm, the contours may be almost normal, there may be no bleeding on careful probing and the patient may not complain of bleeding on brushing. It is as though with the development of the pocket the disease has gone underground.

The presence and severity of gingival inflammation depend upon oral hygiene status; where this is poor, gingival inflammation is evident and bleeding or brushing, or even spontaneous bleeding, is noticed by the patient. When the patient's toothbrushing is good enough to control plaque but where subgingival deposits, because of inadequate scaling, persist, the presence of periodontal disease may not be apparent on superficial examination. If a careful history is taken many such patients report a history of past bleeding which stopped when their toothbrushing technique improved. Periodontal destruction in the average adult is the product of past neglect, not the result of present oral hygiene habits.

Pocketing

Pocket measurement is an essential part of periodontal diagnosis but must be interpreted together with gingival inflammation and swelling, and radiographic evidence of alveolar bone loss. Theoretically, if there is no gingival swelling a pocket over 2 mm deep indicates some apical migration of crevicular epithelium but inflammatory swelling is so common especially in the younger individual that pocketing of 3–4 mm may be entirely gingival or 'false'. Pocketing of 4 mm is likely to indicate an early chronic periodontitis (*Figure 11.2*).

The precise measurement of pockets is difficult because:

1. Probing the pocket can be uncomfortable and even painful if there is frank inflammation.
2. Pocket depth is extremely variable around a tooth. Interproximal pocketing is usually deepest because that is the site of greatest plaque accumulation, while pocketing on the facial aspect of the tooth is usually most

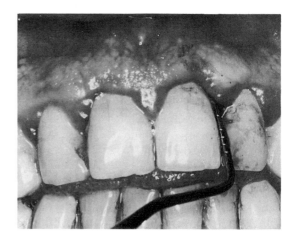

Figure 11.2 Pocket-measuring probe inserted into pocket as parallel to the axis of the tooth as possible

shallow as this is where the toothbrush makes the greatest impact and may even produce gingival recession. This means that four or more measurements may be required on each tooth to give an accurate picture.

3. Where present oral hygiene is good the gingival cuff may be so tight around the neck of the tooth as to resist the insertion of an ordinary periodontal probe without causing pain. The measurement of pockets in anaesthetized tissue often produces quite different results from previous measurement made in sentient tissue.

4. Tooth contour and angulation, subgingival calculus or restorations, as well as carious cavities, may impede the insertion of the probe. The deepest aspect of interproximal pockets usually lie below the contact area. Therefore the probe has to be inclined inwards to reach this point in molar or premolar teeth. Compensation should be made for the effect of this angulation on the probing depth measured, and it is usual to subtract 1 mm from the measurement value in these circumstances.

There are many designs of pocket-measuring probe, some of which are too thick to provide accurate measurement, and some of which are sharp so that the tissue is penetrated unless great care is taken. The special CPITN probe has been described earlier. It has been shown that pockets of over 3 mm are measured with diminishing reliability, and it is unfortunate that much periodontal research is based upon such an unreliable criterion. Sometimes a purulent discharge can be expressed from the pocket by pressure on the pocket wall.

Gingival recession

Gingival recession and root exposure may accompany chronic periodontitis but are not necessarily a feature of the disease. Where recession occurs pocket depth measurement is only a partial representation of the total amount of periodontal destruction. The other causes of gingival recession are discussed in Chapter 8.

Tooth mobility

Some tooth mobility in a labiolingual plane can be elicited in healthy single-rooted teeth, especially lower incisors, being more mobile than multirooted teeth. Increasing tooth mobility is produced by:

1. Spread of inflammation from the gingiva into the deeper tissues
2. Loss of supporting tissue
3. Occlusal trauma.

Mobility also increases after periodontal surgery and in pregnancy. In periodontal pathology tissue destruction is always accompanied by inflammation and frequently by occlusal trauma. Mobility which is produced by inflammation and occlusal trauma is reversible, as demonstrated by the reduction in mobility following scaling and occlusal adjustment; mobility associated with destruction of supporting tissue is not reversible.

Assessment of mobility for research purposes can be made using special apparatus but clinical assessment is usually subjective. It is elicited by exerting pressure on one side of the tooth under examination with an instrument or finger tip while placing a finger of the other hand on the other side of the tooth and its neighbour which is used as a fixed point so that relative movement can be discerned. Another way of eliciting mobility (although not assessing it) is to place fingers over the facial surfaces of the teeth while the patient grinds the teeth.

The degree of mobility may be graded as follows:

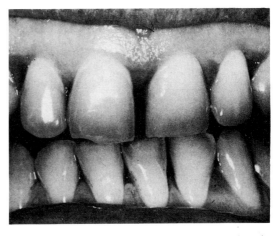

Figure 11.3 Drifting of the upper incisors which alerted the patient to the presence of disease

Grade 1. Just discernible, 0.2–1 mm in a horizontal direction.
Grade 2. Easily discernible, and over 1 mm labiolingual displacement
Grade 3. Well marked labiolingual displacement, mobility of the tooth up and down in an axial direction. There is an element of subjectivity in this grading. No doubt sufficient determination can elicit mobility in perfectly secure teeth!

Tooth migration

Movement of a tooth (or teeth) out of its original position in the arch is a common feature of periodontal disease and one which alerts the patient to the problem. Tooth position in health is maintained by a balance of tongue, lip and occlusal forces. Once supporting tissue is lost these forces determine the pattern of tooth migration. The incisors move most frequently in a labial direction but teeth may move in any direction or become extruded (*Figure 11.3*). Once a tooth migrates the force on that tooth changes and this may promote further stress and further migration. If an upper incisor migrates labially the lower lip may come to lie lingual to the incisal edge of the tooth and produce further migration.

Discomfort

One of the most important features of chronic periodontitis is the almost total absence of discomfort or pain unless acute inflammation supervenes. This is one of the main distinctions between periodontal and pulp disease. Discomfort or pain on percussion of the tooth indicates some active inflammation of the supporting tissues which is at its most acute in abscess formation when the tooth becomes exquisitely sensitive to touch. Sensitivity to hot and cold is sometimes present when there is gingival recession and root exposure. Indeed one common clinical experience is the appearance of sensitivity, especially to cold, when roots once covered in calculus are cleaned. On occasion pulp pathology may be a complication of advanced periodontal disease and severe pain may then develop.

Alevolar bone loss

Resorption of alveolar bone and the associated destruction of periodontal ligament is the most important feature of chronic periodontitis, and the one which leads to tooth loss. There is considerable variation in both the form and rate of alveolar bone resorption and in constructing a treatment plan the amount of bone loss, the rate at which resorption is progressing and the pattern of bone loss need to be accurately established. Radiographic examination is an essential part of periodontal diagnosis and with certain limitations provides evidence of the alveolar bone height, the form of bone destruction, the width of the periodontal ligament space and the density of cancellous trabeculation. Serial radiographs taken over a period of time can provide information about the rate of bone loss. However, radiographic examination without careful clinical examination can be very misleading. A periodontal diagnosis cannot be made from radiographs alone as there is no way of distinguishing on the radiograph past bone destruction from current bone resorption.

Because the images of the facial and lingual plates of bone are largely obscured by the dense image of the tooth, diagnosis depends upon obtaining a clear image of the interdental bone. Careful angulation of the X-ray beam and a standardized routine of exposure and processing the radiographic film is essential.

The first radiographic sign of periodontal destruction is loss of density of the alveolar margin. This is most clearly seen between posterior teeth where in health the broad

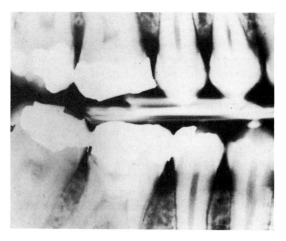

Figure 11.4 Signs of early marginal bone loss shown on a bitewing radiograph. Most bone loss is around the upper molars but note hollowing of septum at 65̄ . The bitewing film is very useful for revealing early bone loss in posterior segments

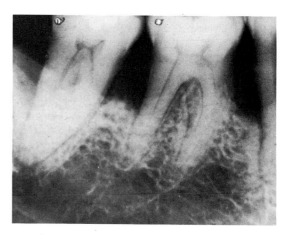

Figure 11.5 Fairly advanced bone loss in a 46 year old woman. Note irregularity of bone margin with vertical defects distal to 7̄ and 5̄

interdental septum projects a dense and well-defined image of the alveolar margin (*Figure 11.4*). The image of the narrow interdental septa between anterior teeth is less well defined in health and early pathological changes are less easy to see. With continuing bone resorption the height of the alveolar bone is further reduced (*Figure 11.5*). Even correctly angulated the radiographs may not disclose the true state of interdental resorption, e.g. an interdental crater between molars can be masked by the images of the facial and lingual walls of the defect. Bone defects which lie over the facial or lingual aspects of the teeth, e.g. marginal gutters, may be completely obscured and revealed only when flaps are raised at surgery. Moreover, distinguishing between facial and lingual defects may not be possible from radiographic evidence alone. Two radiographs taken at slightly different angles often reveal defects undetected by one. This is especially true in the diagnosis of furcation defects. These are usually revealed by radiographic examination but the exact form of the defect may not be discernible. The thick palatal root of an upper molar may mask a trifurcation defect. Widening of the periodontal space in the furcation provides evidence of an early lesion. Widening of the periodontal space on one side or all around a tooth frequently indicates excessive occlusal stress. This is sometimes accompanied by widening or funnelling of the coronal aspect of the socket.

All departures from the normal radiographic appearance must be checked against other clinical features, in particular pocket depth and mobility patterns, and if these do not correspond re-examination should be carried out. Clinical and radiographic features taken together should make a reasonable fit which sheds light on both the pathological condition and its aetiology. Thus, where radio-graphic examination of a mobile tooth reveals that the supporting bone is virtually intact, careful examination of the occlusion is essential. There must always be an identifiable reason for any pathological change.

Halitosis and offensive taste

The metabolism of many of the oral bacteria, in particular Gram negative anaerobics in saliva, the gingival crevice and plaque, when acting on substrates in the mouth, e.g. food debris and plaque, can produce sulphur-bearing compounds such as hydrogen sulphide and methylmercaptan; these can impart an offensive smell to the mouth and exhaled breath.

An offensive taste and smell frequently accompany periodontal disease especially when oral hygiene is poor. Acute inflammation, with the production of pus which exudes from pockets on pressure, also causes halitosis. A source of constant surprise is the lack of awareness of many affected individuals and their spouses to the powerful fetor which like a malignant wind escapes from their mouths when they speak. Lack of sensibility and unconcern about dental health seem to go hand in hand, and as patient cooperation is essential to the success of periodontal treatment this sensibility, or lack of it, can provide a clue to prognosis.

12

Diagnosis, prognosis and treatment plan

Making a diagnosis

The diagnosis should not be limited to giving a name to the condition. If periodontal disease is to be treated and its recurrence prevented, a diagnosis should include the identification of all aetiological factors, i.e. (i) those factors which predispose to plaque deposition and retention, and (ii) those factors, local or systemic, which influence adversely the behaviour of the tissues. It should go without saying that you cannot remove or control factors which have not been identified, yet all too frequently treatment is reduced to the control of signs and symptoms, and inevitably disease recurs.

At the time of the initial examination some attempt should be made to assess the patient's attitude to dental health. Patient cooperation is essential to the success of periodontal treatment and it is this fact which makes the treatment of periodontal disease different from that of caries and other dental diseases when the patient can take a more passive attitude.

Patient examination

The examination should be methodical and comprehensive and should follow the standard pattern of the classic case history.

Present complaint and its history

A patient with periodontal disease may have no complaint at all and be oblivious to the presence of any disease in the mouth; indeed, the patient may be suspicious of any suggestion that disease is present! The most common complaints are bleeding gums, loose teeth, drifting of the teeth (usually the upper incisors), nasty taste, halitosis, swelling of the gums, discomfort and occasionally acute pain.

Few patients at the initial consultation provide concise and completely relevant information. All too often, the necessary information has to be elicited by abstraction from a long, sometimes rambling, account which must be listened to with patience and close attention. In addition, pertinent questions should be asked:

Are you in pain?
Where is the pain?
Is it a throbbing or dull pain?
Does the pain keep you awake?
What brings on the pain – hot, cold, sweet, biting?
Have you had pain in the past or is this the first time?
What treatment have you received for pain?
Do your gums ever bleed?
   When you brush your teeth?
   When you eat hard food?
Did your gums bleed in the past?
What treatment did you receive?
Do any of your teeth feel loose?
Have you always had that space between your front teeth?
Have you had any swelling in your mouth? Where, when, etc.?

Dental history

Do you go to the dentist regularly?
What was the last treatment you received?
When did you last have a scaling, i.e. cleaning by your dentist?
Do you have any dentures (false teeth that you can take out) – how long have you had them?
Have you any false teeth that are fixed in – how long have you had them?

At this stage questioning about home care can be a waste of time. Answers to such questions as 'How often do you clean your teeth?' are often suspect, as the patient is likely to say what he imagines he is supposed to say, i.e. twice a day, night and morning. Even if this happens to be the truth, it gives no indication of the quality of the performance; only an examination of the mouth provides information about that.

At this time, some idea about habits should be gleaned, e.g. smoking, clenching, night-grinding, biting pencils and so on.

Medical history

Although a medical history may not seem relevant to some patients, it is essential to obtain one for a number of reasons:

1. The patient may be suffering from some condition, e.g. cardiovascular disease, renal disease, etc., which will require special precautions and/or modification of the treatment, and will necessitate communication with the patient's physician.
2. Systemic conditions, e.g. pregnancy, diabetes, will alter the way in which the periodontal tissues behave and may demand medical attention before periodontal treatment can be carried out.
3. The mouth may be the site of some manifestation of a systemic condition, e.g. anaemia, which could affect any periodontal treatment.
4. The patient may be receiving medication, e.g. tricyclic antidepressants for depression, which may conflict with medication involved in the periodontal treatment, e.g. general anaesthetics.

A medical history should record any present illness and medication; any past serious illness and medication, e.g. steroids taken in the recent past, allergies, especially any history of penicillin sensitivity, abnormal bleeding tendencies, in particular excessive bleeding after injury or tooth extraction.

The use of a questionnaire may be helpful.

Where some systemic problem exists, communication with the patient's physician is essential.

Patient appraisal

While taking the history, a general appraisal of the patient should be made, and such features as obesity, general posture, pallor, skin rash, heavy breathing, lip posture, should be noted.

Oral examination

The examination of the mouth should be carried out in a methodical and thorough manner; this is the dentist's special area. Halitosis is noted as the mouth is opened, or even earlier when the patient is giving a history.

1. *The oral mucosa*, cheeks, lips, tongue, palate, floor of mouth and vestibules, are examined for ulceration, vesicles, swelling, eroded patches, abnormal colour and white lines or patches.

    Tooth indentations in the margin of the tongue and interdental keratosis, i.e. a white line in the cheek at the level of the occlusion, often indicates a clenching or grinding habit.

    Aphthous ulcers frequently occur in the labial or lingual vestibule or inside the lips. Lichen planus may be seen as fine, interlacing white lines on the cheeks or alveolar mucosa. Vesicles or eroded patches should be fully investigated.

    A sinus on the alveolar mucosa, with or without the discharge of pus on pressure, indicates the presence of an alveolar abscess.

    In the older individual, a squamous-cell carcinoma may appear as a painless swelling, ulcer or eroded white patch in any part of the oral mucosa, but especially in the vestibules. Oral lesions of primary, secondary or tertiary syphilis may appear on the lips, tongue, palate and even the gingivae; widespread candida lesions in a young male could be indicative of HIV infection.

Any departure from the norm must be examined carefully, and if infection or malignant disease is suspected, an examination of the submandibular and cervical lymph nodes will help with a diagnosis. Immediate referral to the physician or appropriate specialist is essential.

2. *Removable appliances*, if present, should be examined for their fit, design and relationship to any inflammation of the oral mucosa and gingiva.

3. *Oral hygiene*. Note presence and position of plaque, supragingival and subgingival calculus. Subgingival calculus can be detected with a probe such as a WHO probe or a Cross calculus probe but may also be seen as a dark blue shadow in the gingival margin. The use of a disclosing agent will help to identify plaque and demonstrate its presence to the patient. Sometimes the location of plaque and calculus points to a predisposing factor, e.g. better oral hygiene on the left side is usually associated with right-handed tooth brushing; interproximal deposits and gingival inflammation may be caused by the overhanging margins of restorations or poor contact relations.

4. *Teeth* are charted and cavities, restorations and malalignments recorded. Attrition may indicate a grinding habit; abrasion a vigorous and damaging toothbrushing technique.

5. *Gingivae* are examined for colour, shape, size and consistency, keeping in mind the picture of health, pink, knife-edged, streamlined and firm, any departure from which could indicate pathology.

6. *Pocket measurement* should be carried out on each tooth and recorded. Ideally, true mesial, distal, facial and lingual measurements are required, but this is possible only where teeth are missing, so that unimpeded access to these surfaces is possible. Where proximal teeth are present, measurement is made at the line angles, and on facial and lingual surfaces. Taking six readings on each tooth is ideal but may be very time consuming, and if diagnosis is made at a reasonably early stage in periodontal breakdown, only one or two measurements made at the mesiobuccal and mesiolingual line angles may be sufficient. Where there appears to be furcation involvement of molars, or drifting of incisors, facial and lingual measurements on these teeth are essential.

A pocket-measuring probe must be fine enough to enter a narrow pocket, but must have a blunt end so that the tissue is not perforated. The sharp-ended probe used for the detection of caries should not be used. The pocket-measuring probe must be inserted into the pocket as near parallel to the axis of the tooth as possible; if inserted obliquely, a false reading will be obtained. However, it is necessary to slightly angulate the probe beneath the contact area on molar and premolar teeth to reach the base of the deepest interdental pockets; the effect of the angulation should be compensated for when recording the measurement. Great care has to be taken to manipulate the probe so that the true depth of the pocket is recorded. Delicate handling of the probe must be employed to negotiate subgingival deposits without impaction against the root surface. Vigorous probing is not only painful but likely to give an inaccurate reading; even gentle probing of inflamed gingivae can be painful. The problems of pocket measurement can be demonstrated by the fact that pocket measurement after local anaesthesia usually gives greater readings than in the unanaesthetized tissue.

Gutta-percha or silver points which may be calibrated may be left in situ during radiographic examination of suspected infrabony pockets.

In addition to recording pocket depth, it is important to assess the probing attachment level, i.e. probing depths measured from the amelocemental junction (CEJ) or some other fixed point. Where there is considerable gingival hyperplasia pocketing may be fairly deep, say 5–7 mm, but attachment loss may be small or nil. Where there has been considerable gingival recession, a shallow pocket may be associated with considerable destruction of the periodontal tissues. Therefore, in order to interpret pocket measurement one must also note (*a*) the position of the gingival margin on the tooth surface, and (*b*) the position of the alveolar crest as seen on the radiograph.

7. *Radiographic examination* will demonstrate the position of the alveolar margin and the condition of the alveolar bone. In a child or adolescent, radiographic examination may not be essential but if any doubt exists about the integrity of the alveolar margin,

bitewing films of posterior teeth and periapical films of the incisors should provide adequate information. If there is evidence of established bone loss, further radiographic examination can then be undertaken.

In the adult, full mouth examination may be necessary. The long-cone paralleling technique provides the most reliable radiographic evidence. The bisecting angle technique is more likely to give a distorted picture of the relationship of the alveolar margin to the CEJ. Rinn bite blocks, film holders and localization devices can be used to ensure that the X-rays pass perpendicular to the teeth and film, preventing any distortion of the bone/teeth relationships. Using these devices can also help to make subsequent radiographs of the same site comparable. Vertical bitewing radiographs are useful for posterior teeth and can be used for teeth with probing depths up to 6 mm; the orthopantomograph (OPG) provides an overall picture, but detail of the alveolar margin is frequently ill defined. Repeat radiographs may be necessary, at intervals (not less than 3 years) determined by patient susceptibility, to show progression. Sophisticated techniques such as subtraction radiography and computer-assisted image analysis (*see below*) have been used as research tools to detect small changes in bone mass, but at present these have no place in clinical practice. It cannot be stressed too strongly that the traditional techniques of clinical radiography can provide a great deal of reliable information, but only if great care is taken in beam angulation, exposure and processing, and in interpretation of the radiographic image.

8. *Occlusion*. The examination of occlusion should include:
   (*a*) The Angle's classification
   (*b*) Overbite and overjet
   (*c*) Tooth relation in protrusive and lateral positions and movements
   (*d*) Any deviation from the normal path of opening and closure
   (*e*) Any temporomandibular joint (TMJ) discomfort of clicking
   (*f*) Any spasm in the masticatory muscles.
   (*g*) Any history of habits, e.g. clenching or grinding the teeth.

The occlusion needs to be examined closely where:
   (*a*) Teeth are mobile or sensitive
   (*b*) There is discomfort, clicking, deviation of the mandible on opening and closing, or limitation of movement
   (*c*) One or more of the masticatory muscles is tender to palpation
   (*d*) Radiographs show widening of the periodontal spaces or vertical bone defects, i.e. possible signs of excessive occlusal stress.

Advances in diagnostic techniques

The methods described above are suitable for most clinical situations but do suffer from a number of drawbacks. These are:

1. Clinical or radiological measurements of attachment loss are not precisely accurate and if not carried out very carefully can be misleading. This is particularly the case for periodontal probing but also affects oral radiography.
2. Full mouth recording is necessary because of the site specific and episodic nature of much periodontal progression.
3. Individual susceptibility to periodontitis, as to all bacterial disease, varies over time and this needs to be determined and taken into account.
4. All clinical diagnostic techniques give us retrospective information about past disease and are unable to diagnose disease activity.
5. If the periodontal examination is required for periodontal research purposes much more accurate diagnostic techniques are necessary.

All of these issues are discussed below.

The episodic nature of chronic periodontitis

A number of longitudinal clinical studies (Socransky *et al.*, 1984) have recorded clinical attachment loss at individual sites in different subjects over time periods ranging from 2–5 years. These have revealed that, despite the presence of inflammation, most sites showed no progression during the study period. Instead, attachment loss occurred at only a few sites and even at these sites was interspersed with long periods of stability or quiescence. This type of episodic, site specific attachment loss has given rise to the burst theory of chronic periodontitis. It has further been proposed that these bursts might occur randomly throughout an individuals life (random burst) or there may be periods when bursts of periodontal breakdown in many sites are more likely (asynchronous multiple burst).

The implications of the burst theories are that:

• Gingival inflammation at a site may not indicate that further periodontal breakdown is occurring or that it will occur at a later date.
• Periodontal disease is site specific and may affect different teeth in the same mouth at different rates.
• Full mouth periodontal charting on a regular basis is necessary to identify sites with attachment loss, to determine the pattern and rate of progression and to determine the patient's susceptibility.
• Each tooth must be considered separately for treatment.

In these studies, only fairly large changes (≥ 3 mm) of clinical attachment level could be reliably measured (see below) and smaller changes could not be detected. Therefore, although these studies show clearly that site specific, episodic disease progression does occur they do not preclude other patterns of progression including slow regular progression also occurring. It seems most likely that episodic progression would predominate in susceptible patients with more rapid rates of progression.

Susceptible and resistant patients

Periodontal attachment loss has been found to be more marked in some patients than others, even when differences of oral hygiene are taken into account (Löe *et al.*, 1978). Studies from a number of different countries have suggested that about 10% of subjects appear to have a high risk of developing destructive periodontal disease and experience severe periodontal destruction with rapid progression and tooth loss. About 80% of subjects are susceptible to periodontitis which progresses rather slowly and rarely results in tooth loss. The remaining 10% appear to be relatively resistant to destructive periodontitis, despite the continued presence of gingivitis (Löe *et al.*, 1978; Page and Schroeder, 1986; Papapanou *et al.*, 1989). Identification of each patient's individual susceptibility to periodontitis is important since this will determine the type and frequency of treatment that they will require.

Advances in measurement of periodontal attachment loss

The main objective of periodontal diagnosis is to detect changes in periodontal attachment level. The traditional methods of recording this are the use of manual probing with a graduated periodontal probe and radiographic examination. The accuracy of probing is affected by a number of factors including the position and angulation of the probe, the probing pressure and the inflammatory state of the tissues. If probing measurements are to be used sequentially to detect progressive loss of attachment these factors need to be controlled where possible and the measurements need to be made from a fixed reproducible point. This cannot be the gingival margin which can change its position as a result of inflammatory swelling or recession and the ideal reference point is the CEJ. However, the CEJ is difficult to locate precisely because it usually lies subgingivally and it may be obscured by calculus or dental restorations. For these reasons other points such as the occlusal surface or a fixed point on a stent are often used in clinical research studies.

Probing measurements even with those controls are not precisely reproducible between different clinicians even when they standardize their procedures. In addition, replicate measurements of the same site at close time intervals are not always reproducible for the same clinician (Haffajee *et al.*, 1983). To overcome these problems in clinical studies they suggested the use of the tolerance method to determine the threshold for confirmed attachment loss based on probing. With this method two replicate measurements of each site are made for each subject and their standard deviation calculated. The subject threshold is considered to be three standard deviations of the mean differences between all paired measurements. The site measurement standard deviation has been calculated as 0.82 mm in the Haffajee studies which makes the subject tolerance 2.46 mm. Thus, using this method any change below 3 mm is considered to be unreliable and this makes it impossible to measure small changes of attachment using manual probing. For this reason, the National Institute for Dental Research (NIDR) of the USA in 1979 requested the development of more sensitive methods (Parakkal, 1979). They wanted:

1. a precision of ±0.1 mm and a range of 10 mm
2. a constant probing force
3. measurement from a fixed reproducible point
4. guidance system to ensure reproducible pathway
5. non-invasive procedure
6. digital output of data.

These criteria were met by the Florida research group (Gibbs *et al.*, 1988) who developed the Florida probe system. This incorporates:

1. constant probing force
2. precise electronic measurement
3. computer storage of data.

It eliminates errors of visual reading which become more important as you age! It consists of a probe handpiece, a digital readout, a foot switch and a computer interface and computer (Magnusson *et al.*, 1988b). It has been found to be significantly superior to manual probing (Magnusson *et al.*, 1988a). Two models have been developed which differ in their fixed reference point. These are the stent and disk models. The probe of stent model has a 1 mm metal collar that rests on a prepared ledge on a prefabricated vacuoform stent. The disk model has a 11 mm disk which rests on the occlusal surface or incisal edge of the tooth (*Figure 12.1a*).

The reproducibility of both types of Florida probe have been compared with conventional manual probing (Low *et al.*, 1989; Osborn *et al.*, 1990). They were both significantly superior to manual probes with a site standard deviation (SD) range of 0.21–0.28 mm. The calculated subject tolerance is 0.63–0.84 mm meaning that changes in attachment of 1 mm can be reliably measured by this method.

The Florida probe can also read probing depths using an interchangeable pocket depth handpiece. This has a collar surrounding the

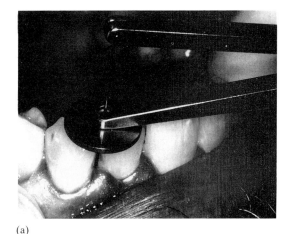

(a)

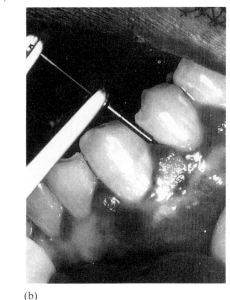

(b)

Figure 12.1 (*a*) A Florida electronic probe with attachment level disk on occlusal surface; (*b*) A Florida electronic probe with sleeve of pocket depth attachment at gingival margin

probe which is related to the gingival margin and the distance from this to the base of the pocket is electronically recorded (*Figure 12.1b*).

All of this data along with other readings such as bleeding on probing can be recorded and saved on a disk or printed on to special charts using a suitable compatible printer.

Other electronic probes have been developed and these include:

- The Interprobe (Goodson and Kondon, 1988)
  This has an optical encoder transduction element.
- The Birek probe (Birek *et al.*, 1987).
  This works by constant air pressure and uses the occlusal surface as its reference point.
  The site SD has been calculated as 0.46 mm and the subject threshold as 1.38 mm.
- The Jeffcoat probe (Jeffcoat *et al.*, 1986, 1989)
  This claims to detect the CEJ automatically and has a calculated site SD of 0.17 mm and a subject threshold of 0.51 mm. This appears to be the lowest subject threshold reported to date.

Radiographic examination

Transmission radiography can show the relationship between the alveolar bone margin and the CEJ and changes in the distance from the bone margin to the CEJ, normally 1–2 mm, are indicative of alveolar bone loss. To achieve an accurate display of this distance the rays must be perpendicular to the tooth and bone surfaces and the tube must also be at the correct antero-posterior angulation. Two types of view can be used in conventional radiography to achieve this:

- Vertical bitewings
- Long cone paralleling views

To detect serial changes in this relationship further controls are necessary and involve a constant film position and constant tube geometry. A constant film position can be achieved by the use of a stent which can be in the form of an acrylic impression of the occlusal surfaces of the teeth on the bite block of the film holder. A mark can also be made to ensure that the film is always placed in the same position in the holder. By these means the holder is accurately located to the teeth and the film to the holder for each serial radiograph. Constant tube geometry can be achieved by relating the tube to positioning devices attached to the film holder (Rinn system) or by the use of a cephalostat (Jeffcoat *et al.*, 1987).

Bone loss can also be expressed as a percentage of the root length to compensate for errors of foreshortening or elongation.

Computer-aided systems

Techniques have recently been developed to aid the detection of small serial changes in bone level. These rely on digitization of the radiographic image to allow computer processing and analysis.

Digital subtraction radiology

The best known of these techniques is digital subtraction radiology (Webber *et al.*, 1982; Gröndahl and Gröndahl, 1983; Jeffcoat *et al.*, 1987). The purpose of this technique is to subtract all unchanged structures from a pair of serial films and display only the areas of change. For periodontal films this means subtraction of the teeth, cortical bone and trabecular pattern leaving only bone loss or gain standing out against a neutral grey background.

The digitization process converts the analogue (nearly continuous grey level information) contained in the transmission radiograph to numbers that are proportional to the brightness of the radiograph at a particular location. This is done by taking a picture of the radiograph with a sensitive black and white video camera. The digitizer automatically superimposes a grid over this picture and converts the grey level of the radiograph within each box in the grid to a number ranging from zero (black) to 255 (white). The fineness of the grid determines the spatial resolution of the digitized image and usually a 512×480 picture element (pixel) grid is used.

This process does not increase the information on the radiograph and in fact decreases it a little. It does, however, put the information in a form that the computer can use so that it can process it in a way in which will aid the dentist or researcher to detect changes in bone level not visible to the unaided eye from the original radiograph. The computer subtracts all structures present in the first radiograph of the serial pair from those in the second radiograph leaving only bone loss (dark) or bone gain (light). Location of bony change can be more readily seen by superimposing the subtracted image over the original radiograph. Subtracted images can also be colour coded by the computer to increase clarity. Bone loss is usually colour coded red and bone gain green.

If this technique were reliable and accurate it could be useful in assessing the natural history of periodontal disease progression and in longitudinal studies of various types including investigations of potential biomarkers of disease activity or proposed new treatment methods. However, the accuracy of digital subtraction radiography has been questioned by Benn (1990) on the basis of his own measurements using this technique. Subtraction radiography depends critically on the very precise registration of the two sequential radiographs. He created two identical digital images of a single radiograph to test the response of the system to small displacements of 0.1–0.42 mm in the X, Y, and XY directions before subtraction. He found that displacements of 0.1–0.14 mm in the Y or XY directions caused 20–25% of crestal pixels to vary by more than ± 2.5% of grey range (2.5% is the noise threshold used for this technique). Larger displacements of 0.3–0.42 mm caused 65% of crestal pixels to vary by more than ± 2.5% of grey range. Such small displacements would be hard to avoid when using this technique with serial radiographs and so false crestal bone gain or loss could regularly result from these causes. The use of a much higher noise threshold of about ± 8% would need to be used to avoid these critical errors.

Computer-assisted linear radiography

Benn (1992) has designed a computer aided method for making linear measurements on serial radiographs using stored regions of interest. In this system, the radiographs are first calibrated and digitized as described above. Under the control of a computer program regions of interest (ROI) of 7.5 mm × 7.5 mm, sufficient to cover the mesial and distal CEJ to alveolar crest margin regions of adjacent teeth, are chosen. The measuring process involves placing the cursor pixel point on the CEJ and clicking the mouse button which records and marks this position. This is then repeated for the alveolar crest after which the distance is calculated and stored by the computer. The ROI with its marked reference points is also stored. The process is then repeated for the first serial radiograph and the ROI of the first measurement with its marked points is redisplayed close to the area to be measured. This reminds the operator of the chosen reference points reducing the chances of error. The computer automatically calculates the distances, the average distances of the two readings and the difference between the two readings. This process is then repeated for the second serial radiograph initially using prompts for the siting of reference points from the displayed ROI from the first radiograph. When the sites for the second radiograph image have been measured twice the computer automatically calculates the differences between the two films and the confidence value attached to the measured change.

The accuracy and reliability of this system were tested with 28 examiners with minimal training (Benn, 1992). They each measured 14 different sites and repeated the process 4 weeks later; 13 out of 14 sites produced an intra-examiner SD threshold of ≤0.15 mm with the ROI method but 0 out of 14 without. The inter-examiner threshold for 13 out of 14 sites was ≤0.22 mm using the ROI method and 0 out of 14 without. Therefore, this system would appear to be accurate to ≤0.22 mm and would seem to be useful for clinical research.

Special tests

If the severity of the inflammation or the degree of periodontal destruction appears to be out of proportion to the observed aetiological factors, or if general appraisal of the patient suggests that some systemic factor may be operating, then blood and urine examination or other special tests may be required. In such cases it is imperative to communicate with the patient's physician prior to the start of treatment.

Making a prognosis

A prognosis is a prediction of the way in which the tissues are likely to respond to treatment. Before a definitive treatment plan can be formulated, a prognosis must be made. This should allow one to establish not merely what treatment can be carried out but, more importantly, what treatment is justified in the attempt to achieve long-term periodontal stability. Frequently the patient will ask that such a prediction be made, and the more complicated the treatment the more important making a prognosis becomes. Looking into the future can be a hazardous exercise but a prediction of the way in which the periodontal tissues will behave can be made on the basis of an understanding of the way in which the tissues of that individual have behaved in the past in the face of disease-producing factors.

A number of parameters need to be considered:

1. The extent of periodontal destruction. This is represented by the amount of alveolar bone loss as seen on the radiograph; obviously the greater the amount of bone loss, the poorer the prognosis.
2. The age of the patient. This, together with the extent of periodontal destruction, provides an idea of the rate at which destruction has taken place. The older the individual, the better the prognosis for any given degree of periodontal destruction.
3. The form of the bone loss. The presence of vertical bone defects must mean a less favourable prognosis than where bone loss is horizontal, for several reasons:
   (*a*) Because the level of attachment is frequently more apical
   (*b*) Because the possibility of fill-in of such defects is uncertain
   (*c*) Because the presence of vertical defects usually indicates that factors other than plaque-induced inflammation are operating. Furcation involvement can present home care problems, even after satisfactory periodontal treatment, and if the furcation lesion is related to pulp pathology, prognosis is compounded by any defects in endodontic treatment.
4. The possibility of removing aetiological factors. The control of aetiological factors is essential to the achievement of long-term health, but control can only be exercised after these factors have been identified. Without such identification, treatment becomes symptomatic. Careful examination and an understanding of clinical features is essential. It is always necessary to ask 'Why are these clinical features present?'

   Patient cooperation is essential for satisfactory plaque control, but is also necessary for the control of predisposing and aggravating aetiological factors, e.g. the replacement of an ill fitting partial denture. Patient cooperation is more likely to be forthcoming after the patient has been given information about the nature of the problem.

Time spent in providing such information and in explaining the rationale behind the treatment plan will improve the chances of achieving a good prognosis.

5. The number, position and form of teeth present. The number of teeth and their position in the arch will determine the occlusal load on each tooth, whether a prosthesis is necessary, and the amount of tooth support for an appliance. In this context, the form of the appliance is extremely important; a removable appliance makes greater demands on the tooth-supporting tissues than a fixed appliance. The symmetrical distribution of the teeth in the arch is likely to provide a better prognosis than where several teeth are placed on one side of the arch. The root base can be a crucial factor in the stability and usefulness of a tooth. An upper molar with widespread roots and therefore a large root base has a much better prognosis than a conical-rooted premolar or incisor with the same amount of bone loss.
6. *General health.* Although certain conditions do affect the periodontal tissue response, e.g. diabetes, Down's syndrome, agranulocytosis, the general health of the patient does not usually affect the periodontal condition directly, but any debility, physical or emotional, can interfere with the patient's oral hygiene regime.
7. *The immunological status in relation to plaque bacteria.* The individual's response is critical to the development and progress of periodontal destruction, and is the subject of much recent research. As described in Chapter 20, a few young individuals appear to suffer some deficiency in the cell-mediated immune response to plaque antigens, which leads to an extremely poor prognosis. It seems likely that other variations in immune response will be identified in the future, and some laboratory tests may be developed which will provide a more objective guide to prognosis than is currently available.

All the factors outlined above must be taken together to provide a periodontal prognosis for that particular individual. This exercise has to be carried out with great care and thought. The assessment of prognosis provides an acid test of the operator's understanding of the biological forces operating in the mouth under examination. Furthermore, the limitations of our understanding of the disease process do handicap our ability to make absolute prognoses.

Treatment plan

The objectives of treatment are:

1. The elimination of disease
2. The restoration of efficient function
3. The production of a satisfactory appearance
One might also add, a contented patient.

It should be evident from the above list that periodontal treatment is not *primarily* concerned with the conservation of individual teeth but with the long-term preservation of a healthy dentition. Indeed, there are situations in which individual teeth have to be sacrificed to the greater good. This concept of treating the dentition as a functioning unit is in conflict with the traditional dental teaching, in which the tooth rather than the dentition is the focus of concern.

Because each patient presents an individual problem, one cannot prescribe a rigid pattern of treatment. Treatment is determined not only by the condition defined by the diagnosis but also by the patient's age, general health and their attitudes and aspirations. Nevertheless, it is important that a well-ordered plan of action is designed at the outset, keeping in mind that departures from this plan may be required as treatment proceeds. No treatment, other than emergency treatment, should be started before a plan is established and explained to the patient.

The following outline should provide a guide to treatment management:

1. Emergency treatment
2. Extraction of teeth with poor prognosis
3. Patient information
4. Plaque control and scaling
5. Initial occlusal adjustment
6. Reassessment
7. Surgery
8. Reconstruction
9. Maintenance.

1. Emergency treatment

The control of pain comes before any other treatment, but to be effective requires accurate diagnosis. An alveolar abscess which is of pulpal origin can be misdiagnosed as a periodontal lesion with consequent errors in treatment and persistence of pain.

Swelling, even without pain, requires immediate attention. Acute infection may require the prescription of antibiotics before further treatment can be carried out, but the use of antibiotics is justified only where pain and infection can be controlled in no other way. A localized and pointing abscess should be treated by incision and drainage rather than by antibiotic.

Large, carious cavities and pulp disease should be treated. Endodontics may be necessary as an emergency measure where there is a pulpitis, apical abscess or a combined periapical–periodontal abscess.

Extremely mobile teeth which seriously interfere with function should be splinted or extracted.

2. Extraction of teeth with very poor prognosis

A decision about extraction should be based not only on the condition of the individual tooth and its supporting tissues but also upon the possible consequences of the extraction. Where periodontal breakdown is advanced, the extraction of weak teeth may create an insoluble prosthetic problem. Such developments need to be anticipated prior to extraction. The provision of removable prostheses may be necessary at this time, and care should be taken with their design, even if temporary.

3. Patient information

Some time should be allowed prior to definitive treatment to explain to the patient the nature of the problem and the kind of treatment needed. Where different lines of treatment are available, these options, with their advantages and disadvantages, should be explained. Frequently, decisions have to be made by the patient, and these can be made intelligently only on the basis of information.

4. Plaque control and scaling

Plaque control and scaling are the most important procedures in periodontal treatment. Where the condition is diagnosed and treated at an early stage, they are the only treatments required. They also provide a clue as to patient attitude, dexterity and level of cooperation. Where that level of cooperation is inadequate, any indicated surgical treatment or other complicated treatment will not be justified. This phase of treatment should also include the correction of filling overhangs and the replacement of defective restorations. It is unrealistic and unjust to expect a high level of plaque control where conditions exist which make that impossible; therefore, all plaque retention factors should be corrected at this stage.

5. Initial occlusal adjustment

This is necessary for repair of the periodontal lesion and may be carried out alongside plaque control. Gross occlusal disharmonies should be eliminated and temporary splints applied to very mobile teeth. At this stage, any minor tooth movement necessary can be carried out. Such movement should be complete and any retention apparatus be in place before any surgery is carried out. A bite-guard is provided in cases of definite bruxism.

6. Reassessment

A reassessment of the periodontal condition should be made at this stage. The tissue response to the treatment already provided may be better than anticipated, so that little or no surgery may be required. Pockets may shrink and mobile teeth become stable after the relatively simple procedures carried out so far. Dramatic stabilization of neighbouring teeth can follow the extraction of an infected tooth.

On the other hand, tissue response or patient cooperation may not be as satisfactory as anticipated and a reappraisal of the case will be needed.

7. Surgery

The management of the surgical phase of treatment depends upon the size of the problem and the patient's domestic and work commitments and their physical and emotional status. Not every patient can cope with several surgical procedures under local anaesthesia over an extended period of time. Furthermore, some patients find it difficult to maintain a satisfactory level of plaque control with a surgical wound, sutures and dressings in their mouth. Therefore any necessary surgery should be carried out in as few stages as possible over as short a time as possible. The options available, i.e. local anaesthesia, general anaesthesia or local anaesthesia plus intravenous sedation, should be offered to the patient with explanations of the obvious advantages and disadvantages, so that decisions can be made which meet their individual needs.

The immediate postoperative phase must be closely supervised for the first 2 postoperative months, after which permanent reconstruction work can be started.

8. Reconstruction

This phase should include fine adjustment of the occlusion and the provision of permanent restorative and prosthetic work. In the design of restorations, subgingival preparation should be avoided, except perhaps (minimally) on the labial aspect of upper incisors, where appearance is important. Embrasure spaces, allowing easy interdental cleaning, are essential. A balanced occlusion should be constructed (Chapter 24).

Any temporary splints can be removed and the need for permanent splinting can be assessed at this stage (*see* Chapter 25).

If they have not already been made, bite-guards for persistent bruxism can be provided.

9. Maintenance

Eternal vigilance is the watchword of successful periodontal treatment and, in that sense, periodontal treatment is never complete. Patients require recall for inspection, oral hygiene monitoring and scaling at 3, 6, 9 or 12 month intervals, depending on their previous disease experience and susceptibility. Individual radiographs may have to be repeated if pocket measurements show that disease is progressing.

One must avoid creating a situation where the patient is totally dependent upon professional care. Some individuals are happy to abdicate responsibility for the state of their mouth to the dentist or hygienist. It is essential to make clear to the patient that in the end the patient must be responsible for his or her own dental health. It is only through a partnership that long-term dental health can be achieved.

References

Benn, D.K. (1990) Limitations of the digital image subtraction technique in assessing alveolar bone crest changes due to misalignment errors during image capture. *Dentomaxillofacial Radiology* **19**, 97–104

Benn, D.K. (1992) A computer assisted method for making linear radiographic measurements using stored regions of interest. *Journal of Clinical Periodontology* **19**, 441–448

Birek, P., McCulloch, C.H. and Hardy, V. (1987) Gingival attachment level measurements with an automated periodontal probe. *Journal of Clinical Periodontology* **14**, 472–477

Haffajee, A.D., Socransky, S.S. and Goodson, J.M. (1983) Comparison of different data analysis for detecting changes in attachment level. *Journal of Clinical Periodontology* **10**, 298–310

Goodson, J.M. and Kondon, N. (1988) Periodontal pocket depth measurements by fiber optic technology. *Journal of Clinical Dentistry* **1**, 35–38

Gröndahl, H-G. and Gröndahl, K. (1983) Subtraction radiology for the diagnosis of periodontal bone lesions. *Oral Surgery, Oral Medicine, Oral Pathology* **55**, 208–213

Gibbs, C.H., Hirschfield, J.W., Lee, J.G. *et al.* (1988) Description and clinical evaluation of a new computerized periodontal probe – The Florida Probe. *Journal of Clinical Periodontology* **15**, 137–144

Jeffcoat, M.K., Jeffcoat, R.L., Jens, S.C. and Captain, K. (1986) A new periodontal probe with an automated cement-enamel junction detection. *Journal of Clinical Periodontology* **13**, 276–280

Jeffcoat, M.K., Jeffcoat, R.L., Captain, K., Reddy, M. and Williams, R.C. (1989) A new periodontal probe with an automated CEJ detection: Clinical trials. *Journal of Dental Research* **68**, 236

Jeffcoat, M.K., Reddy, M. and Webber, R.L. (1987) Extraoral control of geometry for digital subtraction radiology. *Journal of Periodontal Research* **22**, 396–402

Löe, H., Anerud, A., Boysen, H. and Smith, M. (1978) The natural history of periodontal disease in Man. *Journal of Periodontology* **49**, 607–620

Low, S.B., Taylor, M., Marks, R.G. *et al.* (1989) Measuring attachment level with an electronic disk probe. *Journal of Dental Research* **68**, 359

Magnusson, I., Fuller, W.W., Heins, P.J. *et al.* (1988a) Correlation between electronic and visual readings of pocket depth with a newly developed constant force probe. *Journal of Clinical Periodontology* **15**, 180–184

Magnusson, I., Clark, W.B., Marks, R.G. *et al.* (1988b) Attachment level measurements with a constant force electronic probe. *Journal of Clinical Periodontology* **15**, 185–188

Osborn, J., Stoltenberg, J., Huso, B. *et al.* (1990) Comparison of measurement variability using a standard and constant force probe. *Journal of Periodontology* **61**, 497–503

Page, R.C. and Schroeder, H.E. (1986) *Periodontitis in Man and Other Animals*. Basel: Karger

Papapanou, P.N., Wennström, J.J. and Gröndahl, K. (1989) A 10 year retrospective study of periodontal disease progression. *Journal of Clinical Periodontology* **16**, 403–411

Parakkal, P.F. (1979) Proceedings of the workshop on quantitative evaluation of periodontal diseases by physical measuring techniques. *Journal of Dental Research* **58**, 547–553

Socransky, S.S., Haffajee, A.D., Goodson, J.M. and Lindhe, J. (1984) New concepts of destructive periodontal disease. *Journal of Clinical Periodontology* **11**, 21–32

Webber, R.L., Ruttimann, U.E. and Gröndahl, H-G. (1982) X-ray image subtraction as a basis for assessment of periodontal changes. *Journal of Periodontal Research* **17**, 509–511

13

Diagnostic tests of disease activity

The relationship of bacteria and gingival crevicular fluid components to periodontal disease and their possible use in diagnostic tests

One of the liveliest areas of current periodontal research is concerned with the search for diagnostic tests of periodontal disease activity. These tests have potential relevance to both diagnosis and treatment because current clinical diagnostic methods are not precisely accurate and only allow retrospective diagnosis of attachment loss. To improve on this, however, diagnostic tests would need to be predictive of disease activity rather than just correlate with its occurrence.

Potential biomarkers of disease activity would need to be involved in the disease process in some way and therefore need to undergo extensive and careful basic research investigation before undergoing clinical evaluation. Only when the source, precise nature and the role of the potential marker are known and understood can clinical evaluation be meaningful.

The process of developing a predictive diagnostic test

Development of a predictive test based on any of the factors discussed in this section requires a combination of basic and applied research over a long time scale and the stages are listed below:

Basic research

- Separation and characterization
- Investigation of tissue chemistry
- Investigation of its sources in the periodontal tissue
- Investigation of its role in the microbiology or pathology of chronic periodontitis
- Development of a selective and sensitive assay system
- If GCF samples are to be used then verification is necessary that gingival tissue or bacterial components are the same as those found in GCF

Applied clinical research

These investigations involve testing on:

- Experimental gingivitis in humans
- Ligature induced periodontitis in animals
- Natural disease process

Investigations on the natural disease process involve:

- Cross-sectional studies of relationship to disease severity
- Study of the levels before and after successful treatment
- Longitudinal studies of its relation to attachment and bone loss
- Development of simplified test system for chairside use
- Comparison of this system with the laboratory analysis
- Clinical trial

The main candidates in the search for biomarkers have been:

- Bacteria and their products
- Inflammatory and immune products
- Enzymes released from dead cells
- Connective tissue degradation products

Microbiological markers

Bacterial plaque plays a primary role in the initiation and progression of periodontal diseases but the composition of the subgingival flora is complex and may vary from patient to patient and site to site. Despite these differences and the complex interactions that exist between bacteria and the host a number of possible pathogens have been suggested on the basis of their association with disease progression, animal pathogenicity and their possession of virulence factors (Genco *et al.*, 1988; Listgarten, 1992; Socransky and Haffajee, 1992). The main bacteria are shown below and this issue is discussed more fully in Chapters 2 and 4.

Bacterial associated with periodontal diseases

Porphyromonas gingivalis
Prevotella intermedia
Bacteroides forsythus
Actinobacillus actinomycetemcomitans
Capnocytophaga ochracea
Eikenella corrodens
Campylobacter (previously *Wollinella) recta*
Fusobacterium nucleatum
Treponema denticola

There is no evidence for any one specific pathogen in chronic periodontitis and therefore it may be considered as a non-specific bacterial disease (Theilade, 1986). The bacteria listed above tend to be present in higher numbers at active disease sites (Socransky and Haffajee, 1992) and in some cases produce products capable of damaging the tissues either directly or indirectly. However, they may also be present in healthy and inactive sites and the composition of all these sites may vary between patients or even in the same patient. Furthermore, the composition of the pocket depends on many factors including the presence of essential nutrients, the redox potential and the effects of the host defence mechanisms. These considerations may therefore limit the value of diagnostic tests based on bacteria.

Attempts to relate microbiological data to clinical events have proved difficult because of the variability and unreliability of clinical diagnostic methods. Another factor which complicates the quantitative and qualitative assessments of the subgingival flora is the technical problems associated with sampling and processing.

Bacterial species numbers may be determined in a variety of ways which vary in selectivity and sensitivity (Listgarten, 1992). These include:

Darkground or phase contrast microscopy

The main advantage of these techniques is the ability to count all the bacteria in the sample and the main drawbacks are the inability to speciate microorganisms or determine their relative susceptibility to antimicrobial agents. However, studies using these techniques have shown that in gingival health there is a scant subgingival flora of cocci and non-motile rods whilst in gingivitis there is the appearance of motile rods and spirochaetes and in periodontitis a vast increase in these morphotypes with particularly large numbers of spirochaetes (Listgarten and Levin, 1981; Listgarten, 1986).

Culture techniques

These techniques are able to analyse the nature of the microorganisms in a sample since they can be speciated with a variety of laboratory based methods including selective subcultures, biochemical tests, SDS PAGE, gene probes, ribotyping, DNA fingerprinting and cell wall long chain fatty acid analysis (Genco *et al.*, 1986; Greenstein, 1988). Their susceptibility to antimicrobials can also be tested. However, not all bacteria can be readily cultured and the proportional recovery of cultivable species is unlikely to match their proportions in the periodontal pocket. Also the use of selective media will restrict the species that are able to grow (Mandell and Socransky, 1981).

Immunological assays

The use of immunological techniques such as immunofluorescence (Zambon *et al.*, 1985;

Zambon *et al.*, 1986) or enzyme linked immunosorbent assay, ELISA (Ebersole *et al.*, 1984) can detect individual bacterial species. These have proved useful to detect the presence and relative proportions of selected bacterial species. These techniques use specific antibodies which bind to the selected bacterial antigens and are then detected by labelling the primary antibody directly with a fluorescent marker (direct immunofluorescence) or with a fluorescent secondary antibody (indirect immunofluorescence). In the ELISA assay the primary antibody is detected through a colorimetric reaction which is catalysed through an enzyme, usually horseradish peroxidase or alkaline phosphatase, linked to the antibody. These techniques are very specific if controls are used to check for non-specific reactions. They can only detect species for which an antibody is available.

DNA probes

In recent years, DNA probes have been developed to identify nucleotide sequences that are specific for bacteria believed to be of diagnostic significance (Highfield and Dougan, 1985) including suspected periodontal pathogens (French *et al.*, 1986; Savitt *et al.*, 1988; Loesche, 1992). These probes can detect as few as 10^3 cells in a sample and provide information on the presence of selected species in the sample. However, they cannot provide reliable quantitative data and are limited by the availability of probes. They are totally specific and it is possible for a species to be present in large numbers in the sample and not be detected because it was not specifically sought.

Enzyme-based assays

Another approach to the detection of selected bacterial species is to look for an enzyme which is unique to one or more of the relevant bacterial species. The plaque sample is exposed to a substrate that can only be hydrolysed by a specific enzyme. An example of this method is the detection of the trypsin-like protease. This protease is produced mainly by *Porphyromonas gingivalis* and to a much lesser extent by *Bacteroides forsythus* and *Treponema denticola* and is hydrolysed to benzyl arginine naphthylamide, BANA (Loesche, 1986; Loesche *et al.*, 1990; Loesche,

1992). Since some of these species grow poorly in cultures and account for a significant proportion of the protease activity of the subgingival flora, these enzyme assays provide a rapid and inexpensive method of screening samples of these bacteria. The main drawbacks are a lack of quantitative data and the inability to determine which of the 3 bacteria are responsible for the enzyme production. In most cases, however, this will be *Porphyromonas gingivalis* since this produces much more of this protease than the two other bacteria combined (Gazi *et al.*, 1994). Also the BANA system does not include inhibitors of host proteinases which could cleave this substrate and could also contaminate the bacterial sample tested (Cox and Eley, 1989).

Bacterial proteases in GCF

Bacterial proteases are released into the pocket and can be detected in GCF (Cox *et al.*, 1989). Selective biochemical assays have been developed for both bacterial dipeptidylpeptidase (DPP) and trypsin-like proteases and can distinguish them from interfering tissue-derived proteases (Eley and Cox, 1994). The trypsin-like protease detected by this assay is a cysteine proteinase and has the characteristics of the enzyme now called arg-gingivain or arg-gingipain (see Chapter 5). These enzymes correlate positively with clinical indices of disease severity and reduce significantly following periodontal treatment (Eley and Cox, 1995a).

A 2-year longitudinal study of GCF bacterial DPP and arg-gingivain/arg-gingipain in 75 patients has recently been completed and a paper reporting this is in preparation (Eley and Cox, unpublished data). It used both site, patient and population thresholds for probing attachment loss measured with a Florida electronic probe and radiological measurements for confirmed progressive attachment loss. All clinical parameters and enzyme levels significantly reduced following basic periodontal treatment prior to baseline. Over the 2 years there were 124 sites in 49 patients with confirmed attachment loss giving an annual rate of 5.17% of sites. 91 of these sites in 36 patients were rapid episodic attachment loss (RAL) and 33 sites in 22 patients showed gradual progressive attachment loss over a longer time period (GAL). Levels above critical values chosen for both bacterial DPP and arg-gingivain for total enzyme activities and enzyme concentrations were present at all RAL sites both at the time of attachment loss and 3 months previously (predictive time). They were all significantly higher than values at control sites in the same patients. These levels were also shown to be predictive of attachment loss in diagnostic testing. In this regard the values for arg-gingivain were somewhat higher overall than those for bacterial DPP. The values for arg-gingivain were 100% (sensitivity) and 99.93% (specificity) for both total enzyme activity and enzyme concentration. The values for bacterial DPP were 100% (sensitivity) and 99.54% (specificity) for total enzyme activity and 100% (sensitivity) and 99.57% (specificity) for enzyme concentration. The differences can be more clearly seen in the positive and negative predictive values calculated in these tests for the two bacterial proteases. The values were 93.81% (positive prediction) and 100% (negative prediction) for arg-gingivain and 60.81% (positive prediction) and 100% (negative prediction) for bacterial DPP. Also the mean levels over the 2 years and the highest recorded levels at GAL sites were both above their respective critical values and were statistically significantly higher than those values at control sites in the same patients for both enzymes. In addition, all comparisons of mean patient values in patients with or without attachment loss were highly statistically significant.

Thus, GCF arg-gingivain/arg-gingipain appears to be an excellent predictor and GCF DPP a moderately good predictor of future progressive attachment loss. A test system suitable for chairside use has been developed (Cox *et al.*, 1990) and has been shown to produce similar results to the laboratory system.

The relationship of bacteria to periodontal disease progression

A microbiologically based diagnostic system should identify one or more primary pathogens responsible for the disease (Listgarten, 1992). It is, however, impossible to determine in a particular patient which bacteria in the subgingival flora are causing periodontal disease and it seems likely that many species may be involved at different stages of the disease. Nevertheless, some bacterial species have been considered by some workers as markers of disease because of their association with sites with progressive attachment loss. However, it must be appreciated that these bacteria are not always present in all such sites and may also be present at stable sites.

Retrospective studies (Slots *et al.*, 1986; Bragd *et al.*, 1987; Wennström *et al.*, 1987; Slots and Listgarten, 1988) have suggested that microbiological assays for critical levels of the target bacteria *A. actinomycetemcomitans, P. gingivalis* and *P. intermedia* might be of diagnostic value. It should be noted in these studies that the samples were taken after breakdown had occurred and although they showed an association between the number of these bacteria and previous attachment loss at the site they were not shown to be predictive of future attachment loss. In another retrospective study (Schmidt *et al.*, 1988), a group of 23 untreated and 13 maintenance patients were monitored with the BANA test. They reported selectivity and sensitivity values of 83% for negative and positive tests in untreated patients. However, the values were much lower on maintained patients and were not diagnostic. Although these studies showed the ability of the test to correctly identify sites pre-defined as healthy or diseased they were not predictive of future periodontal breakdown.

The numbers of spirochaetes and motile bacteria have been shown to predict future periodontal attachment loss in a 1-year prospective study of patients on maintenance following treatment for periodontitis when no treatment was carried out in the test period (Listgarten and Levin, 1981). However, they were not predictive when patients were scaled every 3 months during a 3-year study (Listgarten *et al.*, 1986). Furthermore, when *A. actinomycetemcomitans, P. gingivalis* and *P. intermedia* were tested as predictors of future periodontal attachment loss in a similar 3-year study of patients on regular maintenance they were not shown to have any diagnostic potential (Listgarten *et al.*, 1991).

In spite of this evidence, diagnostic test kits based on some of these systems have already been marketed. They use either paper point or curette bacterial sampling from the pocket. They include:

Evalusite (Kodak)
Enzyme-linked immunosorbent assays (ELISA) detecting *P. gingivalis, P. intermedius* and *A. actinomycetemcomitans.*
Omnigene (OmniGene, Inc)
BTD (Biotechnica Diagnostics, Inc)
These are DNA probe systems in which paper point sample is placed in container and mailed off to company. Probes are available for *A. actinomycetemcomitans, P. gingivalis, P. intermedius, E. corrodens, F. nucleatum, C. recta, T. denticola, T. pectinovorum.*
Perioscan (Oral-B Laboratories)
BANA (BzArgNA) test for bacterial trypsin-like protease. Mainly from *P. gingivalis* but also *B. forsythus* and *T. denticola.* The commercial firms owning these tests are constantly changing because some of them sell the rights of their products to others. For this reason, the firms cited as owning these tests may not remain accurate.

However, there are serious drawbacks of all these tests, some of which are listed below:

- Expensive
- Some need to be sent away to a special laboratory
- They only detect the bacteria that you look for
- You need to know which site to sample
- Polymicrobial nature of the disease
- Probably not predictive

Inflammatory and immune markers

In periodontal diseases, bacteria trigger inflammatory and immune host responses which, along with the direct effects of the bacteria, cause most of the tissue destruction (Genco, 1992). A number of substances are released from inflammatory and immune cells into the tissues and many of these pass into gingival crevicular fluid (GCF) and are thus easily available for analysis (Page, 1992; Lamster, 1992). Also some enzymes are released from dead cells in the disease process and these also are present in GCF. Samples of these substances can usually be obtained from paper strip GCF samples. Examples of these are:

Immune reponse	Antibody
	Total IgG and IgG subgroups
	Complement
Inflammatory mediators	Arachidonic acid derivatives, e.g. PGE_2
	Cytokines, e.g. IL-1, IL-6
Hydrolytic enzymes associated with inflammatory cells	Collagenase
	Elastase
	Cathepsin B
	Dipeptidylpeptidases
	Other proteases
	Aryl sulphatase
	β-Glucuronidase
	Alkaline phosphatase
	Acid phosphatase
	Myeloperoxidase
	Lysozyme
	Lactoferrin
Enzymes from dead cells (cytosolic enzymes)	Aspartate amino transferase (AST)
	Lactate dehydrogenase (LDH)

Sampling of gingival crevicular fluid

Gingival crevicular fluid (GCF) is an exudate that can be harvested from the gingival crevice or periodontal pocket using either filter paper strips or micropipette tubes. As the fluid traverses the inflamed tissue it may pick up enzymes and other molecules that participate in the disease process. It can also pick up the products of cell and tissue degradation. Therefore, it offers great potential as a source of factors that may be associated with disease activity.

The exact placement of the sampling device and the collection time are of great importance since they influence the composition of GCF collected (Curtis *et al.*, 1988; Page, 1992). Placement of a sampling device into the crevice or pocket induces a steady flow of exudate whilst repeat sampling depletes GCF volume and harvested components per unit of time. Lengthy sampling periods particularly with micropipette tubes will sample mainly inflammatory exudate from vessels rather than the contents of the crevice. The procedure adopted varies for the particular components of interest and its method of analysis but there is general agreement that the method of choice is one which causes the least interference with the site and takes the shortest time to harvest fluid present at the site prior to sampling. Thus, sampling for 30 seconds or less by the placement of paper strips at the orifice of the site seems to be ideal provided it ensures a sample of sufficient size to analyse with the technique used.

Correlation of host factors with disease

Humoral immune response

Patients with various forms of periodontal disease produce antibodies to antigens from periodontopathic bacteria (Lamster, 1992; Page, 1992). These antibodies can be detected in serum, gingival tissue and GCF and the total amount of immunoglobulin (Ig) in GCF positively correlates with that from adjacent gingival tissue. This shows that both serum and locally produced antibody contributes to that in GCF. The relationship of GCF antibodies to periodontal status has been studied in various ways (Page, 1992). These include measuring the total amount of Ig, the relative amounts of IgG subclasses and specific antibody titres to antigens from various periodontal bacteria. These relationships are complex and difficult to interpret.

The total Ig in GCF does not correlate with disease severity or progression and indeed may be lower at progressive sites (Page, 1992; Lamster, 1992). There has been one report (Reinhardt *et al.*, 1989) that compared IgG subclasses in GCF at progressive and stable sites. It found that the concentration of IgG1 and IgG4 subclasses were significantly higher at progressive sites.

Numerous studies (Page, 1992; Lamster, 1992) have compared specific antibodies titres to antigens from periodontal bacteria with periodontal disease status but these have found no correlation between them. The relationship of specific antibodies in GCF to those in serum is also complex, with some being higher and some lower with considerable variation from patient to patient, site to site in sequential measurement at the same site.

Thus, specific antibody or total Ig in GCF appears to be of no use in distinguishing between stable and active sites. Furthermore some evidence suggests that a reduction in

specific antibody in serum and consequently GCF in patients with existing disease can place them at risk for further disease progression (Lamster, 1992). This relationship has been demonstrated in juvenile periodontitis and acute necrotizing ulcerative gingivitis. Specific antibodies in the gingival tissues and serum are important in modulating the pathology of periodontal diseases but with the present level of knowledge do not offer a means of identifying patients at risk for active disease.

Complement

Complement proteins are present in GCF from sites with inflammation and the split fragments C3 and Factor B have been detected during experimental gingivitis (Patters *et al.*, 1989). However, none of these factors has been associated with disease activity.

Cytokines

Interleukin (IL)-1 and tumour necrosis factor alpha (TNF-α) are produced by activated macrophages and other cells and have pro-inflammatory effects of relevance to periodontal pathology which include the stimulation of PGE$_2$ and collagenase production. Since monoclonal antibodies have been produced for these cytokines they can be measured by ELISA and may therefore have diagnostic potential.

IL-1α and β are present in inflamed gingiva (Hönig *et al.*, 1989). They are also present in GCF from patients with periodontitis with extremely low concentrations at healthy sites (Masada *et al.*, 1990). Their levels are reduced following scaling and root planing but did not correlate with probing depth measurements. The amount of IL-1β in GCF also correlated with messenger RNA in adjacent gingival tissue.

TNF-α is also present in GCF but does not correlate with probing depth or gingival inflammation and its total amount was inversely related to tissue inflammation (Rossomando *et al.*, 1990). The levels of IL-1 and IL-6 in refractory periodontitis have also been studied (Reinhardt *et al.*, 1993). There were no significant differences in the mean level of IL-1 in refractory or stable patients but refractory sites produced significantly more IL-6. However, no longitudinal studies have been carried out relating any cytokine to periodontal disease activity and therefore at present they are of no diagnostic use.

Prostaglandins

Prostaglandin E_2 (PGE_2) has pro-inflammatory and immunoregulatory effects and its concentration in gingival tissue is sufficient to elicit significant effects on cell responses and functions (Offenbacher *et al.*, 1993). In bone organ culture (*see* Chapter 5) it stimulates osteoclastic bone resorption. It may thus play a significant role in periodontal pathology.

There is a great deal of evidence which correlates PGE_2 levels in the periodontal tissues and GCF to the severity of periodontal disease. PGE_2 levels are low in health and non-detectable at many sites (Offenbacher *et al.*, 1993). In naturally occurring gingivitis there is a modest rise in GCF PGE_2 levels to about 32 ng/ml and higher (about 53 ng/ml) in experimental gingivitis. Untreated periodontitis patients have significantly higher levels than gingivitis patients. In one study, following scaling and root planing the periodontitis patients were divided into two groups, those that experienced no further attachment loss and those which experienced one or more sites of 3 or more mm of attachment loss (Offenbacher *et al.*, 1986). At this time the group which experienced no further attachment loss in the study period had mean GCF PGE_2 levels which were significantly lower than the group with attachment loss and were similar to those with untreated gingivitis. In contrast, the group which experienced significant attachment loss at one or more sites in the following 6 months had significantly higher mean GCF PGE_2 levels of 113 ng/ml. This observation is the basis of the claim that GCF PGE_2 is predictive for periodontal disease activity (Offenbacher *et al.*, 1986). Levels greater than 66 ng/ml were found to be predictive of further possible loss of attachment and this level was used as a cut off value in a positive and negative screening test. This gave a sensitivity of 0.76, a specificity of 0.96 and an overall predictive value of 0.92–0.95 (Offenbacher *et al.*, 1993).

Although GCF PGE_2 has considerable potential as a screening test for periodontal activity strangely no commercial efforts are currently underway to develop one.

Hydrolytic enzymes of tissue origin

Collagenase and related metalloproteinases

Collagenases are part of a family of metalloproteinases which degrade collagen. They are synthesized by macrophages, neutrophils, fibroblasts and keratinocytes and are secreted by these cells as latent enzymes when stimulated by some bacterial products and cytokines. These cells also produce inhibitors known as tissue inhibitors of metalloproteinases (TIMP). Latent collagenase and related enzymes are activated by a number of proteolytic enzymes including tissue plasmin produced from serum plasminogen by plasminogen activator which is secreted by macrophages. They are inactivated by TIMPs and α_2-macroglobulin (Page, 1991).

Collagenase activity is present in gingival tissue and GCF in naturally occurring and experimental gingivitis and the amounts correlate with the severity of inflammation (Kowashi *et al.*, 1979; Overall and Sodek, 1987). Collagenase levels also correlated with the amount of attachment loss in ligature-induced periodontitis in dogs and latent enzyme predominated at healthy and gingivitis sites (Kryshalskyi *et al.*, 1986; Kryshalskyi and Sodek, 1987). In human periodontitis, GCF collagenase activity has been shown to increase with increasing severity of gingival inflammation and increasing pocket depth and alveolar bone loss (Villela *et al.*, 1987; Larivee *et al.*, 1986; Overall and Sodek, 1987; Golub *et al.*, 1976; Häkkarainen *et al.*, 1988). Total enzyme and active enzyme levels are significantly higher and enzyme inhibitor levels are lower at diseased sites compared with healthy or treated sites (Larivee *et al.*, 1986). At the time of writing there has only been one longitudinal study of GCF collagenase levels and periodontal attachment loss (Lee *et al.*, 1995). This study measured the relative amounts of active and latent collagenase relative to GCF by functional assays in a 12 month longitudinal cohort study. Comparisons were made between 14 subjects with inflammation and a previous history of progressive attachment loss (progressive periodontitis, Group 1), 27 subjects with inflammation and previous attachment loss but now clinical stable (stable periodontitis, Group 2) and 17 subjects with inflammation and no attachment loss (gingivitis, Group 3). Subjects with progressive and stable periodontitis (groups 1 and 2) were given basic periodontal treatment and were then monitored 3 months later. All subjects were then monitored monthly for attachment loss with a constant pressure probe and a threshold of 2 mm was used for confirmed attachment loss. GCF samples were taken from 6 specific sample teeth in each subject and from other teeth that lost attachment of 2 mm or more. Subjects in group 1 were rejected from the study if they did not lose attachment after 1 year and further subjects were recruited until 14 had lost attachment. The samples were all analysed at the end of the study so that all attachment loss sites were included. Inhibitors and blocking antibodies were used to determine the cellular source of GCF collagenase and this was found to be PMNs. There were 14 sites which lost attachment in excess of the tolerance level, one in each of the chosen patients in group 1. Active collagenase activity was pooled from the six sites per subject for the group comparisons and this was significantly higher in group 1 subjects compared to groups 2 and 3. In contrast latent collagenase was 2-fold higher in group 2 than group 1. There was a wide variation in the site specific active collagenase levels in sites with progressive attachment loss and in these sites there was a significant increase with time. However, there were sharp elevations in active enzyme level at the time of attachment loss in only 8 out of the 14 sites which lost attachment. Furthermore, as 7 sites which lost attachment did not show these elevations, although it was not calculated in this study, the diagnostic sensitivity and specificity values for active collagenase as a predictor of attachment loss would have been low. In spite of this, one commercial test kit has been developed (*see below*).

Cysteine proteinases

Cathepsins B, L and H are a family of intracellular cysteine proteinases which can degrade extracellular components including collagen. They act at acid pH and are primarily involved in intracellular degradation but are also active extracellularly when released during inflammation. They are also particularly active during bone resorption (*see*

Chapter 5). They are produced principally by fibroblasts, macrophages (Kennett *et al.*, 1994a) and osteoclasts (Vaes, 1988). They are inhibited by α_2-macroglobulin and the tissue inhibitors known as cystatins (Eley and Cox, 1991). Fibroblasts and some macrophages in human gingiva contain α_2-macroglobulin (Kennett *et al.*, 1994a) and the active cysteine proteinase activity in gingival tissue and GCF is a balance between enzyme and inhibitors.

Cathepsins B, L and H are present in gingival tissue and GCF (Cox and Eley, 1989a; Eley and Cox, 1991) as are also the inhibitors (Eley and Cox, 1991). GCF levels of cathepsins B and L significantly correlate with increasing gingival inflammation, probing depth, probing attachment level and bone loss (Eley and Cox, 1992b, c). In addition, levels of cathepsins B and L significantly reduce following periodontal treatment (Cox and Eley, 1992; Eley and Cox, 1992d). Zero or very low levels are present at healthy sites, low levels at gingivitis sites and high levels at periodontitis sites (Eley and Cox, 1993). Results from a 2-year longitudinal study (Eley and Cox, 1996) have shown that high levels of cathepsin B were present at all sites showing significant periodontal attachment loss. To date there has been only one longitudinal study of GCF cathepsin B activity and periodontal attachment loss (Eley and Cox, 1996). This was a 2 year study of 75 patients using both site, patient and population thresholds for probing attachment loss measured with a Florida electronic probe and radiological measurements to determine confirmed progressive attachment loss. All clinical parameters and enzyme levels significantly reduced following basic periodontal treatment prior to baseline. Over the 2 years there were 121 sites in 49 patients with confirmed attachment loss giving an annual rate of 5.04% of sites. 90 of these sites in 37 patients were rapid episodic attachment loss (RAL) and 31 sites in 21 patients showed gradual progressive attachment loss over a longer time period (GAL). Levels above critical values chosen for total cathepsin B activity and enzyme concentration were present at all RAL sites both at the time of attachment loss and 3 months previous (predictive time). They were all significantly higher than control sites in the same patients. These levels were also shown to be predictive of attachment loss in diagnostic testing. There were values of 100%

(sensitivity) and 99.83% (specificity) for total enzyme activity and 100% (sensitivity) and 99.75% (specificity) for enzyme concentration. Also the mean levels over the 2 years and the highest recorded values at GAL sites were both above their respective critical values and were statistically significantly higher than those values at control sites in the same patients. In addition, all comparisons of mean patient values in patients with or without attachment loss were statistically significant.

Thus, GCF cathepsin B appears to be a good predictor of future progressive attachment loss. A test system suitable for chairside use has been developed (Cox *et al.*, 1990) and has been shown to produce similar results to the laboratory system (see below).

Asparate proteinases

Cathepsin D is found in gingival tissue and GCF and GCF levels have been shown to correlate significantly with increasing gingival inflammation, probing depth, probing attachment level and bone loss (Ishikawa *et al.*, 1972). No longitudinal studies have been carried out relating this proteinase to periodontal attachment loss.

Serine proteinases

Elastase

Elastase in gingival tissue is produced by neutrophil polymorphonuclear leucocytes (PMNs) and is held in the cell in an inactive form probably bound with an inhibitor (Kennett, Cox and Eley, 1995a). It is inhibited in the tissues by α_1-proteinase inhibitor (α_1 PI) and α_2-macroglobulin (α_2-M). α_2-M is found in many fibroblasts and also some macrophages which may also contain α_1 PI (Kennett, Cox and Eley, 1995a). Active elastase can only occasionally be detected in gingival tissue biochemically (Eley and Cox, 1990) or histochemically (Kennett, Cox and Eley, 1995a) and is probably only detectable in an active state where there is an enzyme-inhibitor imbalance and this is usually seen either adjacent to junctional epithelium where PMNs are migrating into the crevice or in granulation tissue at the advancing front of the lesion (Kennett, Cox and Eley, 1995a).

Elastase is able to degrade proteoglycans and can also activate latent collagenase (Eley and Cox, 1990). Collagenases are unable to degrade collagen until the terminal peptide region of the molecule which contains intermolecular cross-links is first cleaved. This can also be carried out by elastase. It may thus have an important role in periodontal pathology.

GCF elastase levels significantly correlate with increasing gingival inflammation, probing depth, probing attachment level and bone loss (Eley and Cox, 1992b, c) and its level also significantly reduces following periodontal treatment (Cox and Eley, 1992; Eley and Cox, 1992d). Zero or very low levels are present at healthy sites, low to moderate levels at gingivitis sites and very high levels at periodontitis sites (Eley and Cox, 1993). A 6-month longitudinal study using a test kit system for elastase measurements has been reported (Palcanis *et al.*, 1992). This study used small thresholds of probing attachment loss of 0.4, 0.6 and 1 mm measured with a Florida probe (*see* Chapter 12) and bone loss detected by subtraction radiology (*see* Chapter 12) to determine when attachment loss occurred. It showed significant differences of total elastase activity at baseline in progressive and non-progressive sites assessed 2–6 months later. Results from a 2-year longitudinal study of 75 patients using both a higher threshold and radiological examination to determine confirmed progressive attachment loss (Eley and Cox, 1995b) showed similar and better results. All clinical parameters and enzyme levels significantly reduced following basic periodontal treatment prior to baseline. Over the 2 years there were 119 sites in 48 patients with confirmed attachment loss giving an annual rate of 4.96% of sites. 89 of these sites in 36 patients were rapid episodic attachment loss (RAL) and 30 sites in 21 patients showed gradual progressive attachment loss (GAL) over a long time period. Levels above critical values chosen for total elastase activity and enzyme concentration were present at all RAL sites both at the time of attachment loss and 3 months previously (predictive time). They were all significantly higher than values at control sites in the same patients. These levels were also shown to be predictive of attachment loss in diagnostic testing. There were values of 100% (sensitivity) and 99.96%

(specificity) for total enzyme activity and 96.63% (sensitivity) and 99.51% (specificity) for enzyme concentration. Also the means levels over the 2 years and the highest recorded values at GAL sites were both above their respective critical values and were statistically significantly higher than those values at control sites in the same patients. In addition, all comparisons of mean patient values in patients with or without attachment loss were highly statistically significant.

Thus, GCF elastase appears to be a good predictor of future progressive attachment loss. A test system suitable for chairside use has been developed (Cox *et al.*, 1990) and has been shown to produce simialr results to the laboratory system. A commercial system based on the same biochemistry has also been developed (Palcanis *et al.*, 1992).

Tryptase

Tryptase activity is present in large amounts in gingival tissue and in small amounts in GCF when measured biochemically (Eley and Cox, 1990; Cox and Eley, 1989a, b, c) and it has been localized to gingival mast cells (Kennett *et al.*, 1993). In the mast cell granules it is stabilized as an active tetramer by association with heparin and is released by these cells on degranulation. Tryptase can cleave the third component of complement and can activate latent collagenase. It can stimulate the release of collagenase from gingival fibroblasts and in inflamed gingival tissues mast cell degranulation occurs in areas of connective tissue breakdown. In dogs an inhibitor of mast cell degranulation has been shown to significantly reduce the rate of alveolar bone loss (Jeffcoat *et al.*, 1985). Thus, tryptase could be involved in the pathogenesis of periodontitis.

In humans, GCF tryptase activity correlates with clinical parameters of disease severity including probing attachment and bone loss (Eley and Cox, 1992b, c) and significantly reduces following periodontal treatment (Cox and Eley, 1992; Eley and Cox, 1992d). Zero to very low levels are present at healthy sites, low levels at gingivitis sites and moderately high levels at periodontitis sites (Eley and Cox, 1993). The test system for chairside use (Cox *et al.*, 1990) described

in the previous section could be used with this enzyme.

Dipeptidylpeptidase (DPPs)

DPP II which is active at acid pH and DPP IV which is active at alkaline pH are present in gingival tissue and GCF (Cox and Eley, 1989; Cox *et al.*, 1992). Within gingival tissue DPP II is a lysosomal enzyme present in fibroblasts (Kennett *et al.*, 1994b, 1996a). In GCF smears it is also present in macrophages (Cox, Kennett and Eley, 1995; Kennett, Cox and Eley, 1996b). This may suggest that this enzyme within macrophages is in an inactive form in gingival tissue, but in an active form in migrated cells in GCF. DPP IV is a lysosomal enzyme present in macrophages, T-lymphocytes and fibroblasts (Kennett, Cox and Eley, 1994b, 1996a). Using immunogold localisation with electron microscopy, DPP IV was present on the surface membrane of T-lymphocytes, macrophages and fibroblasts (Kennett, Cox and Eley, unpublished data). GCF DPP II and IV need to be distinguished from bacterial DPPs and selective assays have been developed for this purpose (Cox *et al.*, 1989; Eley and Cox, 1995a). They are able to cleave glyclyprolyl residues and may play a role in collagen degradation after the action of other enzymes.

Both tissue DPP II and IV correlate with clinical parameters of disease severity and significantly reduce following periodontal treatment (Eley and Cox, 1992a, b, c, d; Cox and Eley, 1992). Zero or very low levels are present at healthy sites, low levels at gingivitis sites and high levels at periodontitis sites (Eley and Cox, 1993). A 2-year longitudinal study of both GCF DPP II and DPP IV in 75 patients has recently been completed and a paper reporting this is in preparation (Eley and Cox, unpublished data). It used both site, patient and population thresholds for probing attachment loss measured with a Florida electronic probe and radiological measurement to determine confirmed progressive attachment loss. All clinical parameters and enzyme levels significantly reduced following basic periodontal treatment prior to baseline. Over the 2 years there were 120 sites in 49 patients with confirmed attachment loss giving an annual rate of 5.0% of sites. 88 of these sites in 35 patients were rapid episodic attachment loss (RAL) sites and 32 sites in 20 patients showed gradual progressive attachment loss (GAL) over a longer time period. Levels above critical values chosen for both DPP II and DPP IV (total enzyme activities and enzyme concentrations) were present at all RAL sites both at the time of attachment loss and 3 months previous (predictive time). They were all significantly higher than controls sites in the same patients. These levels were also shown to be predictive of attachment loss in diagnostic testing. These values were 100% (sensitivity) and 99.58% (specificity) for total enzyme activities and 100% (sensitivity) and 99.34% (specificity) for enzyme concentrations in respect of DPP II and 100% (sensitivity) and 99.48% (specificity) for total enzyme activities and 100% (sensitivity) and 99.17% (specificity) in respect of DPP IV. Also the mean levels over the 2 years and the highest recorded values at GAL sites for both proteases were above their respective critical values and were statistically significantly higher than those values at control sites in the same patients. In addition, all comparisons of mean patient values in patients with or without attachment loss were highly statistically significant.

Thus, both GCF DPP II and DPP IV appear to be good predictors of future progressive attachment loss. A test system suitable for chairside use has been developed (Cox *et al.*, 1990) and has been shown to produce simialr results to the laboratory system.

β-*Glucuronidase and arylsulphatase*

Extensive studies have been carried out on β-glucuronidase and arylsulphatase and this work is reviewed in Lamster (1992) and Page (1992). Both of these enzymes are lysosomal and are found in PMNs. β-glucuronidase is an acid hydrolase which is considered to be a marker for primary granule release by these cells. In cross-sectional studies these enzymes have been correlated significantly with gingival inflammation, pocket depth and alveolar bone loss. The levels of these enzymes are higher in diseased relative to healthy sites and their levels drop following periodontal treatment. During a 4-week period of experimental gingivitis the level of these enzymes increased for the first 3 weeks and then levelled off or dropped. The level of both enzymes increased with increasing pocket depths and β-glucuronidase was also positively associated with spirochaetes, *P. gingivalis*, *P. intermedia* and lactose-negative black pigmenting

bacteria in the subgingival flora and was negatively associated with cocci. There has been one 6-month longitudinal study reported where GCF β-glucuronidase activity was related to disease activity defined as loss of attachment of 2.0 mm or more over that period (Lamster *et al.*, 1988). Those sites which showed the highest β-glucuronidase activity at baseline and again at 3 months had the highest association with loss of attachment. It had a sensitivity and specificity of 89%. In a further study (Lamster *et al.*, 1991) 59 patients were similarly followed for a year and it was shown that persistently elevated β-glucuronidase levels were associated with disease activity that could be predicted from 3–6 months in advance. The sensitivity and selectivity were 92% and 86% respectively. The association with disease activity has been confirmed in a multicentre trial in which 140 patients were followed by 6 months and this showed a total predictive value as high as 90% (Lamster, 1992). This has so far only been reported in oral presentations published as abstracts and reported in the review paper quoted. However, the baseline data for this study has been reported in full (Lamster *et al.*, 1994). A diagnostic kit based on this enzyme is being commercially developed by Abbott Laboratories, North Chicago, USA.

Alkaline phosphatase

Alkaline phosphatase is thought to play a role in bone metabolism and is found in PMNs. A cross-sectional study of GCF alkaline phosphatase in periodontitis patients showed that it positively and significantly correlated with pocket depth but not with bone loss (Ishikawa and Cimasoni, 1970). A longitudinal study (Binder *et al.*, 1987) which related GCF levels to periodontal attachment loss of more than 2 mm showed that active sites yielded 20 times the activity in serum and were significantly associated with periodontal disease activity. When the data was calculated in terms of false positives and negatives using the most favourable cut off point, 73% of active sites were identified although 36% of the inactive sites were included. This would seem to indicate that its predictive value is low.

Acid phosphatase

Acid phosphatase is present in inflammatory cells and has been detected in GCF (Binder *et al.*, 1987). Levels, however do not correlate with measurements of disease severity or activity.

Myeloperoxidase, lysozyme and lactoferrin

Myeloperoxidase, lysozyme and lactoferrin are found in PMNs and can be detected in GCF. GCF myeloperoxidase levels are higher at periodontitis sites than control sites and the levels decrease significantly following periodontal treatment. However, activity did not correlate with clinical indices of disease severity (Smith *et al.*, 1986; Cao and Smith, 1988). An elevation of GCF lysozyme level harvested from diseased sites in patients with localized juvenile periodontitis relative to samples from patients with gingivitis or adult periodontitis has been reported (Friedman *et al.*, 1983). Lactoferrin levels did not differ and the authors suggested that the ratio of lysozyme to lactoferrin could have diagnostic potential.

Enzymes released by dead cells (cytosolic enzymes)

Aspartate amino transferase and lactate dehydrogenase

Aspartate amino transferase (AST) and lactate dehydrogenase (LDH) are soluble cytoplasmic enzymes which are confined to the cell cytoplasm but are released by dead or dying cells. Since cell death is an integral and essential component of periodontal tissue destruction they should be released during this process and should pass with the inflammatory exudate into GCF.

LDH has been correlated with probing depth and related to periodontal activity. In both cases the level of correlation was less than for β-glucuronidase which was included in the same study (Lamster *et al.*, 1988).

Levels of AST in serum and cerebrospinal fluid have been used for a number of years in medicine as an indicator of tissue necrosis and cell death. In dogs, GCF AST levels have been shown to increase during the development of ligature induced experimental periodontitis (Chambers *et al.*, 1984). In experimental gingivitis in humans, levels in GCF samples harvested during the development and resolution of the condition were significantly associated with gingival inflammation (Persson *et al.*, 1990a). In a cross-sectional study GCF AST was shown to correlate with clinical indices of disease severity (Imrey *et al.*, 1991). In longitudinal studies, GCF AST levels were related to confirmed attachment loss (Persson *et al.*, 1990b; Chambers *et al.*, 1991). They found that elevated GCF AST levels were strongly associated with disease active sites in contrast to disease inactive sites. Active sites contained 725 units of AFC more than inactive sites. Sites with severe inflammation also yielded more AST than less inflamed sites. There is as yet no evidence to indicate that GCF AST levels are predictive of disease activity because the positive correlations were made at the time of attachment loss rather than before it. A multicentre trial was performed using a dichotomous colorimetric test which becomes positive when 800 unit or more of GCF AST are present. Samples were taken before and after periodontal treatment and showed that levels were reduced below the detection limit following treatment (Page, 1992). A commercial diagnostic test kit based on GCF AST levels has been developed and is marketed at present by Colgate.

The commercial test kits based on some of the GCF factors described above that are currently available are listed below:

Periocheck (ACTech)	Neutral proteinases in GCF Paper point GCF sample Strip placed in contact with a collagen gel to which a blue stain has been covalently bonded Incubated at 43°C and scored on scale of 0 to 2 by comparing colour intensity and area with standard charts
Prognostik (Dentsply)	Elastase in GCF GCF collected on paper strips which have been impregnated with elastase substrate linked to fluorescent leaving group If elastase present, it reacts with the substrate in 4–8 minutes and the extent of the reactivity is observed under ultraviolet light
Periogard (Colgate)	AST in GCF Test kit using paper point GCF samples and colorimetric detection method under development

The commercial firms owning these tests are constantly changing (as stated earlier) because some of them sell the rights to their products to others. For this reason, the firms cited as owning these tests may not remain accurate.

The main disadvantages of these systems are:

1. The choice of the most appropriate biomarker is difficult at the present state of knowledge.
2. There is difficulty in determining the sites to sample and when to sample them.
3. If a moiety is associated with inflammation this may mask its association with destructive disease.
4. No account of biological control mechanisms is taken in present tests.
5. Cost.

All diagnostic tests should reflect an understanding of the role played by biological control mechanisms in determining the levels of the test substance. For instance, protease levels in gingival tissue are determined partly by a balance between the enzyme and its natural inhibitors. Serine proteinases like elastase are inhibited by the serum inhibitor α_1-proteinase inhibitor and α_2-macroglobulin and cysteine proteases by α_2-macroglobulin and the tissue inhibitors, cystatins. The level of enzyme in the tissues and to some extent GCF must therefore depend upon the enzyme inhibitor balance. In addition, the level of inflammatory cell proteinases in GCF also depends on release from inflammatory cells that have migrated into the crevice.

Markers of connective tissue degradation

During its passage through the inflamed tissue, GCF could pick up normal components of the extracellular matrix or tissue degradation products released during the destructive process. The components that could be involved in this process are listed below:

Soft tissue components

Soft tissue:	Collagens I, III, V
	Proteoglycans
	Hyaluronan
	Fibronectin
Basement membrane:	Collagen IV
	Laminin

Bone components

Bone specific proteins
Collagen I
Proteoglycans

The detection of the breakdown products of these macromolecules could be indicative of tissue breakdown. These include:

Component	Breakdown Product
Collagen	Hydroxyproline
	Collagen cross links
	N-propeptide
Proteoglycan	Glycosaminoglycans (GAGs)
GAGs	Heparan sulphate
	Chondroitin-4-sulphate
	Chondroitin-6-sulphate

Fibronectin, a normal component of serum and the connective tissue matrix, is present in GCF and more intact molecules are present in samples from healthy and treated sites than from diseased sites (Talonpoika *et al.*, 1989; Lopatin *et al.*, 1989). Osteonectin is a normal component of bone matrix and has also been detected in GCF. The total amount of GCF osteonectin has been shown to increase in line with the site probing depth (Bowers *et al.*, 1989).

Proteoglycans incorporating glycosaminoglycans (GAGs) are an integral part of the connective tissue matrix that can be degraded during tissue destruction. Proteoglycan degradation releases GAGs which can then pass into GCF. Hyaluronic acid and chondroitin-4-sulphate have been detected in GCF samples from sites with untreated periodontitis and the amounts of GAGs reduce following treatment. More significantly, chondroitin-4-sulphate was shown to be totally absent from post treatment samples (Embery *et al.*, 1982; Last *et al.*, 1985).

Hydroxyproline-containing peptides are released during collagen degradation. They have been shown to be present in GCF harvested from dogs during the development of experimental gingivitis (Svanberg, 1987). However, the relation of this peptide to human destructive periodontitis has not been studied to date.

The detection of most of these components in GCF requires long collection times of around 15 minutes using micropipettes and this can significantly affect GCF composition. The detection of osteonectin requires the use of nitrocellulose strips as it cannot be recovered from conventional strips (Bowers *et al.*, 1989). In addition, the biochemical techniques used to isolate and detect these components are complex and difficult to modify for chairside use:

Methods of isolation and detection

- Hydroxyproline   High pressure liquid chromatography (HPLC), ion exchange chromatography
- Collagen cross links   HPLC
- GAGs   Cellulose acetate extraction and staining

The problems associated with the possible clinical use of these factors are listed below:

Problems with the possible clinical use of tissue degradation products

1. Most involve complex and expensive techniques to isolate and detect.
2. If present in GCF they usually require long collection times using a micropipette to obtain sufficient quantities to analyse.
3. Long GCF collection times affect its composition.
4. The normal cycle of synthesis and degradation of connective tissue and bone needs to be considered.
5. Most are not suitable for chairside use because it is difficult to develop a simplified detection system.

The use of predictive diagnostic test

If a reliable predictive test were developed it could predict future periodontal activity and thus enable site specific treatment to be given before irreversible damage had occurred.

The possible use of such a test are listed below:

- help to prevent destructive disease
- help to prevent further destructive disease
- identify high risk patients
- target treatment to specific sites
- help to monitor treatment

However, as periodontal disease is site specific and may be episodic, such tests will not tell you which sites to test or when to test them.

References

Binder, T.A., Goodson, J.M. and Socransky, S.S. (1987) Gingival fluid levels of acid and alkaline phosphatase levels. *Journal of Periodontal Research* **22**, 14–19

Bowers, M.R., Fisher, L.W., Termine, J.D. and Somerman, M.J. (1989) Connective tissue-associated proteins in crevicular fluid: Potential markers for periodontal diseases. *Journal of Periodontology* **60**, 448–451

Bragd, L., Dahlén, G., Wikström, M. and Slots, J. (1987) The capability of *Actinobacillus actinomycetemcomitans*, *Bacteroides gingivalis* and *Bacteroides intermedius* to indicate progressive periodontitis. *Journal of Clinical Periodontology* **14**, 95–99

Cao, C.F. and Smith, Q.T. (1989) Crevicular fluid myeloperoxidase at healthy, gingivitis and periodontitis sites. *Journal of Clinical Periodontology* **16**, 17–20

Chambers, D.A., Crawford, J.M., Mukherjee, S. and Cohen, R.L. (1984) Aspartate aminotransferase increases in crevicular fluid during experimental periodontitis in beagle dogs. *Journal of Periodontology* **55**, 526–530

Chambers, D.A., Imrey, P.B., Cohen, R.L. *et al.* (1991) A longitudinal study of aspartate aminotransferase in human gingival crevicular fluid. *Journal of Periodontal Research* **26**, 65–74

Cox, S.W., Cho, K., Eley, B.M. and Smith, R.E. (1990) A simple, combined fluorogenic and chromogenic method for the assay of proteases in gingival crevicular fluid. *Journal of Periodontal Research* **25**, 164–171

Cox, S.W. and Eley, B.M. (1989a) The detection of cathepsin B- and L-, elastase-, tryptase-, trypsin- and dipeptidyl peptidase IV- like activities in gingival crevicular fluid from gingivitis and periodontitis patients using peptidyl derivatives of 7-amino-4-trifluomethylcoumarin. *Journal of Periodontal Research* **24**, 353–361

Cox, S.W. and Eley, B.M. (1989b) Identification of a tryptase-like enzyme in extracts of inflamed human gingiva by effector and gel-filtration studies. *Archives of Oral Biology* **34**, 219–221

Cox, S.W. and Eley, B.M. (1989c) Tryptase-like activity in crevicular fluid from gingivitis and periodontitis patients *Journal of Periodontal Research* **24**, 41–44

Cox, S.W. and Eley, B.M. (1992) Cathepsin B/L-, elastase-, tryptase-, trypsin- and dipeptidyl peptidase IV-like activities in gingival crevicular fluid: a comparison of levels before and after basic periodontal treatment of chronic periodontitis patients. *Journal of Clinical Periodontology* **19**, 333–339

Cox, S.W., Gazi, M.I. and Eley, B.M. (1992) Dipeptidyl peptidase II- and IV- like activities in gingival tissue and crevicular fluid from human periodontitis lesions. *Archives of Oral Biology* **37**, 167–173

Cox, S.W., Kennett, C.N. and Eley, B.M. (1995) Evaluation of the cellular contribution to protease activities in gingival crevicular fluid. *Journal of Dental Research* (in press)

Curtis, M.A., Griffiths, G.S., Price, S.J. *et al.* (1988) The total protein concentration of gingival crevicular fluid; variation with sampling time and gingival inflammation. *Journal of Clinical Periodontology* **15**, 628–632

Ebersole, J.L., Frey, D.E., Taubman, M.A. *et al.* (1984) Serological identification on oral *Bacteroides* sp. by enzyme-linked immunosorbent assay. *Journal of Clinical Microbiology* **19**, 639–644

Eley, B.M. and Cox, S.W. (1990) A biochemical study of serine proteinase activities at local gingivitis sites in human chronic periodontitis. *Archives of Oral Biology* **35**, 23–27

Eley, B.M. and Cox, S.W. (1991) Cathepsin B and L-like activities at local gingival sites of chronic periodontitis patients. *Journal of Clinical Periodontology* **18**, 499–504

Eley, B.M. and Cox, S.W. (1992a) Crevicular fluid dipeptidyl peptidase activities before and after periodontal treatment. *Journal of Dental Research* **71**, 622

Eley, B.M. and Cox, S.W. (1992b) Cathepsin B/L-, elastase-, tryptase-, trypsin- and dipeptidyl peptidase IV-like activities in gingival crevicular fluid: correlation with clinical parameters in untreated chronic periodontitis patients. *Journal of Periodontal Research* **27**, 62–69

Eley, B.M. and Cox, S.W. (1992c) Correlation of gingival crevicular fluid proteases with clinical and radiological parameters of periodontal attachment loss. *Journal of Dentistry* **20**, 90–99

Eley, B.M. and Cox, S.W. (1992d) Cathepsin B/L-, elastase-, tryptase-, trypsin- and dipeptidyl peptidase IV-like activities in gingival crevicular fluid: a comparison of levels before and after periodontal surgery in chronic periodontitis patients. *Journal of Periodontology* **63**, 412–417

Eley, B.M. and Cox, S.W. (1993) Gingival crevicular fluid inflammatory cell proteases at healthy, gingivitis and periodontitis sites. *Journal of Dental Research* **72**, 705

Eley, B.M. and Cox, S.W. (1995a) Bacterial proteases in gingival crevicular fluid before and after periodontal treatment. *British Dental Journal* **178**, 133–139

Eley, B.M. and Cox, S.W. (1995b) A 2-year longitudinal study of elastase in gingival crevicular fluid and periodontal attachment loss. *Journal of Clinical Periodontology* (in press)

Eley, B.M. and Cox, S.W. (1996) The relationship between gingival crevicular fluid cathepsin B activity and periodontal attachment loss in chronic periodontitis patients. A 2-year longitudinal study. *Journal of Periodontol Research* (in press)

Embery, G., Oliver, W.M., Stanbury, J.B. and Purvis, J.A. (1982) The electrophoretic detection of acid glycosaminoglycans in human gingival sulcus fluid. *Archives of Oral Biology* **27**, 177–179

French, C.K., Savitt, E.D., Simon, S.L. *et al.* (1986) DNA probe detection of periodontal pathogens. *Oral Microbiology and Immunology* **1**, 58–62

Friedman, S.A., Mandel, I.D. and Herrera, M.S. (1983) Lysozyme and lactoferrin quantifications in the crevicular fluid. *Journal of Periodontology* **54**, 347–350

Gazi, M.I., Cox, S.W., Clark, D.T. and Eley, B.M. (1994) Cathepsin B, tryptase and *Porphyromonas gingivalis* trypsin-like protease in gingival crevicular fluid. *Journal of Dental Research* **73**, 799

Genco, R.C., Zambon, J.J. and Christersson, L.A. (1986) Use and interpretation of microbiological assays in periodontal diseases. *Oral Microbiology and Immunology* **1**, 73–79

Genco, R.C., Zambon, J.J. and Christersson, L.A. (1988) The origin of periodontal infections. *Advances in Dental Research* **2**, 245–259

Genco, R.J. (1992) Host responses in periodontal diseases: Current concepts. *Journal of Periodontology* **63**, 338–355

Golub, L.M., Siegel, Ramamurthy, N.S. and Mandel, I.D. (1976) Some characteristics of collagenase activity in gingival crevicular fluid and its relationship to gingival disease in humans. *Journal of Dental Research* **55**, 1049–1057

Greenstein, G. (1988) Microbiological assessments to enhance periodontal disease diagnosis. *Journal of Periodontology* **59**, 508–515

Häkkaraianen, K., Uitto, V-J. and Ainamo, J. (1988) Collagenase activity and protein content of sulcular fluid after scaling and occlusal adjustment of teeth with deep periodontal pockets. *Journal of Periodontal Research* **23**, 204–210

Highfield, P.E. and Dougan, G. (1985) DNA probes for microbial diagnosis. *Medical Laboratory Science* **42**, 352–360

Hönig, C., Rordorf-Adam, C., Siegmund, C. *et al.* (1989) Increased interleukin beta (IL-1β)-concentration in gingival tissue from periodontitis patients. *Journal of Periodontal Research* **24**, 362–367

Imrey, P.B., Crawford, J.M., Cohen, R.L. *et al.* (1991) A cross-sectional analysis of aspartate aminotransferase in human gingival crevicular fluid. *Journal of Periodontal Research* **26**, 75–84

Ishiwaka, I., Cimasoni, G. and Ahmad-Zadeh, C. (1972) Possible role of lysosomal enzymes in the pathogenesis of periodontitis. A study of cathepsin D in human gingival fluid. *Archives of Oral Biology* **17**, 111–117

Ishiwaka, I. and Cimasoni, G. (1970) Alkaline phosphatase in human gingival fluid and its relationship to periodontitis. *Archives of Oral Biology* **15**, 1401–1404

Jeffcoat, M.K., Williams, R.C., Johnson, H.G. *et al.* (1985) Treatment of periodontal disease in beagles with lodoxamide ethyl, an inhibitor of mast cell release. *Journal of Periodontal Research* **20**, 532–541

Kennett, C.N., Cox, S.W., Eley, B.M. and Osman, I.A.R.M. (1993) Comparative histochemical and biochemical studies of mast cell tryptase in human gingiva. *Journal of Periodontology* **64**, 870–877

Kennett, C.N., Cox, S.W. and Eley, B.M. (1994a) Comparative histochemical, biochemical and immunocytochemical studies of cathepsin B in human gingiva. *Journal of Periodontal Research* **29**, 203–213

Kennett, C.N., Cox, S.W. and Eley, B.M. (1994b) Histochemical, immunocytochemical and biochemical studies of dipeptidyl peptidases in human gingival tissue. *Journal of Dental Research* (in press)

Kennett, C.N., Cox, S.W. and Eley, B.M. (1995a) Localisation of active and inactive elastase, alpha-1-proteinase inhibitor and alpha-2-macroglobulin in human gingiva. *Journal of Dental Research.* **74**, 667–674

Kennett, C.N., Cox, S.W. and Eley, B.M. (1996a) The histochemical and immunocytochemical localisation and biochemical studies of dipeptidylpeptidase II and IV in human gingiva. *Journal of Periodontology* (in press)

Kennett, C.N., Cox, S.W. and Eley, B.M. (1996b) Investigations into the cellular contribution of host tissue protease activity in gingival crevicular fluid. *Journal of Clinical Periodontology* (in press)

Kowashi, Y., Jaccard, F. and Cimasoni, G. (1979) Increase of free collagenase and neutral protease activities in the gingival crevice during experimental gingivitis in Man. *Archives of Oral Biology* **34**, 645–650

Kryshalskyi, E. and Sodek, J. (1987) Nature of collagenolytic enzyme and inhibitor activity in gingival crevicular fluid from healthy and inflamed periodontal tissues of beagle dogs. *Journal of Periodontal Research* **22**, 264–269

Kryshalskyi, E., Sodek, J. and Ferrier, J.M. (1986) Correlation of collagenolytic enzymes and inhibitors in gingival crevicular fluid with clinical and microscopic changes in experimental periodontitis in the dog. *Archives of Oral Biology* **31**, 21–31

Lamster, I.B. (1992) The host response in gingival crevicular fluid: potential applications in periodontitis clinical trials. *Journal of Periodontology* **63**, 1117–1123

Lamster, I.B., Holmes, L.G., Gross, K.B.W. *et al.* (1994) The relationship of β-glucuronidase activity in crevicular fluid to clinical parameters of periodontal disease. Findings from a multicenter study. *Journal of Clinical Periodontology* **21**, 118–127

Lamster, I.B., Oshrain, R.L., Harper, D.S. *et al.* (1988) Enzyme activity in crevicular fluid for detection and prediction of clinical attachment loss in patients with chronic adult periodontitis. *Journal of Periodontology* **59**, 516–523

Lamster, I.B., Oshrain, R.L., Celenti, R.S. *et al.* (1991) Indicators of the acute inflammatory and humoral immune responses in gingival crevicular fluid: Relationship to active periodontal disease. *Journal of Periodontal Research* **26**, 261–263

Larivee, L., Sodek, J. and Ferrier, J.M. (1986) Collagenase and collagenase inhibitor activity in crevicular fluid of patients receiving treatment for localised juvenile periodontitis. *Journal of Periodontal Research* **21**, 702–715

Last, K.S., Stanbury, J.B. and Embery, G. (1985) Glycosaminoglycans in human gingival crevicular fluid as indicators of active periodontal disease. *Archives of Oral Biology* **30**, 275–281

Lee, W., Aitken, S., Sodek, J. and McCulloch, C.A.G. (1995) Evidence of a direct relationship between neutrophil collagenase activity and periodontal tissue destruction *in vivo*: role of active enzyme in human periodontitis. *Journal of Periodontal Research* **30**, 23–33

Listgarten, M.A. (1986) Direct microscopy of periodontal pathogens. *Oral Microbiology and Immunology* **1**, 31–36

Listgarten, M.A. (1992) Microbial testing in the diagnosis of periodontal disease. *Journal of Periodontology* **63**, 332–337

Listgarten, M.A. and Levin, S. (1981) Positive correlation between proportions of subgingival spirochaetes and motile bacteria and susceptibility of human subjects to periodontal deterioration. *Journal of Clinical Periodontology* **8**, 122–138

Listgarten, M.A., Schifter, C.C., Sulivan, P. *et al.* (1986) Failure of a microbial assay to reliably predict disease recurrence in a treated periodontitis population receiving regularly scheduled prophylaxes. *Journal of Clinical Periodontology* **13**, 768–773

Listgarten, M.A., Slots, J., Nowotny, A.H. *et al.* (1991) Incidence of periodontitis recurrence in treated patients with and without cultivable *Actinobacillus actinomycetemcomitans*, *Porphyromonas gingivalis* and *Prevotella intermedia*: a prospective study. *Journal of Periodontology* **62**, 377–386

Loesche, W.J. (1986) The identification of bacteria associated with periodontal disease and dental caries by enzymatic methods. *Oral Microbiology and Immunology* **1**, 65–70

Loesche, W.J. (1992) DNA probe and enzyme analysis in periodontal diagnosis. *Journal of Periodontology* **63**, 1102–1109

Loesche, W.J., Bretz, W., Lopatin, D. *et al.* (1990) Multicenter clinical evaluation of a chairside method for detecting certain periodontopathic bacteria in periodontal disease. *Journal of Periodontology* **61**, 189–196

Lopatin, D.E., Caffessee, E.R., Bye, F.L. and Caffessee, R.G. (1989) Concentrations of fibronectin in the sera and crevicular fluid in various stages of periodontal disease. *Journal of Clinical Periodontology* **16**, 359–364

Mandell, R.L. and Socransky, S.S. (1981) Selective medium for *Actinobacillus actinomycetemcomitans* and the incidence of the organism in juvenile periodontitis. *Journal of Periodontology* **52**, 593–598

Masada, M.P., Persson, R., Kenney, J.L. *et al.* (1990) Measurement of interleukin-1α and 1β in gingival crevicular fluid: implications for the pathogenesis of periodontal disease. *Journal of Periodontal Research* **25**, 156–163

Offenbacher, S., Heasman, P.A. and Collins, J.G. (1993) Modulation of host PGE_2 secretion as a determinant of periodontal disease expression. *Journal of Periodontology* **64**, 432–444

Offenbacher, S., Odle, B.M. and Van Dyke, T.E. (1986) The use of crevicular fluid prostaglandin E_2 levels as a predictor of periodontal attachment loss. *Journal of Periodontal Research* **21**, 101–112

Overall, C.M. and Sodek, J. (1987) Initial characterization of a neutral metalloproteinase, active on 3/4-collagen fragments, synthesized by ROS 17/2.8 osteoblastic cells, periodontal fibroblasts, and identified in gingival crevicular fluid. *Journal of Dental Research* **66**, 1271–1282

Page, R.C. (1991) The role of inflammatory mediators in the pathogenesis of periodontal disease. *Journal of Periodontal Research* **26**, 230–242

Page, R.C. (1992) Host response tests for diagnosing periodontal diseases. *Journal of Periodontology* **63**, 356–366

Palcanis, K.G., Larjava, I.K., Wells, B.R. *et al.* (1992) Elastase as an indicator of periodontal disease progression. *Journal of Periodontology* **63**, 237–274

Pattres, M.R., Niekrash, C.E. and Lang, N.P. (1989) Assessment of complement cleavage in gingival fluid during experimental gingivitis. *Journal of Clinical Periodontology* **16**, 33–37

Persson, G.R., De Rouen, T.A. and Page, R.C. (1990a) Relationship between levels of aspartate aminotransferase in gingival crevicular fluid and gingival inflammation. *Journal of Periodontal Research* **25**, 17–24

Persson, G.R., De Rouen, T.A. and Page, R.C. (1990b) Relationship between gingival crevicular fluid levels of aspartate aminotransferase and active tissue destruction in treated chronic periodontitis patients. *Journal of Periodontal Research* **25**, 81–87

Reinhardt, R.A., McDonald, T.L., Bolton, R.W. *et al.* (1989) IgG subclasses in gingival crevicular fluid from active versus stable periodontal sites. *Journal of Periodontology* **60**, 44–50

Reinhardt, R.A., Masada, M.P., Kaldahl, W.B. *et al.* (1993) Gingival fluid IL-1 and IL-6 levels in refractory periodontitis. *Journal of Clinical Periodontology* **20**, 225–231

Rossomando, E.F., Kennedy, J.E. and Hadjimichael, J. (1990) Tumor necrosis factor alpha in gingival crevicular fluid as a possible indicator of periodontal disease in humans. *Archives of Oral Biology* **35**, 431–434

Savitt, E.D., Strzemoko, M.N., Vaccaro K.K. *et al.* (1988) Comparison of cultural methods and DNA probe analysis for the detection of *A. actinomycetemcomitans, P. gingivalis,* and *B. intermedius* in subgingival plaque samples. *Journal of Periodontology* **52**, 431–438

Schmitt, E.F., Bretz, W.A., Hutchinson, R.A. and Loesche, W.J. (1988) Correlation of the hydrolysis of benzoyl-arginine-naphthylamide (BANA) by plaque with clinical parameters and subgingival levels of spirochaetes in periodontal patients. *Journal of Dental Research* **67**, 1505–1509

Smith, Q.T., Hinrichs, J.E. and Melnyk, R.S. (1986) Gingival crevicular fluid myeloperoxidase at periodontitis sites. *Journal of Periodontal Research* **21**, 45–55

Socransky, S.S. and Haffajee, A.D. (1992) The bacterial etiology of destructive periodontal disease: current concepts. *Journal of Periodontology* **63**, 322–337

Slots, J., Bragd, L., Wikström, M. and Dahlén, G. (1986) The occurrence of *Actinobacillus actinomycetemcomitans, Bacteroides gingivalis* and *Bacteroides intermedius* in destructive periodontal disease in adults. *Journal of Clinical Periodontology* **13**, 570–577

Slots, J. and Listgarten, M.A. (1988) *Bacteroides gingivalis, Bateroides intermedius* and *Actinobacillus actinomycetemcomitans* in human periodontal diseases. *Journal of Clinical Periodontology* **15**, 85–93

Svanberg, G.K. (1987) Hydroxyproline determination in serum and gingival crevicular fluid. *Journal of Periodontal Research* **22**, 133–138

Talonpoika, J., Heino, J., Larjava, H. *et al.* (1989) Gingival crevicular fluid fibronectin degradation in periodontal health and disease. *Scandinavian Journal of Dental Research* **97**, 415–421

Theilade, E. (1986) The non-specific theory in microbial etiology of inflammatory periodontal diseases. *Journal of Clinical Periodontology* **13**, 905–911

Vaes, G. (1988) Cellular biology and biochemical mechanism of bone resorption. *Clinical Orthopaedics and Related Research* **231**, 239–271

Villela, B., Cogan, R.B., Bartolucci, A.A. and Birkedal-Hansen, H. (1987) Collagenolytic activity in crevicular fluid from patients with chronic adult periodontitis, localised juvenile periodontitis and gingivitis, and from healthy control subjects. *Journal of Periodontal Research* **22**, 381–389

Wennström, J.L., Dahlén, G., Swensson, J. and Nyman, S. (1987) *Actinobacillus actinomycetemcomitans, Bacteroides gingivalis* and *Bacteroides intermedius*: Predictors of attachment loss? *Oral Microbiology and Immunology* **2**, 158–163

Zambon, J.J., Reynolds, H.S., Chen, P. and Genco, R.J. (1985) Rapid detection of periodontal pathogens in subgingival plaque. Comparison of indirect immunofluorescence microscopy with bacterial cultures for detection of *Bacteroides gingivalis. Journal of Periodontology* **56**, 32–40

Zambon, J.J., Bochacki, V. and Genco, R.J. (1986) Immunological assays for putative periodontal pathogens. *Oral Microbiology and Immunology* **1**, 39–44

14

Basic treatment of chronic gingivitis and periodontitis

Chronic gingivitis

Treatment has three components which are carried out concurrently:

1. Instruction in home care
2. Removal of plaque and calculus by scaling
3. Correction of plaque-retention factors

These three exercises are interdependent. The removal of plaque and calculus cannot be completed without the correction of plaque-retention factors; rendering the mouth plaque free provides no benefit if no effort is made to prevent the recurrence of plaque deposition or ensure its swift removal after deposition.

In some patients, especially the young, calcified deposits may be negligible and the treatment of gingival inflammation is largely a matter of plaque control, described in Chapter 10. Where calcified deposits are present scaling is needed. When deposits of calculus are heavy it is rarely possible to remove them completely in one appointment; Furthermore, resolution of gingival inflammation, especially when longstanding, may take a number of weeks. These facts must be explained to the patient. It is essential to establish a partnership of effort to restore gingival health (*Figure 14.1*).

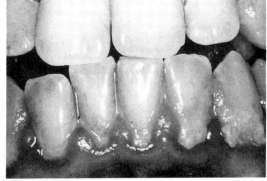

(a)

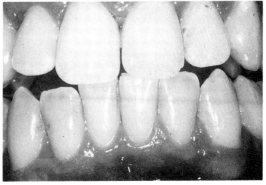

(b)

Figure 14.1 (*a*) Gingival inflammation associated with poor oral hygiene prior to treatment. (*b*) The gingival condition after scaling and instruction in home care over the course of 8 weeks

Instruction in home care

Patients bear the major responsibility for their own dental health, and where disease is present the patients have a special duty to themselves. The presence of disease indicates (i) past neglect, and (ii) vulnerability to disease. The truth of the situation must be explained to the patient.

The organization of treatment needs to be very carefully planned but it is impossible to prescribe a general timetable which could apply to every patient; each individual requires a personal schedule but it is as well to make clear at the outset that gingival health will not be achieved overnight and that treatment is likely to take several months. Depending on the severity of the gingival inflammation, the state of oral hygiene, the presence of aggravating factors and the patient's perceived concern a series of appointments can be made. Some instruction in home care must be given on the first visit when scaling is started.

Where oral hygiene is poor subsequent appointments may need to be made at weekly intervals especially where there is a great deal of subgingival calculus. The proportion of time spent on scaling and on oral hygiene instruction must vary with individual needs but in most cases the earlier appointments are largely given over to scaling and as the patient feels and sees the improvement in gingival health which this brings about his home care efforts can be stimulated. The patient is always advised to bring his toothbrush with him and visits can be started by using a disclosing agent and enjoining the patient to 'get the stain off'. At this time difficult areas are defined and modifications to his technique devised. Encouragement is always helpful, criticism rarely; a positive approach is essential to patient cooperation.

Treatment should continue until both oral hygiene and gingival condition are satisfactory. Recall appointments are then made at suitable intervals dictated by the patient's condition (*see* p. 142).

Scaling

This is the removal of all tooth depsosits, supragingival calculus, subgingival calculus, plaque and stains. It must be carried out

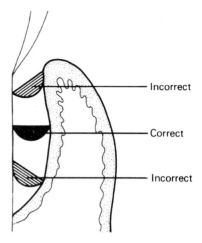

Figure 14.2 Diagram to show the angulation of a curette blade against the tooth surface. Incorrect positioning may make use of the instrument either ineffective or damaging

thoroughly; inflammation persists if all tooth deposits are not removed. Scaling technique can be learned only by constant practice but a number of conditions are essential to an effective technique.

1. The operation must be undertaken methodically, working around the mouth and around each tooth in an orderly manner.
2. The correct instrument should be used, i.e. one which fits well against the tooth surface to be cleaned. A fairly large bladed instrument can be used to remove supragingival calculus; a much smaller one is necessary for the removal of subgingival calculus.
3. Each stroke of the instrument should be deliberate and effective. It is very easy to scratch around ineffectively or to use the instrument so that it actually damages the tooth surface (*Figure 14.2*).

A firm finger rest on the teeth is essential for controlled use of the instrument.

The movement of the instrument can be divided into two phases:

(*a*) The exploratory stroke in which the apical limit of deposits is defined. In the removal of subgingival calculus this is a blind procedure and one carried out entirely by tactile sensation. The exploratory stroke must be gentle but deliberate so that the tissue, hard or soft, is not damaged.

(*b*) The working stroke which removes the deposits. In this action the instrument blade is pressed against the tooth surface and brought deliberately and slowly in a coronal direction bringing the deposits with it.

4. The tooth surface should be rendered clean and smooth. The surface can be examined with a suitable instrument, e.g. the Cross calculus probe, to detect any residual deposits. Sometimes the gingival margin can be retracted and the subgingival tooth surface visualized by blowing warm air gently into the gingival crevice.

Scaling instruments

Hand instruments

A large number of instruments are available and each operator will choose those which he or she finds most effective in his (or her) hands. The names of the instruments describe the design of the instrument and their mode of action: curettes, hoes, files, sickles and chisels. The instruments have three parts: a handle, a shank and blade. The handle needs to fit into the hand so that it is stable and cannot slip under pressure. The 'balanced grip' handle meets these requirements. The shank of the instrument varies in length and angulation so that all tooth surfaces are accessible to the blade, thus a short shank may be used in shallow pockets and a long shank in deep pockets and for interproximal sites at the back of the mouth. The blade has one or more edges designed to remove deposits from the tooth surface or soft tissue from the crevicular face of the gingiva. The edges of the blade must be kept sharp if the instrument is to be effective. Several instruments are now available with tungsten carbide blades which do not need to be sharpened but need to be replaced when blunt.

Curettes (Figure 14.3a) Curettes have a double-edged, spoon-shaped blade which is curved to conform to the tooth surface. Most surfaces can be reached with a pair (left and right) of curettes. Because of the small size and shape of the blade it can be inserted under the gingival margin and if necessary can be used to clean the tooth surface and curette the gingival soft tissue simultaneously. The two most common types of curette are the McCall and the Younger-Goode.

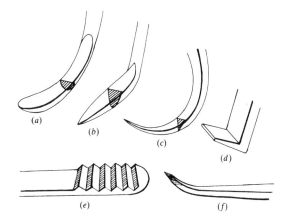

Figure 14.3 Diagram to show the blades of various scaling instruments: (*a*) curette, (*b*) Jaquette scaler, (*c*) sickle, (*d*) hoe, (*e*) file (much enlarged), (*f*) chisel

Jaquette scalers (Figure 14.3b) The blade of this instrument is triangular in cross-section and it has two cutting edges. It is available in different sizes; the large blade is used for superficial scaling, the smaller blade for subgingival scaling. It comes in a set of three with differently angulated shanks for use in different parts of the mouth.

Sickle scalers (Figure 14.3c) These have a sickle-shaped blade which is triangular in cross-section so that there are two cutting edges. The blade may also be curved in a lateral plane so that it fits against the tooth surface. Sickles are available in several sizes, the larger ones being used for superficial scaling.

Hoes (Figure 14.3d) As the name implies these are hoe-shaped instruments which are available as a set of four, each shank angulated differently so that all tooth surfaces may be reached. They are available with tungsten carbide blades. In use the blade is inserted lightly under the gingival margin keeping the shank parallel to the axis of the tooth; the blade is then pressed against the tooth surface apical to the deposits of calculus and pulled in a coronal direction detaching the calculus.

Files (Figure 14.3e) These are indeed files which because of their very small dimensions can be inserted extremely easily into the gingival crevice or pocket. They are used like hoes.

Chisels (Figure 14.3f) (watch-spring, push or Zerfing scaler) These scalers are designed for the removal of interproximal deposits and are especially useful in the front of the mouth.

The ultrasonic scaler

Ultrasonic vibrations, i.e. above the range of normal hearing (above 20 000 Hz), can be used to remove tooth deposits and curette the soft tissue. Vibrated at about 25 000 Hz the instrument tip fragments surfaces against which it is placed. Special tips, usually curette shaped, are used under a cooling water spray as the vibration creates heat. The water spray also has a detergent effect which helps cleaning.

The instrument is applied to the tooth with soft stroking movements. Unlike a hand instrument, in using the ultrasonic scaler there is no tactile sensation in the operator's fingers, therefore it is essential to avoid excessive pressure.

The ultrasonic scaler can also be used to remove tooth stains and cement. It must be used with great care against ceramics. It can also discolour composite restorations as the metal tip can be abraded by the composite so that metal particles become incorporated in its surface. Some patients find that ultrasonic scaling is very painful and in these cases it should not be used. It is best to use the ultrasonic instrument to remove supragingival and the more superficial subgingival deposits and then to complete the scaling with hand instruments. It can also be used effectively for repeat scaling of periodontal pockets at maintenance visits, provided that all subgingival calculus deposits have been removed previously by hand instruments at the first treatment visits. Special tips are available for subgingival scaling.

Tooth polishing

Rough surfaces become sites of plaque and calculus deposition, therefore the tooth surface must be made smooth as well as free of calculus, plaque and stain. After scaling any residual plaque and stain should be removed using rotating cup-shaped brushes or rubber cups and a small amount of abrasive polishing paste. The brush should be rotated fairly slowly and applied intermittently to the tooth surface to avoid overheating. An advantage of the rubber cup is that it can be taken below the gingival margin. Linen polishing strips can be used to polish interproximal tooth surfaces.

Correction of plaque-retention factors

Faulty restorations

Restorations may be rough and badly contoured but the most frequent and important fault is the overhanging cervical margin which collects plaque and prevents its removal. Very small overhangs may be removed using polishing burs or strips but in most cases it is necessary to replace the restoration, with careful attention given to the placement of the matrix band and the use of interdental wedges.

Marginal ridges and contact points must be properly designed. Under-contoured restorations should be replaced. Any caries under the margin of the restoration must be identified and a new restoration placed. Where possible the margins of restorations should be placed coronal to the gingival margin (see Chapter 27).

Faulty appliances

Appliances irritate the tissues in several ways (*see* Chapter 4). They can compress or rub the gingiva directly or act to retain plaque against the gingiva. A removable partial denture should be designed so that as far as possible it is tooth borne and gingiva free. Where contact with the gingiva is unavoidable the fit should be good and pressure on the tissue should be avoided. The model should never be carved to produce lines of pressure, nor should relief areas be provided in an attempt to avoid pressure, as these provoke gingival hyperplasia which fills the relief chamber.

Appliances must be kept scrupulously clean and *not* worn at night.

Fixed appliances must be designed so that they do not promote plaque stagnation or impede plaque removal. To this end certain rules should be followed (see Chapter 27):

1. Restoration margins should be supragingival except on the labial face of upper incisors where cosmetic considerations dictate that the crown margin should be just hidden.
2. The provision of adequate embrasure spaces is imperative; when crowns or pontics are being waxed up a woodstick should be used to create a cleanable embrasure space. The design of pontics is particularly important; the ridge-lap pontics should be avoided and where possible sanitary pontics used.

3. Overcontouring restorations should be avoided. It is safer to err on the side of undercontouring crowns as this makes them easier to clean.

Fixed orthodontic appliances can present a difficult problem for the young patient to keep clean and the patient must be taught how to look after the appliance without at the same time damaging it. Fortunately young tissues recover quickly when the appliance is removed and thorough oral hygiene measures instituted.

Lack of lip-seal

Although not a plaque-retention factor, lack of lip-seal does seem to render the exposed gingiva more vulnerable to plaque irritation. Once upon a time, the oral screen was prescribed to wear during sleep, the theory being that it would seal the mouth, prevent evaporation of saliva and dehydration of the tissues. Smearing the gingiva with petroleum jelly was a popular practice and even Sellotaping the lips was recommended! None of these measures was aimed at the cause of the problem, the plaque. Patients with lack of lip-seal need to have their particular vulnerability carefully explained so that they can cooperate intelligently. With a clean mouth the patient can breathe through any available orifice without jeopardizing gingival health.

Tooth malalignment

Frequently orthodontic treatment is carried out to correct tooth malalignment which appears to be associated with gingival inflammation. A large proportion of this effort is wasted because the patient's home care is inadequate to clean even well-aligned teeth. On the other hand, some patients' efforts are effective enough to clean malaligned teeth and therefore do not need orthodontic treatment. Such treatment is justified where the patient is obviously trying to control plaque deposition and fails only in areas of malalignment.

Gingivoplasty

Gingival swelling creates gingival or 'false' pockets. When hyperplastic gingivitis has

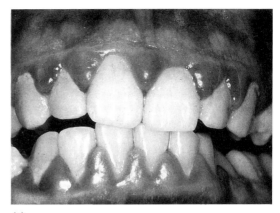

(a)

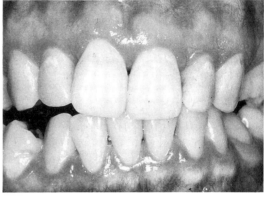

(b)

Figure 14.4 (*a*) Hyperplastic gingivitis which did not resolve following a prolonged period of scaling and home care. (*b*) Gingival condition following surgical reshaping, i.e. gingivoplasty

been present for a relatively short time the main component of the swelling is inflammation and given adequate scaling the inflammation resolves and the swelling reduces. In the case of longstanding irritation most frequently but not exclusively seen in the adult patient, there is a great deal of fibrous tissue formation which does not resolve on scaling. The pocket persists and plaque redeposits so that inflammation is maintained. If pocketing and gingival swelling persist after repeated scaling and assiduous patient effort over a period of several months, surgical reshaping of the gingiva, i.e. gingivoplasty, is indicated. It may also be needed after recurrent episodes of acute ulcerative gingivitis where tissue destruction has resulted in the saucer-shaped gingival defects characteristic of this disease.

Gingivoplasty is a gingivectomy with the limited aim of improving gingival contour, i.e. producing a streamlined contour with a knife-edged and scalloped margin and interdental sluice-ways (*Figure 14.4*).

Details of the technique are given in Chapter 16.

Chronic periodontitis

Although chronic gingivitis may remain contained for many years, in many people failure to control the inflammation will lead to periodontitis. The susceptibility to periodontitis is variable and its rate of progression varies from one person to another and from one tooth to another. Traditionally chronic periodontitis has been thought to advance slowly and progressively but, as described earlier, a number of longitudinal clinical studies of untreated chronic periodontitis have produced results that are inconsistent with this view (Goodson *et al.*, 1982; Socransky *et al.*, 1984). They suggest that the disease progresses by short and recurrent bursts of activity, probably of acute inflammation at specific sites, which are followed by long but variable periods of remission. Many tooth sites within an affected individual may remain free of destructive periodontal activity and indeed some patients remain free from destructive periodontal disease throughout their lives. It is also suggested that destructive periodontal disease activity may occur more frequently during certain periods of an individual's life.

At the time of an examination many periodontal pockets may be inactive, so that periodontal examination will reveal evidence of past disease rather than present activity. Since there are currently no certain means either to diagnose current activity or to predict when disease activity will occur; the only way to be sure that periodontal disease is actually progressing is to keep it under careful longitudinal observation. This method, however, has the obvious disadvantage that further periods of destruction will have to occur before they can be detected and treated. Therefore it is important to treat all periodontal pockets when they are first detected, and to aim at the removal of

all soft and hard deposits from the root surface, to create conditions which allow the patient to perform efficient plaque control, and to eliminate all factors which would prevent the patient from maintaining that plaque control.

The objectives of periodontal treatment are:

1. The resolution of the disease process.
2. The creation of conditions that will mitigate against recurrence of disease.
3. If possible, the regeneration of lost periodontal attachment.

The methods of treatment are described below.

Treatment of acute conditions

Acute conditions associated with chronic periodontitis should be treated without delay. The treatment of an acute lateral periodontal abscess and acute ulcerative gingivitis is described in Chapters 18 and 24.

In addition, a careful watch should be kept for sites of active disease which should be treated immediately. Patients may complain of local symptoms at these sites, such as discomfort, itching or gingival bleeding, and they will usually show signs of acute inflammation with redness, swelling and bleeding on probing. These sites should be treated by immediate, careful subgingival scaling and root planing under local anaesthesia. The pocket can be washed out by subgingival irrigation with a 0.2% chlorhexidine solution or gel using a blunt needle and a 5 ml syringe.

Treatment of chronic conditions

Scaling and root planing

All patients, other than those with acute problems, should first receive thorough supragingival scaling as this will reduce gingivitis and bleeding. It is important to have a full pocket chart before starting subgingival scaling.

Subgingival scaling is the most conservative method of pocket reduction and, where pocketing is shallow, it is the only treatment required. However, when pockets deepen to 4 mm or more, additional measures are required. The commonest of these is root planing.

Subgingival calculus is hard and tenaciously adherent to the root surface and CEJ and is difficult to remove. It is firmly attached to the root because the calcification process involves filamentous bacteria which may themselves penetrate into the surface cementum. Surface irregularities, such as the small pits previously occupied by Sharpey's fibres, are penetrated by apatite crystals firmly locking the calculus to the root surface. It can be particularly adherent in areas with difficult access such as furcations between multirooted teeth and in grooves and concavities on the root surface.

The object of root planing is to remove necrotic cementum and embedded calculus and to smooth the root surface. It is also concerned with the removal of cementum infiltrated with toxic material of bacterial origin such as endotoxin (LPS). Recently it has been found that this material is only loosely associated with the root surface (Moore *et al.*, 1986) and can be removed by hand or ultrasonic scaling without the need for cementum removal. This indicates that the aim of scaling and root planing should be to produce a smooth, deposit-free root surface with the minimal removal of cementum.

Subgingival scaling and root planing significantly alter the bacterial composition of the pocket. Using dark ground microscopy techniques it has been shown that this treatment results in a marked decrease in the number of motile rods and spirochaetes and a corresponding increase in cocci (Listgarten *et al.*, 1978). The time taken for bacterial repopulation to occur is variable and ranges from 1 to 6 months (Listgarten *et al.*, 1978; Mousques *et al.*, 1980). Cultural studies have also shown significant reductions in the numbers of obligate anaerobes and black pigmented *Bacteroides* (Walsh *et al.*, 1986). These significant and prolonged reductions in the numbers of Gram negative anaerobic bacteria and spirochaetes probably result from changes in the pocket environment, brought about by subgingival scaling which makes it less favourable for the growth of these fastidious bacteria. The rate of recolonization is affected by the standard of oral hygiene since a regrowth of supragingival plaque will favour recolonization of the pocket (Magnusson *et al.*, 1984).

Scaling and root planing are effective at reducing gingival inflammation and reducing pocket depth. When combined with good oral hygiene and regular maintenance these effects

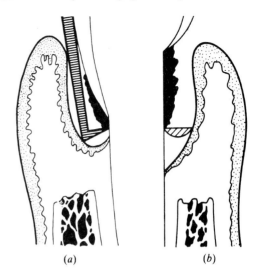

Figure 14.5 Diagram to show the use of instruments and their correct placement in subgingival scaling and root planing: (*a*) a hoe is used to remove resistant deposits; (*b*) a curette is used to remove fine deposits and to root plane

can be prolonged over several years (Pihlstrom *et al.*, 1983; Ramfjord *et al.*, 1987; Badersten *et al.*, 1987). These studies indicate that these measures alone can be effective in treating and maintaining patients with moderate and even advanced chronic periodontitis but it must be remembered that treatment is very time consuming and demanding, particularly in patients with deep pocketing, and requires frequent maintenance visits. In the studies quoted above, the time taken for scaling and root planing ranged from 5 to 8 hours and the patients were recalled for maintenance treatment every 2–4 months. Relapses did occur in some patients despite these measures. Obviously the patient's susceptibility to periodontal disease is a factor but it is also becoming clear that it is very difficult to remove all calculus deposits from deep pockets by 'blind' subgingival scaling. Several studies have shown that some calculus frequently remains after careful subgingival scaling and the incidence increases with increasing pocket depths (Rabbani *et al.*, 1981; Eaton *et al.*, 1985). This is less common following surgical exposure by flap procedures (Caffesse *et al.*, 1986).

Subgingival scaling and root planing are indicated for periodontal pockets >4 mm and

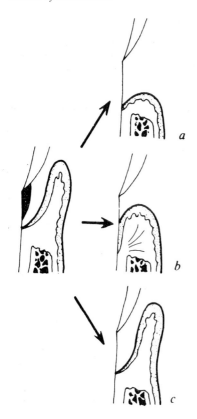

Figure 14.6 Diagram to show some possible tissue changes which may follow scaling: (*a*) complete shrinkage of the pocket wall with resolution of inflammation; (*b*) reformation of gingival fibres plus some shrinkage of pocket wall to form wide gingival cuff with long epithelial attachment; (*c*) little shrinkage of the pocket wall and the pocket remains patent. The tissue change following scaling frequently represents a combination of these possibilities

if necessary, should be carried out under local anaesthesia. Although ultrasonic scalers are equally effective as hand scaling in removing calculus and root associated LPS, they have more limited access to deep pockets. The main hand instruments used for scaling and root planing are hoes and curettes and it is essential that these instruments are sharp. This usually means that they have to be sharpened immediately before use, which can be done with a set of sterile stones.

Hoes are used to remove resistant deposits of calculus but care should be taken to avoid excessive pressure or incorrect positioning of the instrument as this may groove the root surface (*Figure 14.5a*). Sharp curettes are used

to remove residual fine deposits and to plane and smooth the root surface (*Figure 14.5b*). In many situations it is easier to use curettes for the whole process. If the intention is to avoid trauma to the soft tissue, single-sided curettes such as the Gracy curettes can be used. These are particularly good instruments for finishing and smoothing the root surface.

The patient may experience some discomfort following root planing and it may be wise to prescribe a mild analgesic following this procedure. Healing will take place over several days and will be aided by meticulous oral hygiene.

Tissue response to scaling and root planing

The tissue response to even perfect scaling is variable. There are several possible consequences:

1. The pocket wall may shrink completely. This is most likely to happen when the pocket is fairly shallow and the inflammatory element in the pocket wall dominates over the fibrous tissue component. This is usually the case in young people where the walls of pockets as deep as 6 mm may shrink completely (*Figure 14. 6a*).
2. With resolution of inflammation the collagen bundles of the gingival fibre system are reformed so that the gingival cuff contracts against the tooth surface and the crevicular epithelium heals to form a long epithelial attachment which may become connected to the tooth surface by hemidesmosomes. Thus a wide gingival cuff is formed which is not supported by bone (*Figure 14. 6b*). The integrity of this cuff depends on the length of the attachment, its strength of attachment to the tooth, the strength of the collagen bundles of the gingival fibres and the level of oral hygiene. If plaque-induced inflammation recurs the cuff collapses readily.
3. Little shrinkage of the pocket wall may take place and the pocket may remain patent. This occurs most commonly when the pocket is deep and its wall is composed predominantly of fibrous tissue (*Figure 14. 6c*).
4. Frequently the gingival response represents a combination of these possibilities.

Summary

Subgingival scaling and root planing are difficult procedures, and ones which require considerable practice, skill and patience. The complete removal of soft and hard deposits from the root surface is difficult enough when the root is visible – as it is when surgically exposed – but when the procedures have to be undertaken 'blind' tactile sensibility has to be well developed to achieve anything approaching an immaculate and smooth root surface. Root proximity and rotation, concavities and ridges, grooves and pits, all compound cleaning problems. This is especially the case in the furcations of multirooted teeth. These problems can only be overcome by careful instrumentation. Hill *et al.* (1981) spent 5–8 hours over the course of 3–8 appointments, and Stambaugh *et al.* (1981) spent between 25 and 39 minutes on each posterior tooth to achieve root surfaces free of detectable roughness.

In a comparative study of open (surgical) versus closed scaling and root planing on multi-rooted teeth, Wylam *et al.* (1993) showed that although the open approach was more effective on external root surfaces, heavy residual deposits remained in furcation areas after both open and closed procedures. They conclude that hand instrumentation is inadequate for the debridement of furcations, and suggest that the use of ultrasonic instruments or rotary burrs is necessary.

The deeper the pocket the smaller the chance of complete debridement. It is possible to detect residual deposits with a special 'calculus probe', but using this presents the same problems as using a scaling instrument, and the persistence of gingival inflammation after scaling remains the best indicator of residual deposits, which can then be removed at successive scalings. Each scaling helps to reduce inflammatory swelling and allows continuingly improved access to the root surface. It is essential to inform the patient at the outset that subgingival scaling and root planing require a commitment to multiple appointments.

The degree of pocket reduction following scaling and root planing must be carefully assessed before any decision about surgical treatment is made. Several months should elapse before reassessment of the patient, with a view to surgery, takes place.

References

Badersten, A., Nilveus, R. and Egelberg, J. (1987) 4 year observations of basic periodontal therapy. *Journal of Clinical Periodontology* **14**, 438–444

Caffesse, R.G., Sweeney, P.L. and Smith, B.A. (1986) Scaling and root planing with and without periodontal flap surgery. *Journal of Clinical Periodontology* **13**, 205–211

Eaton, K.A., Kieser, J.B. and Davies, R.M. (1985) The removal of root surface deposits. *Journal of Clinical Periodontology* **12**, 141–152

Goodson, J.R., Turner, A.C.R., Haffajee, A.D. *et al.* (1982) Patterns of progression and regression of advanced destructive periodontal disease. *Journal of Clinical Periodontology* **9**, 472–481

Hill, R.W., Ramfjord, S.P., Morrison, E.C. *et al.* (1981) Four types of periodontal treatment compared over 2 years. *Journal of Periodontology* **52**, 655–622

Listgarten, M.A., Lindhe, J. and Hellden, L. (1978) Effects of tetracycline and/or scaling on human periodontal disease. Clinical microbiological and histological observations. *Journal of Clinical Periodontology* **5**, 246–271

Magnusson, I., Lindhe, J., Yoneyama, T. and Liljenberg, B. (1984) Recolonisation of the subgingival microbiota following scaling in deep pockets. *Journal of Clinical Periodontology* **11**, 193–207

Moore, J., Wilson, M. and Kieser, J.B. (1986) The distribution of bacterial lipopolysaccharide (Endotoxin) in relation to periodontally involved root surfaces. *Journal of Clinical Periodontology* **13**, 748–751

Mousques, T., Listgarten, M.A. and Phillips, R.W. (1980) Effect of scaling and root planing on the composition of the human subgingival microbial flora. *Journal of Periodontal Research* **15**, 144–151

Pihlstrom, B.L., McHugh, R.B., Oliphant, T.H. and Ortiz-Campos, C. (1983) Comparison of surgical and non surgical treatment of periodontal disease. A review of current studies and additional results after 6.5 years. *Journal of Clinical Periodontology* **10**, 524–541

Rabbani, G.M., Ash, M.M. and Caffesse, R.G. (1981) The effectiveness of subgingival root planing in calculus removal. *Journal of Periodontology* **52**, 119–123

Ramfjord, S.P., Caffesse, R.G., Morrison, E.C. *et al.* (1987) 4 modalities of periodontal treatment compared over 5 years. *Journal of Clinical Periodontology* **14**, 445–452

Socransky, S.S., Haffajee, A.D., Goodson, J.M. *et al.* (1984) New concepts of destructive periodontal disease. *Journal of Clinical Periodontology* **11**, 21–32

Stambaugh, R.V., Dragoo, M., Smith, D.M. and Carasali, L. (1981) The limits of subgingival curettage. *Journal of Periodontal Restorative Dentistry* **1**, 31–41

Walsh, M.M., Buchanan, S.A., Hoover, C.I. *et al.* (1986) Clinical and microbiological effects of single dose metronidazole on scaling and root planing in treatment of adult periodontitis. *Journal of Clinical Periodontology* **13**, 151–157

Wylam, J.M., Mealey, B.L., Mills, M.P. *et al.* (1993) The clinical effectiveness of open versus closed scaling and root planing on multi-rooted teeth. *Journal of Periodontology* **64**, 243–253

15

The chemotherapeutic approach to periodontal treatment

Conference centre.

Actisyte Tetracyclines.
Dentomycin minocycline
Elzyl metronidazol.

As periodontal disease is caused by bacteria the use of antibacterial agents would appear to be reasonable in both prevention and treatment (*Table 15.1*). However, for their use to be effective certain conditions need to be fulfilled:

1. They should be effective against the bacteria involved in the lesion.
2. They should reach the site of infection in sufficient concentration for an adequate length of time.
3. Their efficiency should outweigh all contraindications, e.g. side effects.

A number of chemotherapeutic agents have been studied, including antibiotics, antiseptics, metal ions and oxygenating agents.

Antibiotics and periodontal treatment

Until recently there has been a justifiable reserve in the dental profession regarding the use of antibiotics to treat periodontal disease. However, in the past few years, interest in the use of antibiotics for this purpose has increased and many clinical trials of their use have been published.

Several criteria must be met before the use of antibiotics can be justified. These are, first, that the nature of the bacteria flora associated with periodontal disease must be amenable to control by antibiotics. Second, antibiotics must be shown either to be superior in controlling the disease than traditional clinical treatment

or to act as useful adjuvants to it. Third, antibiotics used must be free from adverse side effects and from the induction of hypersensitivity or bacterial resistance. Finally they must achieve effective concentrations in the periodontal pocket where the causative bacteria reside.

Mode of action of antibiotics

The precise chemical mode of action varies from one antibiotic to another and will not be considered here. Antibiotics are either bactericidal, i.e. they kill sensitive bacteria, or bacteriostatic, i.e. they inhibit multiplication of sensitive bacteria. Bactericidal antibiotics are usually the first choice in treating infections but in general, provided that an adequate concentration of the antibiotic is achieved at the site of infection and the host defences are normal, there is little difference in the effectiveness of both types. Penicillin and metronidazole are examples of bactericidal antibiotics and tetracycline and erythromycin examples of bacteriostatic ones.

The spectrum of action of antibiotics varies considerably. It is obviously necessary for the antibiotic of choice to be strongly active against the causative bacteria of the disease. An example of this affecting the choice of an antibiotic for periodontal purposes is in the use of metronidazole, which is active against strictly anaerobic bacteria but not against facultative, capnophilic aerobes such as *Eikenella corrodens, Capnocytophaga* species

Table 15.1 Chemical supragingival plaque control

Antibiotics	Enzymes	Bisbiguanides	Quaternary ammonium compounds	Phenolic compounds
Penicillin	Protease	Chlorhexidine	Cetypyridinium chloride	Thymol
Vancomycin	Lipase	Alexidine	Benzalconium chloride	4-Hexylresorcinol
Kanamycin	Nuclease	Octenidine		2-Phenylphenol
Erythromycin	Dextranase			Eucalyptol
Niddamycin	Mutanase			
Spiromycin				
	Glucose oxidase			
	Amyloglucosidase			

Natural products	Fluorides	Metal ions	Oxygenating agents	Other antiseptics
Sanguinarine	Sodium fluoride	Copper	Peroxide	Iodine
	Sodium monofluoro-phosphate	Tin		Povidone iodine
		Zinc		Chloramine-T
	Stannous fluoride			Sodium hypochlorite
	Amine fluoride			Hexetidine
				Triclosan

(Reproduced from the *Journal of Clinical Periodontology* (1986) by kind permission of Dr M. Addy and the Editor)

and *Actinobacillus actinomycetemcomitans.* Generally antibiotics with a low potential for sensitization and bacterial resistance should be preferred for treating periodontal diseases.

Antibiotics are primarily used for treating specific bacterial infections where the infection can be treated with an antibiotic, with a narrow spectrum, specifically directed against the foreign pathogen. During treatment the susceptible pathogens and any indigenous bacteria sensitive to the antibiotic will be either killed (bactericidal antibiotic) or stopped from multiplying (bacteriostatic antibiotic). Bacteriostatic antibiotics depend upon the host defence mechanisms to rid the body of the suppressed pathogens. The success of the treatment depends on which bacteria regrow after the treatment is stopped. If the indigenous bacteria regrow rapidly after treatment they will prevent the re-establishment of the pathogens (Van Palenstein Helderman, 1986).

The nature of periodontal infections

Although the primary cause of inflammatory periodontal disease is bacterial, no single causative pathogen has been found (Chapter 4). Thus, chronic periodontitis seems best regarded as a non-specific bacterial disease caused by a local imbalance in the local indigenous bacterial population (Theilade, 1986). Certain indigenous bacteria may play a more important role in the disease process because they possess virulence factors that may enable them to damage host defences or degrade host tissues. However, there is no evidence that eradication of suspected pathogens of chronic periodontitis without the suppression of other members of the flora is effective in treating chronic periodontitis. If, as seems to be the case, all the suspected pathogens are members of the normal oral flora their permanent eradication by antibiotics will not be possible because they will reestablish themselves after treatment.

However, it is known that transient shifts in the subgingival bacterial flora can be produced both by scaling and root planing and the systemic administration or local application of some antibiotics. A number of studies have been carried out into the most promising antibiotics, tetrecycline and metronidazole, and these will be described below.

There is a much stronger case for using antibiotics to treat acute necrotizing ulcerative gingivitis (Chapter 22) and juvenile periodontitis (Chapter 20) as they appear to be associated with selective growth of a narrower range of bacteria.

The site of action of antibiotics for periodontal treatment

The site of action for an antibiotic treating periodontal disease is the periodontal pocket and it is essential that it should achieve a high concentration at this site (Van Palenstein Heldermann, 1986).

Antibiotics for treating periodontal disease can be administered either systemically or locally. The local method seems better for achieving high local concentrations of the drug and for minimizing the risks of developing bacterial resistance. This method should not be used with antibiotics such as penicillin that carry a high risk of sensitization. The inaccessibility of the pocket is a problem in this regard and cannot be reached by antibiotics in mouthrinses, ointments, toothpastes or chewing gum. This problem can be overcome by subgingival irrigation but daily irrigation is not practical since it is patient dependent. To avoid this problem, slow release devices have been developed that can be inserted by the dentist into the pocket, extending down to its base. These currently include hollow and monolithic fibres (Goodson *et al.*, 1979, 1983) and acrylic strips (Addy, 1986) and slow release gels (Norling *et al.*, 1992).

Systemically administered antibiotics can also reach the pocket in gingival crevicular fluid, which is an exudate. This has been shown to occur with tetracyclines (Gordon *et al.*, 1981), clindamycin (Walker *et al.*, 1981a) and metronidazole (Notten *et al.*, 1982). Tetracycline and its derivates achieve higher concentrations in crevicular fluid than in serum, possibly by binding to calcium-containing substances (Baker *et al.*, 1983). The antibiotic concentrations in crevicular fluid, achieved using either the systemic route or local delivery systems, are higher than those necessary to inhibit the sensitive bacteria *in vitro* (Van Palenstein Helderman, 1986).

Clinical trials of antibiotics in the treatment of chronic periodontitis

A number of clinical trials of the use of antibiotics for the treatment of chronic periodontitis have been carried out. They have used antibiotics either as the sole treatment, or in combination with scaling and root planing, and in both cases have compared the results obtained with scaling and root planing alone. All of these have involved the use of either a tetracycline or metronidazole.

Local application of antibiotics into the periodontal pocket would seem to have some advantages over systemic administration. Local application can produce a much higher concentration in the pocket with a much lower total dose and very low systemic levels. This reduces the risk of resistant bacteria emerging and the risks of the development of hypersensitivity. However, local application does not affect the reservoirs of bacteria at other sites in the mouth and only maintains bactericidal levels for about 24 hours. It is also much more expensive.

The effects of antibiotics as the sole agent

Short-term use of systemic or local tetracycline and metronidazole produce a marked reduction in Gram negative anaerobes and spirochaetes and improvements in the clinical condition, i.e. reduction in probing pocket depth (PPD) and bleeding on probing (BOP). Similar results have been shown with the local delivery of tetracycline in hollow or solid fibres (Goodson *et al.*, 1979, 1983; Lindhe *et al.*, 1979) or metronidazole in acrylic strips (Addy, 1986). Re-establishment of the pocket flora after antibiotic treatments occurs between 8 and 12 weeks (Lindhe *et al.*, 1979).

These studies show that, whilst marked reductions in the number of subgingival bacteria can be achieved with these antibiotics, these are often less than can be achieved by scaling and root planing and tend to persist for shorter periods.

The effects of antibiotics as adjuvants to scaling and root planing

Since it is impossible to remove the whole pocket flora by scaling and root planing, the use of antibiotics as adjuvants to these procedures might enhance their effects. To test this possibility a number of studies have been carried out to compare the combined effects of antibiotics and scaling and root planing with the effects of scaling and root planing alone (Lindhe *et al.*, 1979, 1983). In both groups the changes in the flora were maintained for up to 25 weeks.

Long- and short-term systemic treatment with tetracyclines in combination with scaling and root planing have not shown any more benefit over scaling and root planing alone. The effect of local tetracycline and metronidazoles with local administration or slow release devices as an adjuvant to scaling and root planing has also been studied. Similar changes were seen with and without the adjuvants and thus no additional benefit appeared to accrue (Lindhe *et al.*, 1979, 1983; Addy, 1986).

The results of some studies using systemic metronidazole in combination with scaling and root planing were similar to scaling and root planing alone (Lindhe *et al.*, 1983). However, there are other studies which show more marked and prolonged improvements in the clinical condition using systemic metronidazole as an adjuvant to scaling and root planing (Loesche *et al.*, 1985, 1991; Joyston-Bechal *et al.*, 1984, 1986; Söder *et al.*, 1990). In one study, these improvements disappeared 3 years after treatment (Joyston-Bechal *et al.*, 1986).

Loesche and his co-workers have carried out three double-blind clinical trials of systemic metronidazole in the treatment of periodontal disease and have observed each time a significant clinical improvement in the group receiving metronidazole (Loesche *et al.*, 1985, 1991, 1992). In these patients there was a significant rapid decline or disappearance of spirochaetes. Systemic metronidazole as an adjuvant to to scaling was also found significantly to reduce the need for periodontal surgery (Loesche *et al.*, 1992). However, a few patients in the metronidazole groups appeared to be non-responsive to the drug. In another study (Loesche *et al.*, 1993), the compliance in taking the drug was investigated by measuring the reduction in spirochaetes and it was found that only 10 patients out of 18 in the study were compliant in regularly taking the drug. These 10 patients experienced a significantly greater clinical benefit than the 8 non-compliant patients.

Further studies on local delivery using slow release gels

Further studies on local delivery of tetracycline and metronidazole have been carried out more recently following the incorporation of these antibiotics into biodegradable slow-release gels (Norling *et al.*, 1992). Studies of the release characteristics from these gels have shown that both the 2% minocycline (Dentomycin) gel (Satomi *et al.*, 1987) and the 25% metronidazole (Elyzol) gel (Stoltze, 1992) produce levels above the MIC for suspected pathogens for 12–24 hours after treatment. It has also been shown that the systemic absorption, including that from swallowed excess gel, was less than that absorbed from one 200 mg metronidazole tablet taken orally (Stoltze and Stellfeld, 1992).

Further studies in human patients with these agents for 2% minocycline gel (Van Steenberge *et al.*, 1993) and 25% metronidazole gel (Klinge *et al.*, 1992a; Ainamo *et al.*, 1992; Pedrazzoli *et al.*, 1992) produced similar findings to those reported for other local delivery agents in the previous section. It has also been shown that 25% metronidazole gel improved the clinical features of experimental periodontitis in dogs and eliminated some of the bacteria associated with the condition (Klinge *et al.*, 1992b). Good results have also been achieved with topical irrigation with tetracycline-HCl solution (100 mg/ml) and this might in part be due to absorption of the compound on to root dentine and its subsequent release (Christersson *et al.*, 1993). Irrigation for long periods (5 minutes) is, however, necessary to achieve release of therapeutic concentrations of active antibiotic.

Thus, it seems from current available evidence that although systemic administration and local application of tetracycline and metronidazole can produce similar clinical and bacteriological effects to scaling and root planing they appear to offer no significant advantages. However, the use of the adjuvant antibiotic gels may be advantageous in a few situations.

These are:

- deep pocket with very difficult access for scaling and root planing
- localized pockets in juvenile periodontitis (instead of systemic tetracycline)
- pockets which fail to respond to scaling and root planing
- deep pocket sites in refractory or rapidly progressive periodontitis
- pockets exuding pus
- sites with acute lateral periodontal abscess (instead of systemic antibiotic)

Other uses of antibiotics in periodontal treatment

In the light of the studies described above the use of antibiotics in periodontal treatment should be restricted to those cases where it will give benefits over and above those of conventional treatment. At the present time its use cannot be justified in the routine treatment of chronic periodontitis. Antibiotics should be restricted in the treatment of non-specific infections, particularly where other treatments are effective, since their prolonged use could give rise in some cases to hypersensitivity reactions, toxic reactions, the development of bacterial resistance and of superinfections with resistant organisms such as *Candida*. In spite of these restrictions, antibiotics could be of use in the following situations:

1. To protect against the possible effects of a transient bacteraemia in susceptible patients.
2. The treatment of acute ulcerative gingivitis.
3. The treatment of acute abscesses of periodontal origin.
4. The treatment of juvenile periodontitis.
5. The initial treatment of severe generalized periodontitis.

Protection against the effects of transient bacteraemia

The cardiac lesions which are known to predispose to infective endocarditis and those which do not are shown in Table 15.2. Antibiotic prophylaxis should be given in these cases for extractions, scaling and periodontal surgery (Eley, 1983). Transient bacteraemia may also arise from normal functional activity and tooth cleaning when gingivitis is present and is best prevented by the maintenance of dental health and the prevention and early treatment of periodontal diseases.

Antibiotic prophylaxis can either be 3 g amoxycillin orally 60 minutes before the procedure or one vial of Triplopen intramuscularly (i.m.) 30 minutes before the procedure. Patients who are allergic to penicillin may be given erythromycin stearate 2 g orally, 2 hours before the procedure. Orally administered regimens are obviously more convenient for dental practice. High risk cases, such as patients with a history of previous infective endocarditis or with prosthetic heart valves, should be treated in hospital and should be given either Triplopen (1 vial i.m.) plus gentamicin (120 mg i.m.) or erythromycin lactobionate (300 mg intravenously (i.v.) over 5 minutes) plus gentamicin (120 mg i.m.). In addition a chlorhexidine mouthwash should be given prior to treatment in all cases.

Treatment of acute abscesses of periodontal origin

The treatment of an acute lateral abscess may include the use of an antibiotic (Chapter 19). These infections are usually sensitive to penicillin and can be controlled with oral penicillin V 250 mg four times daily for 5 days. If the patient is allergic to penicillin, oral erythromycin stearate can be used in the same dosage. Local treatment with a slow-release gel could be considered instead of systemic administration if the infection is completely localized. Either 2% minocycline or 25% metronidazole gel could be used.

Treatment of acute ulcerative gingivitis

Acute ulcerative gingivitis (Chapter 22) is an endogenous fusospirochaetal infection and may be treated with penicillin or metronidazole.

Treatment of juvenile periodontitis

Juvenile periodontitis (Chapter 20) is associated with capnophilic, facultatively aerobic subgingival flora and is best treated with either metronidazole 250 mg and amoxycillin 375 mg, 3 times daily for 7 days (van Winkelhoff *et al.*, 1989), or tetracycline 250 mg 4 times per day for 14 days (Slots and Rosling, 1983) before or during periodontal treatment. Ideally antibiotic sensitivity of the bacteria, in particular *Actinobaccillus actinomycetemcomitans*, should be determined in a microbiology laboratory.

The local application of 2% minocycline gel to the affected pockets could be considered. However, in this regard it should be noted that the results may not be as effective (Mandell *et al.*, 1986). This could possibly be related to the local invasive properties of *A. actinomycetemcomitans* resulting in local colonization of the periodontal tissues (Christersson *et al.*, 1987). Bacteria in the tissues may not be reached by antibiotic in the pocket.

Table 15.2

Cardiac conditions requiring antibiotic cover	Cardiac conditions not requiring antibiotic cover
Ventricular septal defect (VSD)	Angina
Primum atrial septal defect (ASD)	Myocardial infarction
ASD repaired with prosthetic patch	Ventricular aneurysm
Post valvotomy	Innocent systolic murmur
Prolapsing mitral valve	Permanent pacemaker
Pulmonary stenosis	Ligated ductus arteriosus
Patent ductus arteriosus	ASD – unrepaired or repaired without patch
Coarctation of aorta	Coronary artery bypass graft unless within 6 months
Tetralogy of Fallot	Rheumatic fever without history and evidence of
Arteriovenous (AV) shunt	valvular disease – needs cardiac examination to confirm
Bicuspid aortic valve	
Murmurs of doubtful origin	
Rheumatic valvular stenosis or incompetence	
AV malformation or fistula	
History of infective endocarditis*	
Prosthetic valve replacement*	
Recent coronary artery bypass	
Hip prosthesis	

* High risk

Initial treatment of generalized severe periodontitis

Sometimes patients will present with a severe active generalized periodontitis with marked gingival swelling and bleeding, deep pocketing and possibly multiple lateral abscesses. In some cases these may be initially treated with full-mouth ultrasonic scaling, reaching as deep as possible into the pockets. However, in many such cases the gingivae are acutely sensitive and localized areas of acute infection are present which prevent immediate scaling and adequate brushing by the patient. The condition may also occur as a complication of systemic disease and in these circumstances immediate scaling treatment may be difficult or impossible. Since it is known that systemic antibiotics can reduce the subgingival flora to an extent comparable to subgingival scaling, they can be of great use in this situation. The two most useful antibiotics are tetracycline and metronidazole, either of which can be administered orally for 1–2 weeks prior to conventional periodontal treatment. Obviously any local abscesses present should be drained.

The use of chemical antibacterial agents

The association of bacteria with periodontal disease has given rise to considerable interest in the development and use of non-antibiotic antimicrobial agents for its management (Table 15.1). Interest has mainly centred on their use as adjuvants to scaling and root planing. Antimicrobials can be divided into two main uses:

1. Agents directed against supragingival plaque development.
2. Agents directed against subgingival bacteria.

Supragingival plaque control

The agents studied for this purpose can be divided into enzymes, bisguanide antiseptics, quaternary ammonium antiseptics, phenolic antiseptics, other antiseptics, oxygenating agents, metal ions and natural products (Addy, 1986).

Enzymes: Two approaches to plaque control with enzymes have been tried: (i) studies of enzymes interfering with bacterial attachment, including dextranases and proteolytic enzymes, the results of which have been inconclusive in humans (Addy, 1986); (ii) potentiation of host defences, which involves potentiation of salivary antibacterial activity using the enzymes amyglucoxidase and glucose oxidase to produce hydrogen peroxide from dietary fermentable carbohydrates. This in turn converts thiocyanate to hypothiocyanite in the presence of salivary lactoperoxidase, which then acts as a bacterial inhibitor by interfering with cell metabolism. There is *in vitro* evidence for this process but such activity in the mouth has not yet been demonstrated. Clinical studies of the use of this system as a mouthwash and a toothpaste (Zendium) have given conflicting results.

Bisguanide antiseptics Several bisguanide antiseptics possess antiplaque activity, including chlorhexidine, alexidine and octenidine (Addy, 1986). Of these the most effective is chlorhexidine gluconate. These antiseptics are able to kill a wide range of microorganisms by damaging the cell wall. The antiplaque properties of chlorhexidine are unsurpassed by other agents and it has much greater effects than other antiseptics of similar or greater antibacterial activity. This appears to be due to the absorption of the dicationic chlorhexidine molecule on to oral surfaces and its release at bacteriostatic levels for prolonged periods. It has been shown that a 0.2% chlorhexidine gluconate mouthwash will prevent the development of experimental gingivitis after the withdrawal of oral hygiene procedures. When used as an adjunct to normal oral hygiene measures, variable results are achieved, suggesting that chlorhexidine is more effective in preventing plaque accumulation than in reducing pre-existing plaque deposits. Although chlorhexidine is not toxic, it has an unpleasant taste, alters taste sensation and produces brown staining on the teeth which is difficult to remove. This can also affect the mucous membranes and the tongue and may be related to the precipitation of chromogenic dietary factors on to the teeth and mucous membranes. Other much rarer side effects are mucosal erosion and parotid swelling. For these reasons the prolonged use of chlorhexidine should be avoided in normal periodontal patients. It is useful for short periods (up to 2 weeks) when oral hygiene may be difficult or impossible, such as during acute oral infections or following periodontal surgery. It may occasionally be used as an adjunct to mechanical oral hygiene in initial periodontal treatment and during periods of intermaxillary fixation following the treatment of fractures or skeletal surgery. Its more prolonged use may be justified in physically and mentally handicapped patients, in medically compromised

patients predisposed to oral infections and as an adjunct to oral hygiene in fixed orthodontic appliance wearers. In many of these special cases the mouthwash or gel will be used over a prolonged period and severe staining will be a problem. This can be minimized by using concomitant toothbrushing and by avoiding the intake of certain foods and drinks such as tea and coffee.

It has been shown that chlorhexidine is less active in toothpastes and gels than in mouthwashes. This is probably because the binding of chlorhexidine by other components in the toothpaste reduces its activity (Addy *et al.*, 1989).

Quaternary ammonium compounds Quaternary ammonium compounds such as cetylpyridinium chloride have moderate antiplaque activity. Although they have greater oral retention and equivalent antibacterial activity to chlorhexidine, they are less effective in inhibiting plaque and preventing gingivitis. One reason for this may be that these compounds are rapidly desorbed from the oral mucosa. It has also been found that the antibacterial properties of these compounds are considerably reduced once absorbed on to a surface and this may be related to the monocationic nature of these compounds.

Phenolic antiseptics Phenols have been used in mouthwashes for a considerable time. When used at high concentrations relative to other compounds they have been shown to reduce plaque accumulation.

Other antiseptics A number of other antiseptics have been tried for their antiseptic activity. Hexetidine has some activity but this is small in comparison with chlorhexidine. It can cause oral ulceration at concentrations greater than 0.1%. Povidone iodine appears to have no significant antiplaque activity when used as 1% mouthwash and may cause a problem of iodine sensitivity in some individuals.

Triclosan is a non ionic antiseptic used recently in a number of the commercial toothpastes and mouthwashes. It has a useful antibacterial effect but in 0.2% concentration in toothpastes with or without 0.5% zinc citrate it has plaque inhibitory effects which are little different from other detergent based commercial toothpastes (Jenkins *et al.*, 1989).

Oxygenating agents Oxygenating agents such as hydrogen peroxide and sodium peroxyborate mouthrinses have a beneficial effect on acute ulcerative gingivitis, probably by inhibiting anaerobic bacteria. As obligate anaerobes are important in the development of gingivitis and periodontitis these effects could be useful.

Metal ions A number of metal ions have been studied for their effects on plaque: zinc, copper and tin have antiplaque activities. Both copper and tin suffer from the local side effect of staining. Some fluoride compounds have antiplaque effects but not as a result of the fluoride ion itself. Stannous fluoride is due to the effect of stannous ion; amine fluoride is due to the surface-active amine portion of the molecule.

Natural products Preliminary studies on the plant extract sanguinarine chloride have shown that it produces moderate reductions in plaque and gingivitis. The zinc present in the formulations could be partly responsible for the effect.

Subgingival plaque control

The gingival crevice or periodontal pocket is not reached by chemical agents in mouthwashes or toothpastes, which have their effect purely on supragingival plaque. This is the main reason that such mouthwashes have no place in the treatment of established gingivitis or periodontitis. More recently local drug delivery systems have been developed to carry antibiotics into the pocket area and some of these have been used to deliver antiseptics. Chlorhexidine is the most common antiseptic to be used in this way. It can be irrigated into the pocket using a 5 ml syringe and blunt needle in either a liquid or gel form. It can also be incorporated into acrylic strips (Addy, 1986) and other slow releasing devices but none of these are commercially available. Using an acrylic strip delivery system, chlorhexidine was shown to change markedly the subgingival bacterial composition as measured by dark ground microscopy. Comparative studies of the effect of subgingival delivery of either chlorhexidine or antibiotics have shown that it is less effective than tetracycline or metronidazole in changing the bacterial flora and reducing gingivitis (Addy,

1986). It does not, however, suffer from the potential drawbacks of inducing bacterial resistance and may therefore be more suitable for repeated use. In particular, chlorhexidine pocket irrigation is a useful and practical adjuvant to scaling and root planing deep pockets, particularly when marked inflammation is present.

The Keyes technique The Keyes technique consists of packing a mixture of $NaCl$, $NaHCO_3$ and H_2O_2 (3%) subgingivally and then irrigating the pockets with an antiseptic solution such as iodine solution, e.g. 0.5% povidone iodine (Betadine). Used in combination with scaling this has been reported to improve marginally the clinical effects of scaling and root planing alone (Rosling *et al.*, 1983). The mixture can also be used by patients during brushing but this does not seem to produce any benefit over brushing alone. The use of the Keyes technique on its own is much less effective than scaling and root planing; therefore the technique does not seem to offer any significant advantage in periodontal treatment.

Use of agents to raise redox potential

The growth of anaerobic bacteria in an ecosystem such as the periodontal pocket is dependent in part of the redox potential (Eh) (Finegold, 1989). It has been shown that redox potentials as low as $-300mV$ may exist in some parts of deep periodontal pockets and this may enable strictly anaerobic bacteria to survive in this environment (Kenney and Ash, 1969). These researchers have also shown that the redox potential of the healthy gingival crevice (Eh $+70mV$) with its very low proportion of anaerobes, is significantly higher than the average potential of the periodontal pocket (Eh $-48mV$). By raising the redox potential it may be possible to create an environment which is incompatible with the growth of anaerobic periodontal pathogens.

A variety of substances including redox dyes and transitional metal ions can raise the redox potential in an ecosystem without producing molecular oxygen. One of the most promising of these is the redox dye methylene blue which was partly chosen because of its low toxicity for humans (Gibson *et al.*, 1994).

This was first studied in a pilot study using chronic periodontitis patients (Wilson *et al.*, 1992). Methylene blue was applied by subgingival irrigation and was shown after 28 days to have reduced gingival crevicular fluid flow and to have produced a shift in the bacterial flora towards one more compatible with health.

A recent study (Gibson *et al.*, 1994) compared subgingival methylene blue application with a negative control and scaling and root planing using a split mouth design; 24 chronic periodontitis patients were chosen because they had matched periodontal pockets in all four quadrants of 5 mm or more. One quadrant received subgingival irrigation of 0.1% methylene blue irrigation at baseline, 1 and 4 weeks; the second received sterile water irrigation (negative control); the third received scaling and root planing; the fourth received a single subgingival application of methylene blue in a slow release device consisting of a biodegradable collagen alginate vicryl composite.

After four weeks, there were no significant differences in the clinical measurements although the gingival index and pocket depth reduced for all groups. Darkground microscopy showed an increase in cocci and a decrease in motile organisms for all groups. There were also reductions in the numbers of spirochaetes and these were statistically significant for both methylene blue by slow release and scaling and root planing. Bacterial cultures showed an increase in the aerobic/anaerobic ratio for all groups with significant changes in both the methylene blue groups and scaling and root planing. Methylene blue, irrigation and slow release also showed significant reductions in the numbers of black-pigmented anaerobics and this was not produced by either water irrigation (negative control) or scaling and root planing. Furthermore, in contrast with scaling and root planing, very few patients complained of discomfort with methylene blue applications.

These results indicate that methylene blue, by raising the redox potential, is able to alter the microflora in the periodontal pocket to one more compatible with periodontal health. In most respects these changes are comparable to those achieved with scaling and root planing but are in some respects better. It has none of the disadvantages associated with the use of antibiotics either given locally or systematically such as the emergence of resistant bacterial strains and the development of hypersensitivity. Methylene blue may therefore have potential as a therapeutic agent in the treatment of chronic periodontitis.

It is not precisely known what dose of methylene blue is necessary in the periodontal pocket for the optimal effect of redox potential. However, *in vitro* studies have shown that *Porphyromonas gingivalis* is killed by the change in redox potential produced by methylene blue at 1.0 mg/ml (Fletcher and Wilson, 1993).

References

Addy, M. (1986) Chlorhexidine compared with other locally delivered antimicrobials. *Journal of Clinical Periodontology* **13**, 957–964

Addy, M., Jenkins, S. and Newcombe, R. (1989) Studies of the effect of toothpaste rinses on plaque regrowth. (1) Influence of surfactants on chlorhexidine efficiency. *Journal of Clinical Periodontology* **16**, 380–384

Ainamo, J., Lie, T., Ellingsen, B.H. *et al.* (1992) Clinical responses to subgingival application of metronidazole 25% gel compared to the effect of subgingival scaling in adult periodontitis. *Journal of Clinical Periodontology* **19**, 723–729

Baker, P. J., Evans, R. T., Coburn, R. A. and Genco, R.J. (1983) Tetracycline and its derivatives strongly bind to and are released from the tooth surface in an active form. *Journal of Periodontology* **54**, 580–585

Christersson, L.A., Albini, B., Zambon, J.J. *et al.* (1987) Tissue localization of *Actinobacillus actinomycetemcomitans* in human periodontitis. (I) Light, immunofluorescence and electronmicroscopic studies. *Journal of Periodontology* **58**, 529–539

Christersson, L.A., Norderyd, O.M. and Puchalasky, C.S. (1993) Topical application of tetracycline-HCl in human periodontitis. *Journal of Clinical Periodontology* **20**, 88–95

Eley, B.M. (1983) Infective endocarditis: a dentist's view. 1. Aetiology and dental treatment. *Cardiology in Practice* **1**(7), 35–38

Finegold, S.M. (1989) Classification and taxonomy of anaerobes. In: Finegold, S.M. and George, W.L. (eds) *Anaerobic Infections in Humans*. San Diego: Academic Press, pp. 23–26

Fletcher, J.M. and Wilson, M. (1993) The effectiveness of a redox agent, methylene blue, on the survival of *Porphyromonas gingivalis in vitro*. *Current Microbiology* **26**, 85–90

Gibson, M.T., Mangat, D., Gagliano, G. *et al.* (1994) Evaluation of the efficiency of a redox agent in the treatment of chronic periodontitis. *Journal of Clinical Periodontology* **21**, 690–700

Goodson, J.M., Haffajee, A.D. and Socransky, S.S. (1979) Periodontal therapy by local delivery of tetracycline. *Journal of Clinical Periodontology* **6**, 83–92

Goodson, J.M., Holborow, D., Dunn, R. *et al.* (1983) Monolithic tetracycline containing fibres for control delivery to periodontal pockets. *Journal of Periodontology* **54**, 575–579

Gordon, J.M., Walker, C.B., Murphy, J.C. *et al.* (1981) Tetracycline levels achievable in gingival crevice fluid and *in vitro* effect on subgingival organisms. Part 1. Concentrations in crevicular fluid after repeated doses. *Journal of Periodontology* **52**, 609–612

Jenkins, S., Addy, M. and Newcombe, R. (1989) Studies of the effect of toothpaste rinses on plaque regrowth (II) Triclosan with and without zinc citrate formulations. *Journal of Clinical Periodontology* **16**, 385–387

Joyston-Bechal, S., Smales, F.C. and Duckworth, R. (1984) Effect of metronidazole on chronic periodontal disease in subjects using a topically applied chlorhexidine gel. *Journal of Clinical Periodontology* **11**, 53–62

Joyston-Bechal, S., Smales, F.C. and Duckworth, R. (1986) A follow-up study 3 years after metronidazole therapy for chronic periodontal disease. *Journal of Clinical Periodontology* **13**, 944–949

Kenney, E.B. and Ash, M. (1969) Oxidation-reduction potential of developing plaque, periodontal pocketing and gingival sulci. *Journal of Periodontology* **40**, 630–633

Klinge, B., Kuvatanasuhati, J., Attström, R. *et al.* (1992a) The effect of topical metronidazole therapy on experimentally-induced periodontitis in the beagle dog. *Journal of Clinical Periodontology* **19**, 702–707

Klinge, B., Attström, R., Karring, T. *et al.* (1992b) Three regimes of topical metronidazole therapy compared with subgingival scaling on periodontal pathology in adults. *Journal of Clinical Periodontology* **19**, 708–714

Lindhe, J., Heijl, L., Goodson, J.M. and Socransky, S.S. (1979) Local tetracycline delivery using hollow fibre devices in periodontal therapy. *Journal of Clinical Periodontology* **6**, 141–149

Lindhe, J., Liljenberg, B., Adielson, B. and Börjesson, I. (1983) Use of metronidazole as a probe in the study of human periodontal disease. *Journal of Clinical Periodontology* **10**, 100–111

Loesche, W.J., Syed, S.A., Morrison, E.C. *et al.* (1985) Metronidazole in periodontitis (I) Clinical and bacteriological results after 15 to 30 weeks. *Journal of Periodontology* **55**, 325–335

Loesche, W.J., Schmidt, E., Smith, B.A. *et al.* (1991) Effects of metronidazole on periodontal treatment needs. *Journal of Periodontology* **62**, 247–257

Loesche, W.J., Giordano, J.R., Hujoel, P.P. *et al.* (1992) Metronidazole in periodontitis: Reduced needs for surgery. *Journal of Clinical Periodontology* **19**, 103–112

Loesche, W.J., Grossman, N. and Giordano, J.R. (1993) Metronidazole in periodontitis (IV): The effect of patient compliance on treatment parameters. *Journal of Clinical Periodontology* **20**, 96–104

Mandell, R.C., Tripodi, L.S., Savitt, E. *et al.* (1986) The effect of treatment on *Actinobacillus actinomycetemcomitans* in localized juvenile periodontitis. *Journal of Periodontology* **57**, 94–99

Norling, T., Lading, P., Engström, S. *et al.* (1992) Formulation of a drug delivery system based on a mixture of monoglycerides and triglycerides for use in the treatment of periodontal disease. *Journal of Clinical Periodontology* **19**, 687–692

Notten, F., Koek-van Oosten, A. and Mikx, F. (1982) Capillary agar diffusion assay for measuring metronidazole in human gingival crevicular fluid. *Antimicrobial Agents and Chemotherapy* **21**, 836–837

Pedrazzoli, V., Kilian, M. and Karring, T. (1992) Comparative clinical and microbiological effects of topical subgingival application of metronidazole 25% dental gel and scaling in the treatment of adult periodontitis. *Journal of Clinical Periodontology* **19**, 715–722

Rosling, B.G., Slots, J., Webber, R.L. *et al.* (1983) Microbiological and clinical effects of topical subgingival antimicrobial treatment on human periodontal disease. *Journal of Clinical Periodontology* **10**, 487–514

Satomi, A., Vraguchi, R., Ishikawa, I. *et al.* (1987) Minocycline hydrochloride concentration in periodontal pockets after administration of LS-007. *Journal of Japanese Association of Periodontology* **29**, 937–943

Slots, J. and Rosling, B. (1983) Suppression of periodontopathic microflora in localized juvenile periodontitis by systemic tetracycline. *Journal of Clinical Periodontology* **10**, 465–486

Söder, P.Ö., Frithiof, L., Wikner, S. *et al.* (1990) The effect of systemic metronidazole after non-surgical treatment in moderate and advanced periodontitis in young adults. *Journal of Periodontology* **61**, 281–288

Stoltze, K. and Stellfield, M. (1992) Systemic absorption of metronidazole after application of a 25% metronidazole dental gel. *Journal of Clinical Periodontology* **19**, 693–697

Stoltze, K. (1992) Concentration of metronidazole in periodontal pockets after application of a 25% metronidazole dental gel. *Journal of Clinical Periodontology* **19**, 698–701

Theilade, E. (1986) The non-specific theory in microbial etiology of inflammatory periodontal diseases. *Journal of Clinical Periodontology* **13**, 905–911

Van Palenstein Heldermann, W. H. (1986) Is antibiotic therapy justified in the treatment of human chronic inflammatory periodontal disease? *Journal of Clinical Periodontology* **13**, 932–938

Van Steenberge, D., Bercy, P., Hohl, J. *et al.* (1993) Subgingival minocycline hydrochloride ointment in moderate to severe chronic adult periodontitis: randomised, double-blind, vehicle-controlled, multicentre study. *Journal of Periodontology* **64**, 637–644

Van Winkelhoff, A.J., Rodenberg, A.J., Goené, R.J. *et al.* (1989) Metronidazole plus amoxicillin in the treatment of *Actinobacillus actinomycetemcomitans* associated periodontitis. *Journal of Clinical Periodontology* **16**, 128–131

Walker, C.B., Gordon, J.M., Cornwall, H.A. *et al.* (1981) Gingival crevicular fluid levels of clindamycin compared with its minimal inhibitory concentrations for periodontal bacteria. *Antimicrobial Agents and Chemotherapy* **19**, 867–871

Wilson, M., Gibson, M., Strahan, J.D. and Harvey, M. (1992) A preliminary evaluation of the use of a redox agent in the treatment of periodontal disease. *Journal of Periodontal Research* **27**, 522–527

16

Surgical periodontal treatment

Introduction

As described in Chapter 14, there are limitations to what can be achieved by subgingival scaling and root planing. Increased relationships, and the presence of defective restorations especially overhanging margins, limit what can be accomplished by this 'blind' procedure. It has been claimed that a pocket depth of about 5 mm represents the limit for efficient debridement, but there is much debate about this. Many studies have compared the results of surgical (open) and non-surgical (closed) procedures (among them, Hill *et al.*, 1981; Brayer *et al.*, 1989; Wylam *et al.*, 1993). The Wylam study is especially interesting as it compared the clinical effectiveness of the open and closed techniques on multi-rooted teeth and demonstrated heavy residual deposits in furcations after both procedures; better results were obtained on external root surfaces using the open procedures. These workers state that hand instrumentation alone is inadequate for debridement in furcations, and they suggest that ultrasonic instrumentation or rotating burrs are necessary. Kaldahl *et al.* (1993) have reviewed over twenty longitudinal studies that compared the results of surgical and non-surgical treatment, and they conclude that:

1. Both surgical and non-surgical procedures produce improvement in clinical parameters, i.e. gingival inflammation and bleeding, and reduction in pocket depth.

2. Surgical procedures produced greater short-term reduction in probing depth, but long-term results were mixed.

3. Comparison of those surgical procedures that did not include manipulation of alveolar bone with those that included bone resection showed mixed results.

One must conclude from the very mixed results of so many studies that much rests on:

1. The appropriateness of the technique used to the pathological situation. This highlights the crucial nature of precise diagnosis and the identification of all the factors involved in the production of the lesion.

2. The competence of the operator in executing different procedures.

3. The production of a tissue anatomy which facilitates the patient's home care efforts which, whatever the operator may do, remain central to long-term success.

The type of surgical treatment necessary depends upon the form of the lesion, which can be described as:

1. Simple or suprabony, in which all the walls of the lesion are in soft tissue and are uncomplicated by mucogingival problems.

2. Intrabony lesions where the base of the pocket is apical to the bone margin and therefore one or more of the pocket walls are bounded by bone.

3. Pockets complicated by mucogingival problems such as high muscle attachments or the absence of attached gingiva.

The most difficult lesions to treat are those intrabony defects associated with mucogingival problems and furcation involvement.

Contraindications to surgery

These may be oral or systemic.

1. In patients of advanced age where teeth may last for life without resort to radical treatment. Procedures indicated in someone of 60 may not be justified in someone of 70.
2. The presence of systemic disease, such as severe cardiovascular disease, malignancy, kidney and liver disease, blood diseases and bleeding disorders, uncontrolled diabetes, etc. Consultation with the patient's physician is essential.
3. Where thorough subgingival scaling and conscientious home care will remove or control the lesion.
4. Where patient motivation is obviously inadequate.
5. In the presence of acute infection.
6. Where the postoperative appearance would be so poor as to cause patient distress.
7. Where the prognosis is so poor that tooth loss is inevitable.

Some situations may require delay or special preoperative attention. An inadequately controlled diabetic patient will need to be stabilized. Surgery in the pregnant patient is best delayed until after parturition, except where acute lesions develop.

Patients with a history of valvular disease, open heart surgery and hip prostheses must have preoperative antibiotic cover (*see* Chapter 15). Patients on various drugs, anticoagulants, steroids and antidepressants require special attention as directed by their physician. A thorough medical history is always essential.

Preparation for surgery

Patients should have completed basic treatment and reassessment and have good oral hygiene before being considered for surgery. They must be provided with information about what surgery can achieve in their case, about prognosis, limitations or complications and the problems of the postoperative period.

Information also must be provided about the available anaesthesia and analgesia. The most common method of organization of the surgery is to carry this out in stages on sections of the mouth, either a segment or quadrant at one time, under local anaesthesia in the dental chair. Where full-mouth surgery is required this will involve the patient in several procedures over many weeks. Alternatively, full-mouth surgery can be carried out under general anaesthesia in hospital. As full-mouth surgery can be an extremely lengthy procedure, involving a long general anaesthetic, postoperative overnight stay in hospital is recommended. A third option, where several surgical stages are to be avoided, is to carry out surgery under local anaesthesia plus intravenous sedation. Whichever of the alternatives is used depends on patient preference, their emotional state, work and domestic commitments. Comprehensive information and discussion are essential to meet the patient's needs.

Periodontal surgical techniques

The aims of periodontal surgery are:

1. To arrest the progress of periodontal disease and prevent its recurrence, and
2. To attempt to produce regeneration of tissue destroyed in the disease.

Thus, the various surgical techniques may also be divided into these same two groups. These are:

1. Those that are limited to eliminating disease and producing conditions which obviate against its recurrence. These can be further divided into two subgroups:
   i. Procedures aimed at pocket elimination or reduction:
      • Gingivectomy
      • Inverse bevel gingivectomy
      • Apical reposition flap.
   ii. Procedure to expose the root surface for open scaling and root planing:
      • replaced flap (modified Widman flap)
   This procedure should produce a long junctional epithelium.
2. Those that eliminate disease and also aim to produce regeneration of periodontal tissue which has been destroyed by disease, and thereby produce increased attachment level:
   • Guided tissue regeneration (GTR)
   • Bone grafting

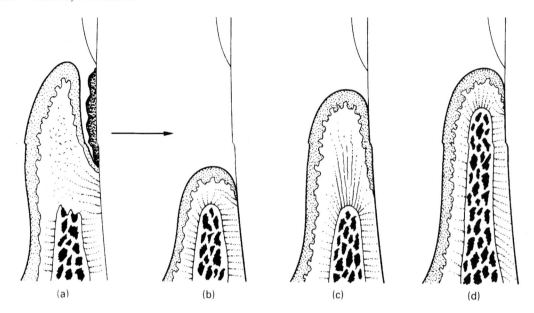

Figure 16.1 (*a*) Periodontal lesion; (*b*) The result of radical elimination of the lesion, e.g. by gingivectomy or apically repositioned flap; (*c*) The result of less radical procedure with long epithelial attachment; (*d*) Regeneration of alveolar bone plus fibrous attachment

In this context it is important to distinguish two forms of healing:

  i. The adherence of a long junctional epithelium to the root surface so that clinical probing depth may be reduced.
 ii. The formation of new connective tissue attachment consisting of periodontal ligament fibres embedded into bone and cementum.

These end-results are illustrated in *Figure 16.1*.

Simple suprabony pockets can be treated by any of these procedures, choosing whichever is most appropriate. Compound infrabony pockets require access by means of a flap procedure and their treatment is discussed in Chapter 17. Mucogingival problems associated with periodontal pockets which extend close to or beyond the mucogingival junction must be treated by an apically repositioned flap in order to increase the zone of attached gingiva.

Procedures for pocket elimination

Gingivectomy

Gingivectomy is the complete removal of the soft-tissue wall of the pocket.

Indications for gingivectomy

1. The presence of suprabony pockets >5 mm which persist despite repeated subgingival scaling and root planing and conscientious home care, and where gingivectomy would leave an adequate zone of attached gingiva.
2. The presence of persistent gingival swelling where 'real' pocketing may be shallow but there is considerable gingival enlargement and deformity. If the gingival tissue is fibrous, gingivectomy may be the treatment most likely to produce a satisfactory result.
3. The presence of furcation involvement (without associated bone defects) where there is a wide zone of attached gingiva.
4. A gingival abscess, i.e. an abscess contained entirely by soft tissue.
5. A pericoronal flap.

Gingivectomy is a radical procedure which has been largely replaced by more conservative flap techniques. However, it remains the treatment of choice where recontouring of deformed tissue is needed, and where access and a precise and predictable anatomy are required to facilitate restorative treatment.

The procedure is given in detail as it provides a model for other surgical procedures.

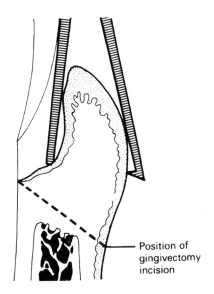

— Position of
gingivectomy
incision

Figure 16.2 Pocket-marking forceps defining the
approximate depth of the pocket. Note that the position
of the gingivectomy incision is apical to the marking and
that the angle of the incision is about 45°

Procedure

Pocket marking For complete removal of the
pocket wall the apical limit of the pocket must
be identified and marked using either pocket
marking forceps (*Figure 16.2*) or a periodontal
probe. A series of such markings on both facial
and lingual gingivae provides a guide for
gingivectomy incision.

The gingivectomy incision The incision can be
made with several knives: e.g. Swann–Morton
Nos 12 or 15 on a conventional scalpel handle;
the Blake knife which uses disposable blades;
special gingivectomy knives, such as the
Kirkland, Orban or Goldman–Fox knives which
have to be sharpened. The choice of knife is
entirely personal but where possible the use of
disposable blades is to be recommended.

The incision must be made apical to the
markings, i.e. apical to the base of the pocket,
and at an angle of 45° so that the blade
completely perforates the gingiva to the base
of the pocket (*Figure 16.2*). A continuous
incision (*not* an interrupted scalloped incision)
which follows the base of the pockets is made.
The correct incision will both remove the
pocket wall and produce a streamlined tissue
contour; if the incision is too flat the postoperative contour will be unsatisfactory. The

most common fault is to incise in a coronal
position so that the base of the pocket wall is
retained with the possibility of disease recurrence. Following the bevelled incisions,
horizontal incisions are made between each
interdental space, with a No. 12 blade on a
conventional scalpel handle, in order to
separate the remaining interdental wedges of
tissue.

Tissue removal If the incision has completely
separated the pocket wall from the underlying
tissue, the pocket wall can be removed easily
with a large curette or scaler, e.g. the Cumine
scaler. Remnants of fibrous connective tissue
and granulation tissue are removed thoroughly
with sharp curettes to reveal the root surface.
Efficient suction is essential but once granulations have been removed bleeding reduces
significantly.

Root scaling and planing The root surfaces
should be inspected for evidence of residual
calculus deposits and where necessary the root
surfaces should be scaled and root planed.

If necessary, further trimming and reshaping
of the gingivae can be carried out using
scalpel, fine scissors or diathermy. Sterile
swabs are placed over the wound to control
bleeding so that the periodontal dressing can
be applied to a relatively dry wound area.

The periodontal dressing A dressing to cover
the wound serves a number of purposes:

1. To protect the wound from irritation.
2. To keep the wound clean.
3. To control bleeding.
4. To control exuberant granulation tissue
   production.

The dressing thereby promotes healing and
provides postoperative comfort.

The requirements of a satisfactory periodontal dressing are as follows:

1. It should be non-irritant and should not
   induce an allergic response.
2. It should be adaptable to the teeth and
   tissues and flow between the teeth so that
   it is well retained. A slow setting-time
   allows manipulation.
3. It should exclude food and saliva.
4. It should have antibacterial properties to
   inhibit bacterial growth.

5. It should set fairly hard so that it is not easily displaced.
6. Its taste should be acceptable.

It is essential to apply the dressing carefully so that it covers the wound and fills the interdental spaces completely. It should be muscle trimmed by movement of the cheeks, lips and tongue, and all excess dressing on occlusal surfaces removed.

A number of dressings based on zinc-oxide–eugenol are available but many people find the taste of eugenol unacceptable and some reports of contact allergy to eugenol have been made. For these reasons eugenol-free dressings have been devised, e.g. Coe-Pack, Peripak, Septopak. These are easy to apply and well tolerated by the patients.

Postoperative care

It is very important to provide the patient with comprehensive information about postoperative care. The following advice in writing should be given.

1. Avoid eating or drinking for one hour.
2. Avoid hot drinks and alcohol for 24 hours. Do not rinse mouth for first day.
3. Avoid eating hard, sharp or sticky foods and eat on the unoperated side.
4. Take an analgesic if there is pain when the anaesthetic wears off. Aspirin is contraindicated for 24 hours.
5. Use warm saline mouthwashes after the first day. A 0.2% chlorhexidine mouthwash is used morning and night as mechanical plaque control is not possible. This can be used on the first day provided it is not swished around the mouth. Tea, coffee and smoking should be avoided when using a chlorhexidine mouthwash to reduce staining.
6. If there is bleeding, exert pressure on the dressing for 15 minutes with a clean, boiled handkerchief; do not rinse; contact the surgery if the bleeding does not stop.
7. Use the toothbrush only on unoperated parts of the mouth.
8. If the immediate postoperative phase is uneventful but pain and swelling occur 2 or 3 days later, report immediately to the surgery.

A postoperative antibiotic is only prescribed in certain cases, e.g. a diabetic or any individual who may be debilitated. For routine purposes the dressing is usually removed after one week. All debris must be completely removed and the wound irrigated with warm water. If the wound is not sufficiently well epithelialized and is tender, a new dressing is applied for a further week.

After the dressing has been removed, further instruction in home care is needed. The chlorhexidine mouthwash can be used morning and night for a further week only, as prolonged use will cause staining which is very difficult to remove. The patient is encouraged to start gentle toothbrushing with a soft toothbrush in warm water that evening. Either a gentle roll or Charter's technique is used at this stage. The Bass technique and interdental cleaning are avoided for a week. The patient is advised to avoid cold and hard food.

After 2 weeks the wound is inspected and the teeth cleaned. The patient's oral hygiene must be reviewed until entirely satisfactory and the healing is complete, after which a 3–6 monthly recall regime, as appropriate, is established.

Healing after gingivectomy

The connective tissue wound is covered by a blood clot. The area beneath this undergoes a brief phase of acute inflammation, which is followed by demolition and organization. Epithelial cells migrate from the edge of the wound beneath the clot. They cover the wound in 7–14 days and keratinize in 2–3 weeks. The formation of a new epithelial attachment may take as long as 4 weeks. Good oral hygiene is essential during the healing period.

The limitations and drawbacks of gingivectomy

1. The gingivectomy procedure creates an open wound which heals by secondary intention.
2. Tissue is wasted which could be used to close the wound and obtain healing by primary intention.
3. Alveolar bone defects are not revealed and therefore cannot be treated adequately.
4. The zone of attached gingiva may be eliminated.
5. The clinical crown may be lengthened considerably and in the front of the mouth this may be unsightly and unacceptable to

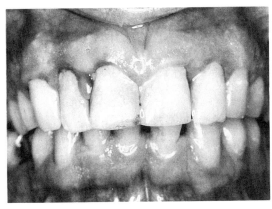

(a)

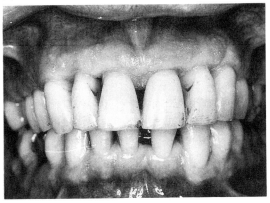

(b)

Figure 16.3 (*a*) Before gingivectomy; (*b*) after gingivectomy, showing the increase in clinical crown length

the patient. It is important to explain before surgery that 'the teeth will look longer' (*Figure 16.3*).

6. Exposed root may be sensitive. Some sensitivity to cold and sweet immediately after gingivectomy is extremely common but this symptom is usually transient. If it persists it will require the use of desensitizing agents (*see* pp. 216–217).

Despite the above limitations the gingivectomy technique has a place in periodontal treatment. It is extremely easy to carry out and gives an excellent result in the appropriate cases.

Flap techniques

The flap techniques have several obvious advantages over gingivectomy:

1. They allow access to the root and alveolar bone.
2. Tissue is conserved which can be used to close the wound.
3. The soft tissues can be manipulated if necessary to achieve an improved soft tissue morphology.

In raising a flap certain basic requirements must be satisfied:

1. The flap must be big enough to expose any underlying bone defects.
2. The base of the flap must be wide enough to maintain an adequate blood supply.
3. The incisions must allow movement of the flap without tension.
4. No important vessels or nerves should be damaged in raising the flap.

There are three basic flap shapes:

1. The full flap made by a gingival incision and two releasing incisions.
2. The triangular flap with a gingival incision and one releasing incision.
3. The modified flap with only a gingival incision and no releasing incisions.

Flaps have also been divided into two types:

1. A full-thickness flap, which consists of the complete mucoperiosteum and is raised by a periosteal elevator.
2. The split-thickness flap, in which the gingiva is dissected from the underlying periosteum which is left on the bone. This type of flap is more difficult to raise and its use is restricted to special situations described below.

Flaps are further divided into those which are raised and replaced into their original position, and flaps which are moved into apical, coronal or lateral positions.

Flap procedures used to treat chronic periodontitis are described below.

The replaced flap (modified Widman technique)

The debate about 'open' and 'closed' approaches to subgingival scaling and root planing represents the most recent aspect of a historical conflict in periodontics between the conservative and radical approaches to treatment. In the early part of this century, as a reaction to gingivectomy, a mucoperiosteal flap approach to the periodontal lesion was described by Neuman (1912) and Widman (1918). This technique involved raising a full-thickness flap which , after scaling and root planing, was replaced in its original position to produce a closed wound which was more comfortable and healed more rapidly than the open wound produced by gingivectomy.

Morris (1965) introduced the internal bevel incision which separated the pocket wall from the rest of the mucoperiosteal flap and produced a healthy, thin and flexible margin to the flap. This was used by Ramford and Nissle (1974) in what they called the 'modified Widman flap' procedure, which allowed open access to the periodontal lesion and then much closer adaptation of the replaced flap to the tooth surface than had been possible with the unmodified full-thickness flap. The flap approach also allows access to alveolar bone defects (Chapter 17). A further advantage is that there is less postoperative root exposure than after gingivectomy, which is especially important in the front of the mouth.

When introduced it was thought that the technique would produce a physiological dentogingival junction, and therefore lead to permanent pocket elimination, but this is not possible (Caton and Nyman, 1980).

The long junctional epithelium produced by this procedure is inherently less stable than the physiological junctional epithelium and demands much higher standards of plaque control and higher frequencies of recall for maintenance than pocket elimination procedures.

However, it has been shown that this technique can successfully treat and stabilize cases with moderate and advanced chronic periodontitis. There have been many longitudinal studies, over periods ranging from 2 to 6 years, which have compared non-surgical and surgical treatment techniques including both replaced and pocket elimination flap techniques (Pihlstrom *et al.*, 1983; Ramfjord *et al.*, 1987). These all show that both non-surgical scaling/root planing and surgical replaced flap/pocket elimination techniques can effectively control moderate to advanced chronic periodontitis, preventing further attachment loss. However, all of these workers used regular and often long maintenance visits at intervals of 3 months or less throughout the

period of study; this factor could have been at least as important as the technique itself in preventing relapse. The effect of maintenance in preventing deterioration following treatment has been clearly shown in a number of studies (Nyman *et al.*, 1975). These studies also showed that cases with deep pockets needed retreatment more often when treated with scaling alone. This is consistent with reports that residual deposits of subgingival calculus are commonly left in deep pockets following subgingival scaling and that this is significantly less common when surgical techniques are used (Chapter 14). Therefore this would seem to justify the use of periodontal flap techniques for open scaling and root planing which is the main purpose of the replaced flap technique.

Procedure

1. Incision An inverse bevel incision is made up to 1 mm from the gingival margin on both the facial and lingual sides of either the upper or lower arches. The aim of this incision, as with other flap techniques, is to separate the pockt epithelium and inflamed connective tissue (cervical wedge) from the flap (*Figure 16.4a*). No vertical relieving incisions are made unless necessary for reflection purposes. Two further incisions were described by Ramfjord and Nissle (1974). The first is an incision made from the base of the pocket to the bone crest. The second, which is made after flap reflection, is a horizontal incision made from the crest of the bone to the tooth surface. The purpose of these additional incisions is to allow the cervical wedge to be removed easily and to minimize damage to the underlying periodontal ligament. These incisions are not totally necessary and obviously serve no purpose if infrabony defects are present which have to be curetted.

Another suggested modification is to exaggerate the scalloping of the palatal inverse bevel incision in order to lengthen the interdental papillae so that they completely cover the interdental space on closure.

2. Reflection of flap A full-thickness mucoperiosteal flap is reflected with a periodontal elevator in order to expose the roots of the teeth and the bone margin (*Figure 16.4b*).

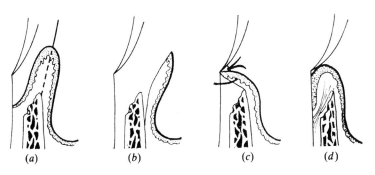

Figure 16.4 Diagram to show the replaced flap procedure: (*a*) inverse bevel incision; (*b*) the flap is reflected to reveal the alveolar margin; (*c*) the flap is replaced and sutured in its original position; (*d*) long junctional epithelium following healing

3. Curettage, scaling and root planing The cervical wedge is removed and the root surfaces are scaled and root planed. Great care should be taken with this process as a totally clean and smooth root surface is necessary to ensure that the long junctional epithelium, which will form following healing, will adhere to it. Failure of this adherence will lead to the re-establishment of pocketing. Any bony craters and deeper defects should be totally cleared of granulation tissue to create the best conditions for bone regeneration (Chapter 17).

4. Suturing The flaps are then replaced in their original position and secured by tight interdental suturing (*Figure 16.4c*). Every effort is made to ensure total interdental coverage and to avoid any root exposure. There is no need to place a periodontal dressing as it has no supporting function in this procedure. However, it can be placed if required for patient comfort and in this case it need cover only the gingival margin.

5. Postoperative management Postoperative instructions are the same as those for the gingivectomy. Postoperative swelling with this procedure is usually slight because of the smaller amount of flap retraction involved. Sutures are removed after a week and the chlorhexidine mouthwash is continued for a further week. Brushing is started with an extra soft brush. Flossing is usually started a week postoperatively, although some discretion needs to be exercised in this regard. It must be carried out with great care to avoid gingival trauma. The patient should be seen every 4 weeks until healing is complete and plaque control perfect. Maintenance visits will be necessary every 3 months thereafter as the long junctional epithelium is more liable to breakdown and a very careful check must be kept for pockets reforming. This procedure is likely to be more stable around single-rooted anterior teeth since they are more accessible for home care and for professional maintenance. Posterior teeth are likely to be complicated by furcation involvements which are extremely difficult to maintain if situated subgingivally.

6. Healing Following acute inflammation healing will begin by the organization of the blood clot between the flap and the tooth into granulation tissue. This is then slowly replaced by collagenous connective tissue over the next 2–5 weeks. Epithelium proliferates over the connective-tissue wound to its preoperative position. If the root surface is free of irritant the long junctional epithelium can adhere to it. However, the longer the junctional epithelium, the more unstable this situation becomes and the greater the risk for the re-establishment of pocketing. A mature long epithelial attachment may take several weeks to form and care should be taken not to disrupt it by probing during this period. Quite frequently gingival recession will occur following replaced flaps and this has the effect of both producing some root exposure and reducing the length of the long junctional epithelium (*Figure 16.4d*).

Root conditioning with citric acid

Recently a fresh approach to obtaining new connective tissue attachment has been attempted using citric acid conditioning of the root surface (Polson and Proye, 1982). Root cementum is first removed from the affected part of the root by planing with curettes. Citric acid at pH 1 is then applied to the dentine surface for 3 minutes. The superficial zone of the dentine becomes demineralized, leading to the exposure of collagen fibrils in the matrix. It has been claimed that a connective tissue attachment will reform by the interdigitation of new and existing collagen fibres on the root surface but if this occurs at all the amount is limited. The usual result is the development of a long junctional epithelium and this method does not therefore seem to offer any advantage over flap techniques alone (Moore *et al.*, 1987).

Apically repositioned flap

This procedure was first described by Friedman in 1962. It is indicated for the elimination of periodontal pocketing and increasing the zone of attached gingiva. Pocketing separates the attached gingiva from the tooth and deep pockets may extend below the mucogingival junction, i.e. through the whole width of the attached gingiva. In these circumstances gingivectomy techniques would leave either a narrow zone of attached gingiva or none at all and are contraindicated. Replaced flap techniques (*see* above) cannot increase the zone of attached gingiva and are thus not indicated for pockets extending to or beyond the mucogingival junction.

The apically repositioned flap achieves pocket elimination by moving the flap in an apical direction. Adequate mobility of the flap is necessary for this and is obtained by extending the releasing incisions to the base of the vestibule and further dissection of the flap from the underlying tissues. Apical repositioning will leave the flap just covering the alveolar crest, thus eliminating the pocketing. During healing the merging of the connective tissue on the inner surface of the flap with the bone will recreate a mucoperiosteal attached gingival zone.

Procedure

1. Incisions Two vertical releasing incisions are made through to bone at either end of the operative area. They should be made mesial or

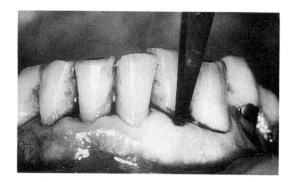

Figure 16.5 Position of blade for inverse bevel incision. The incision is discontinuous and scalloped, following the contour of each tooth

distal to the last interdental periodontal pocket to be treated and must not be positioned interdentally. They should be parallel to each other and should extend into the alveolar mucosa at the base of the vestibule.

An inverse bevel incision is made along the gingival margin (*Figure 16.5*). It should start up to 1 mm from the gingival margin and extend down to the crest of the alveolar bone (*Figure 16.6a*). It is discontinuous and scalloped around the neck of each tooth and may be made in two stages, a superficial outlining incision and deepening incision. This allows the interdental papilla to be deflected outwards when making the deepening incision, which allows the blade to be angled more acutely. The aim of these incisions is to separate the pocket lining and inflamed connective tissue from the inner wall of the flap. This tissue is left on the surface of the tooth when the flap is raised and is referred to as the cervical wedge.

In the lower jaw care should be taken lingually with the distal relieving incision to ensure that there is no risk to the lingual nerve. Care should also be taken not to damage or bruise the submandibular ducts in raising the flap. Palatal gingiva is treated by means of an inverse bevel gingivectomy incision, as obviously palatal tissue cannot be apically positioned. The angle of the incision can be varied according to the thickness of the tissue and may be used to fillet out hyperplastic tissue.

2. Raising the flap A periosteal elevator is used to separate attached gingiva from the alveolar process so that a full-thickness flap is

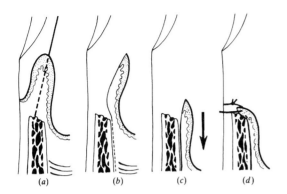

Figure 16.6 The apically repositioned flap procedure: (*a*) inverse bevel incision; (*b*) the flap is reflected and dissected from the alveolar process, so that (*c*) it can be moved in an apical direction; (*d*) the flap is sutured in an apical position, just covering the bone margin

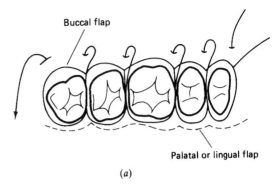

Buccal flap

Palatal or lingual flap

(*a*)

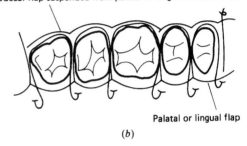

Buccal flap suspended from palatal or lingual root surfaces

Palatal or lingual flap

(*b*)

Figure 16.7 Diagram to show the continuous suspensory suturing technique: (*a*) a single tie is made at the anterior papilla and the buccal flap is suspended from the lingual root surfaces; (*b*) following adjustment of the apical position the palatal or lingual flap is suspended against the buccal root surfaces. The suture is tied off at the end left on the single tie at the anterior papilla

lifted (*Figure 16.6b*). It should peel away easily from the tooth and bone and clearly separate from the cervical wedge. If it does not separate easily the marginal inverse bevel incision should be deepened.

The flap may be released in two stages, the first just to expose the bone to allow curettage and the second to detach the flap further, just before apical positioning. In this way bone exposure is reduced to the minimum.

In the case of upper teeth, the palatal tissue is raised to expose the margin of the bone and to give sufficient access for the removal of the large wedge of tissue produced by the inverse bevel gingivectomy incision.

3. Removing the cervical wedge and granulation tissue The separated cervical wedge is removed with curettes and scalers. All granulation tissue attached to the tooth surface, bone margin or within bone defects should be carefully and comprehensively curetted away to leave a clean tooth and bone surface. Efficient aspiration is necessary to ensure good visibility. Bleeding will reduce dramatically when this tissue has been removed. The treatment of infrabony pocketing and furcation involvement is discussed in Chapter 17.

4. Root scaling and planing The exposed roots must be scaled to remove any residual calculus and planed.

5. Apical repositioning The flap is reflected to the base of the vestibule: Once released the

flap tends to contract and fold up so that apical positioning often takes place spontaneously. One should ensure that the flap is displaced apically so that its edge just covers the alveolar crest (*Figure 16.6c*).

6. Suturing It is important to be sure that the flap is not pulled coronally when suturing. Sutures should be placed first at the mesial and distal vertical incisions. The suture should be placed near to the margin of the free flap and sufficiently apically on the attached gingiva of the fixed tissue to ensure the degree of apical positioning required.

The margin of the flap can be secured with either loose separate interdental sutures or by means of a continuous suspensory suture (*Figure 16.7a,b*). Continuous suspensory suturing is useful in allowing manipulation of the flap margin where the bone margin is irregular and where the width of attached gingiva varies. Care should be taken not to pull the suture too tight as this will drag the flap coronally. The tension on the suture can be adjusted at each loop, rather like loosening or tightening the lace of a shoe. The tension should be adjusted so that the flap margin just covers the bone margin (*Figure 16.6d*). It must be remembered that the continuous suture does not hold the flap in an apical position but simply suspends it from the necks of the teeth. The degree of apical positioning will be maintained by the correct placement of the periodontal pack.

7. Placing the periodontal dressing   It is usual to use Coe-Pack. Close adaptation of the flap to the underlying bone can be assured by pressing damp swabs over the flap while the periodontal dressing is being mixed. The dressing must be placed when it is freely mouldable. It should occupy the area between the flap margin and the crowns of the teeth so that it prevents any coronal displacement of the flap. It should also extend down to the base of the vestibular to maintain the vestibular depth and should be carefully muscle trimmed.

8. Healing   The inner surface of the flap in contact with the bone and tooth undergoes inflammation, demolition, organization and healing. The blood clot, which should be thin, is replaced by granulation tissue in about a week. This matures into collagenous connective tissue in 2–5 weeks. The inner surface of the flap will unite with the bone to produce a mucoperiosteum which increases the attached gingival zone. About 2 days after surgery the epithelium will begin to proliferate from the flap margin over the connective tissue wound. It will migrate apically at the rate of 0.5 mm per day to produce a new junctional epithelium. As the margin of the flap just covers the bone this will be of physiological length. A mature epithelial attachment takes about 4 weeks to form. Some resorption of the alveolar bone margin will occur as the result of raising a flap but with careful management this will be in the order of 0.5 mm. Connective tissue attachment will reform between the marginal tissues and the root cementum from the bone margin to the base of the junctional epithelium. It will prevent further apical migration of the junctional epithelium.

9. Postoperative care   The postoperative care is the same as for gingivectomy. The patient should however be additionally warned of facial swelling. This will develop over the first 3 postoperative days and then slowly reduce. The dressing and sutures are removed after one week and the chlorhexidine mouthwash is usually discontinued a further week after this. The patient should be encouraged to return to normal brushing and flossing as soon as possible and certainly no longer than 7 days after suture removal. An extra soft toothbrush should be used for 2–3 weeks. Particular care is necessary with plaque control during the first few weeks after surgery since the tissues will be healing during this period and are particularly vulnerable to damage. Modification of these regimes must be made to take into account individual variation in healing.

Careful maintenance is necessary after this procedure. However, once immaculate plaque control is achieved recall periods can be extended to 6 months as all pockets have been eliminated and a physiological length of junctional epithelium results.

Because apical repositioned flaps are often carried out in cases where bone loss is quite advanced, it is inevitable that the clinical crown will be lengthened. Patients must be warned of this beforehand.

This procedure can give excellent long-term results providing that good oral hygiene is carried out by the patient and regular maintenance is carried by the dentist and hygienist.

Comparison of apical repositioning and replaced flap techniques

It can be seen from the foregoing that the apically repositioned flap results in pocket elimination and the formation of a normal or physiological length of junctional epithelium whereas the replaced flap results in the formation of a long junctional epithelium which may adhere to the root surface (*Figure 16.4d*).

A long junctional epithelium must be regarded as inherently unstable because it lacks the mechanical support of gingival fibres passing into it from the crest of the bone and adjacent cementum. The stability of the delicate biological seal between the junctional epithelium and the root would seem to depend on a very high standard of oral hygiene and frequent regular maintenance visits. If any

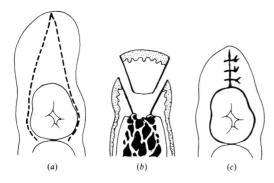

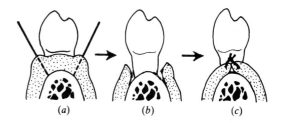

Figure 16.9 The treatment of an edentulous ridge is similar to the distal wedge. (*a*) Incisions mark out flabby ridge tissue which is removed (*b*). The wound is sutured (*c*)

Figure 16.8 Diagram to illustrate distal wedge dissection of a tuberosity: (*a*) incision lines; (*b*) vertical section to show the wedge of tissue; (*c*) wound sutured

plaque is allowed to mature at the margin there is the risk that subgingival plaque will become re-established and will proliferate apically to detach the epithelium and reform the pocket.

The result of an apically repositioned flap is much more stable since pockets are eliminated and the dentogingival junction is normal. This is particularly important for posterior teeth with furcation involvement.

Treatment of the tuberosity

The maxillary tuberosity may be large, flabby, unsupported by bone and related to a distal pocket on the last molar. It can be removed by making a radical gingivectomy incision but this creates a large open wound which bleeds readily, can be painful and heals slowly. The retromolar pad in the lower jaw can present similar problems. Both situations can be dealt with by using the 'distal wedge' technique (*Figure 16.8*). Facial and lingual incisions are made through the tuberosity or retromolar pad to form a triangular wedge. The incisions must be deep enough to allow clean separation of the soft-tissue wedge from the underlying bone. When the wedge is removed, any loose tags of tissue are trimmed and the distal root surface of the adjacent tooth cleaned. The edges of the wound are then sutured and the wound closed as completely as possible.

This procedure works well where the tissue is firm and fibrous, as it usually is with the maxillary tuberosity. However, it may be difficult or impossible to produce the desired result in the lower retromolar area when the tissue is soft and flabby.

Treatment of the edentulous ridge

If teeth involved in surgery are adjacent to an edentulous ridge that is covered by fibrous or flabby tissue, this can be removed by gingivectomy but the situation is better managed using a flap technique. Inverse bevel incisions are continued from around the teeth along the facial and lingual aspects of the edentulous ridge to dissect out a wedge of tissue with its base on the bone. This wedge of tissue is removed with curettes from the surface of the ridge. Then the edges of the flaps are trimmed and sutured (*Figure 16.9*). The apical movement of the flaps will remove soft-tissue pocketing mesial and distal to the two bordering teeth.

References

Brayer, W.K., Mellonig, J.T., Dunlap, R.M. *et al.* (1989) Scaling and root planing effectiveness: The effect of root surface access and operator experience. *Journal of Periodontology* **60**, 67–72

Caton, J. and Nyman, S. (1980) Histometric evaluation of periodontal surgery. 1. The modified Widman flap procedure. *Journal of Clinical Periodontology* **7**, 212–223

Caton, J., Nyman, S. and Zander, H. (1980) Histometric evaluation of periodontal surgery. II. Connective tissue attachment levels after four regenerative procedures. *Journal of Clinical Periodontology* **7**, 224–231

Friedman, N. (1962) Mucogingival surgery: the apically repositioned flap. *Journal of Periodontology* **33**, 328–340

Hill, R.W., Ramfjord, S.P., Morrison, E.C. *et al.* (1981) Four types of periodontal treatment compared over two years. *Journal of Periodontology* **52**, 655–662

Kaldahl, W.B., Kalkwarf, K.L. and Patil, K.D. (1993) A review of longitudinal studies that compared periodontal therapies. *Journal of Periodontology* **64**, 243–253

Lindhe, J. and Nyman, S. (1984) Long-term maintenance of patients treated for advanced periodontal disease. *Journal of Clinical Periodontology* **11**, 504–514

Moore, J.A., Ashley, F.P. and Waterman, C.A. (1984) The effect on healing of the application of citric acid during replaced flap surgery. *Journal of Clinical Periodontology* **14**, 130–135

Morris, M.L. (1965) The unrepositioned mucoperiosteal flap. *Periodontics* **3**, 141–151

Neumann, R. (1912) *Die Alveolar-Pyorrhea und ihre Behandlung.* Berlin: H. Meusser

Nyman, S., Rosling, B. and Lindhe, J. (1975) Effect of professional tooth cleaning after periodontal surgery. *Journal of Clinical Periodontology* **2**, 80–86

Pihlstrom, B.L., McHugh, R.B., Oliphant, T.H. and Ortiz-Campos, C. (1983) Comparison of surgical and non surgical treatment of periodontal disease. A review of current studies and additional results after 6.5 years. *Journal of Clinical Periodontology* **10**, 524–541

Polson, A.M. and Proye, M.P. (1982) Effect of root surface alterations on periodontal healing. II. Citric acid treatment of the denuded root. *Journal of Clinical Periodontology* **9**, 441–454

Ramfjord, S.P. and Nissle, R.R. (1974) The modified Widman flap. *Journal of Periodontology* **45**, 601–607

Ramfjord, S.P., Caffesse, R.G., Morrison, E.C. *et al.* (1987) 4 modalities of periodontal treatment compared over 5 years. *Journal of Clinical Periodontology* **14**, 445–452

Widman, L. (Dec. 1918) The operative treatment of pyorrhea alveolaris. A new surgical method. *Svensk Tandlakare-Tidskrift* (special issue)

Wylam, J.M., Mealey, B.L., Mills, M.P. *et al.* (1993) The clinical effectiveness of open versus closed scaling and root planing on multi-rooted teeth. *Journal of Periodontology* **64**, 1023–1028

17

Management of bone defects and furcation involvement

As the periodontal lesion advances the alveolar crest is resorbed and cancellous spaces are opened up. To compensate for resorption some deposition may take place at sites more distant from the inflammation. The result of this remodelling process is the formation of bone defects or 'intrabony' defects of an infinite number of shapes. In Chapter 8 these have been classified as marginal defects, intra-alveolar defects, furcation defects and perforations, and can be further subdivided according to the number of bone walls bounding the defect.

The objectives of treatment of these defects are:

1. To eliminate the periodontal lesion.
2. To achieve a tissue shape which will allow the patient to carry out efficient plaque control.
3. If possible to obtain some bone formation, increase in tooth attachment and improved tooth support.

Careful radiographic examination is essential to diagnosis but even good radiographs may not reveal the presence of a bone defect or its precise morphology. This limitation can be overcome only by direct examination of the alveolar process and all bone lesions are approached by lifting full-thickness mucoperiosteal flaps. In all cases granulations are curetted and root surfaces planed clean. When these procedures have been carried out it

should be possible to examine the alveolar crest, define the morphology of any bone defect and decide on the mode of treatment.

Three basic options are available:

1. To shape the bone so that after healing and remodelling the resultant alveolar architecture will allow effective oral hygiene measures to be carried out (*Figure 17.1a*). This procedure, osteoplasty, must be undertaken with great care. Attempts to impose a stereotype of 'normal anatomy' are not justified. Cutting bone induces subsequent bone resorption so that the final result could be loss of tooth support. Therefore osteoplasty should be resorted to only where gross bone deformity is present, e.g. buccal ledges often associated with craters which extend into furcation areas.
2. To attempt to obtain some fill-in of the bone defect. This may be achieved with or without bone graft (*Figure 17.1b*).
3. To attempt to obtain new connective attachment. To date, this has been obtained only by guided tissue regeneration techniques.

In practice options 1 and 2 are frequently used together depending on the morphology of the bone defect. A three-walled intrabony defect offers a better chance of bony in-fill than a two-walled defect. A narrow, deep defect is more likely to be bridged by bone than a wide, shallow defect.

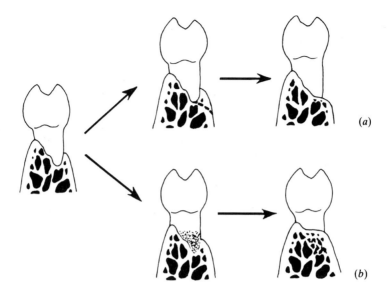

Figure 17.1 A bone defect may be treated by (*a*) bone reshaping to produce a cleanable tissue contour, or (*b*) an attempt to obtain fill-in (with or without graft) and reattachment

Bone reshaping

Osteoplasty is the term used for shaping bone that is not directly attached to the tooth. Ostectomy (osteo-ectomy) is the removal of bone that is directly involved in tooth support. Frequently these two procedures are carried out together. Bone may be removed by chisels or by rotating instruments, burs or diamond stones. If a rotating instrument is not adequately cooled, excessive bone loss may follow. If chisels are used to remove bone, the fragments may be used to fill in the bone defects. Small chisels, e.g. the Ochsenbein chisel, can be used with hand pressure. In attempting to obtain an acceptable bone shape, especially where there is a great deal of bone loss, a compromise must often be made to effect a balance between adequate tooth support and a cleanable tissue shape. No attempt should be made to reproduce some ideal bone architecture as bone remodelling *always* follows surgery.

Bone reshaping is usefully applied to thickened and uneven alveolar margins, to marginal gutters providing they are not very deep, interdental craters and two-walled infrabony defects. When carrying out bone resection the removed fragments may be used as an autograft in an attempt to obtain some fill-in of the defect.

Bone 'swaging' is the name given to a technique whereby a piece of bone is incompletely detached from its base (by a chisel) and swung into a neighbouring bone defect with some of its blood supply maintained. There is some clinical evidence of success following this procedure.

Periodontal tissue regeneration

The term 'reattachment' is used to describe the reunion of root and connective tissue separated by incision or injury and the term 'new attachment' to describe the union of connective tissue with a previously pathogenically altered root surface. The cells with regenerative potential in the periodontal wound are junctional epithelial cells, gingival connective tissue cells, bone cells and periodontal ligament cells. The role of these tissues has been studied by clinical investigations and by the use of animal models, in particular the technique of producing experimental periodontitis in monkey teeth by placing orthodontic elastics into the gingival crevice (Caton and Zander, 1975).

Clinical investigations have shown that:

1. Alveolar bone has good regenerative capacity within two- and three-walled intrabony defects following inverse bevel flap surgery

and curettage to remove all granulation tissue. Claims of success in obtaining bony in-fill of such defects vary greatly from 15% to 70%. These assessments are based, however, upon measurements of clinical attachment levels, radiographic measurements and clinical observation following re-entry procedures, all of which are unreliable to varying degrees (Nyman *et al.*, 1990).

2. Bone regeneration may be encouraged or enhanced by the use of autograft cancellous bone or red bone marrow implants. With the latter material this may be complicated in some cases by root resorption and ankylosis unless it is frozen before use (Nyman *et al.*, 1990).

Melcher (1976) postulated that the cells which populate the root surface after surgery determine the nature of the healing process. These tissues will now be considered separately.

1. Junctional epithelium Junctional epithelium has a high regenerative capacity and will rapidly proliferate over the connective tissue wound surface. Using the monkey, Caton *et al.* (1980) studied the effect of four surgical procedures on the healing of experimental periodontal lesions: (i) root planing and curettage; (ii) replaced flap and curettage; (iii) replaced flap followed by implantation of previously frozen autograft red marrow and (iv) replaced flap followed by implantation of a bone substitute – beta tricalcium phosphate. They found that all four procedures resulted in the formation of a long junctional epithelium to the presurgical level and extending to the base of the intrabony defects. Where bone regeneration occurred in intrabony defects, which was a frequent occurrence with all the open techniques, the epithelium always interposed itself between the new bone and the root surface. No new connective tissue attachment occurred.

2. Gingival connective tissue and bone The effect of gingival connective tissue and bone on the healthy exposed root surface and the diseased root surface was studied in monkeys by Nyman *et al.* (1990). Extracted, partially periodontally diseased roots were buried below the surface of the edentulous ridge with one surface in contact with gingival connective tissue and one with bone. Reattachment

occurred around the healthy portion of the root but no reattachment occurred around the diseased portion. Both the bone and gingival connective tissue induced resorption of the diseased root surface. These experiments showed that granulation tissue derived from bone or gingival connective tissue does not have the capacity to form new connective tissue attachment to diseased root surfaces. It also shows that in the clinical situation the formation of a long junctional epithelium protects the root surface from resorption.

3. Periodontal ligament cells The fact that new cementum with connective tissue attachment may occasionally form at the most apical portion of the periodontal wound suggests that coronal migration of periodontal ligament cells may be responsible for this (Melcher, 1976). This was confirmed by Nyman *et al.* (1990) using a monkey model which prevented junctional epithelial cells and gingival connective tissue cells from populating the wound. A portion of the buccal root surface of the canine tooth was exposed between the apex and the margin, then root planed to remove the cementum. The preservation of the marginal tissues prevented interference from apical migration of junctional epithelium and the placement of a plastic filter barrier over the bony fenestration prevented ingress of gingival connective tissue cells when the wound was closed. After 3 months new attachment had spread over the root surface from the margins of the fenestration and included new cementum, fibrous attachment and bone. This suggests that periodontal ligament cells have the capacity to develop new attachment if epithelium and gingival connective tissue are excluded from the wound during healing (Nyman *et al.*, 1990).

Methods aimed at the regeneration of periodontal tissues

Curettage for bony in-fill

The complete removal of inflammatory tissue from bony defects and careful root planing will often result in some bone in-fill produced by the activity of osteoblasts from the surrounding marrow spaces. No new cementum will form on the root surface, which will be covered by the junctional epithelium, and this will interpose itself between the new bone and the root, preventing resorption. A number of factors can prevent this from happening:

1. Choosing the wrong type of defect, i.e. one that is too wide and shallow, with too few bone walls. The ideal is the deep three-walled defect.
2. Failure to curette away all inflamed connective tissue and granulations.
3. Failure to clean the root surface completely.
4. Failure to close the flaps completely over the bone defect.
5. Infection and disintegration of the blood clot.
6. Excessive tooth mobility which can disturb the healing tissues. Temporary immobilization of a very mobile tooth will help to protect the lesion from mechanical stress.

The surgical procedure may be an apically repositioned or replaced flap procedure (Chapter 16). Particular attention is paid to closing the soft-tissue wound over the bone lesion.

Eliminating the bone defect by reshaping is a more predictable procedure than curettage; therefore in a situation where there is doubt about the treatment of the bone defect the position of the lesion may well provide an answer to the dilemma. However, it must be borne in mind that in many cases bone resection will further reduce tooth attachment and therefore be contraindicated. In the posterior segment it may be better to treat the bone defect definitively by bone reshaping, whereas in anterior segments one needs to conserve bone to preserve the appearance.

Bone grafts

Attempting to obtain some fill-in of the bone defect and reattachment by simple curettage of the bone defect is an unpredictable procedure and a number of different types of graft material have been tried. Graft materials are of four general types: (i) the autograft which is bone from the same individual, (ii) the allograft which is from an individual of the same species, (iii) xenografts which are bone from a different species, treated with ethylene diamine to remove the organic and antigenic fraction and (iv) grafts of bone substitutes and synthetic materials. There are four types of alloplastic synthetic grafts which are available

for clinical use. These are beta tricalcium phosphate, porous hydroxyapatite, non-porous hydroxyapatite and HTR polymer (Mellonig, 1990). One of these 'Periograft' or 'Durapatite', a non-porous hydroxyapatite is illustrated in *Figure 17.2*.

The essential requirements of a graft material are:

1. It should be immunologically acceptable.
2. It should have osteogenic potential, i.e. it should contain viable bone cells which become active in the new site, or contain some chemical factor with osteogenic potential.

It would seem that graft materials which lack osteogenic potential act simply as a replacement for the blood clot which usually breaks down, or as an inert scaffold on which some bone formation takes place prior to the resorption of the graft. This is because cellular events of periodontal regeneration involve the controlled integration of a number of cell signalling systems for bone, cementum and periodontal ligament. Unless these are present in the graft material and/or the adjacent tissues in the right proportions, controlled regeneration cannot take place. However, regeneration of new cementum, periodontal ligament and alveolar bone can be achieved to some degree in infrabony defects with some grafting techniques including autograft bone and marrow (Hiatt and Schallhorn, 1973; Rosenberg, 1971), human freeze-dried, demineralized bone allograft (Mellonig *et al.*, 1976; Rummelhart *et al.*, 1989) possibly with bone substitutes such as HTR polymer (Stahl, Froum and Tarnom, 1990) and with guided tissue regeneration, GTR (*see below*).

Bone autografts using iliac crest marrow (Hiatt and Schallhorn, 1973) or cancellous bone from oral sites (Rosenberg, 1971) have been used with some success. Cancellous bone and marrow can be obtained from a number of sites in the mouth such as the tuberosity, extraction sockets or the edentulous ridge. The ideal autograft is obtained from the iliac crest but it is doubtful whether tapping this site is justifiable. Also, fresh marrow tissue often produces root resorption and ankylosis; it must be frozen before use to prevent this. Shavings of cortical bone obtained from the neighbourhood of the bone defect, although not as useful or as effective as cancellous

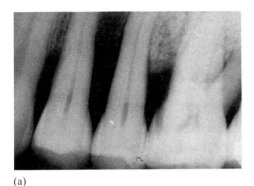

(a)

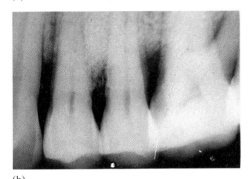

(b)

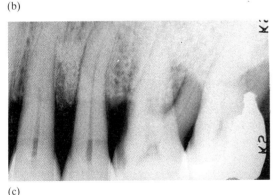

(c)

Figure 17.2 Three radiographs showing a man of 50:
(*a*) bone lesion between $\underline{45}$ caused by a lateral abscess;
(*b*) postoperative radiograph showing graft (Periograft);
(*c*) one year postoperative radiograph showing graft
partly resorbed

bone, may also be used. Unless bone formation is very rapid, as with fresh bone marrow tissue, junctional epithelium will usually migrate apically over the connective tissue wound to cover the root surface and protect it from root resorption.

More recently freeze-dried bone allograft has been used to treat periodontal osseous defects. Two types of bone allograft are in

clinical usage. These are freeze-dried unde-mineralised bone allograft (FDBA) and freeze-dried demineralised bone allograft (FDDBA). Originally introduced as a periodontal material in 1976 it has been used successfully in clinical medicine for more than 4 decades (Mellonig, 1990). The freeze drying permits storage within a vacuum for an indefinite shelf life and also markedly reduces the antigenicity of the graft (Friedlaender, 1987; Turner and Mellonig, 1981; Quattlebaum, Mellonig and Hansel, 1988). Clinical studies have shown that the use of the graft in intra-bony defects following debridement produces more than 50% bony in-fill in 63% of the defects (Sanders *et al.*, 1983). Using a combination of FDBA and autograft bone to produce a composite graft produces this result in over 80% of defects (Sanders *et al.*, 1983). Although there is relatively little difference in the clinical results with FDBA and FDDBA, the latter has largely superseded the former as a periodontal grafting material (Rummelhart *et al.*, 1989). FDDBA appears to have superior bone induction properties and clinical studies indicate that sites grafted with this material produce more than 50% bony in-fill in 78% of sites comparing with only 38% of sites for debridement alone (Urist, 1965; Urist and Strates, 1971; Mellonig *et al.*, 1976; Mellonig, Bowers and Baily, 1981; Quintero, Mellonig and Gambill, 1982). In addition, human histo-logical studies (Bowers *et al.*, 1989a,b,c) have provided evidence for regeneration of new bone, ligament and cementum using this material (see below). Furthermore, it has been shown that bone matrix contains bone inductive proteins (Sampath and Reddi, 1983) and several osteoinductive signal molecules have been purified from FDDBA powder. These include bone morphogenic proteins (BMP) 2 and 7 (Sampath *et al.*, 1990) and six other distinct bone derived growth factors (Hauschka *et al.*, 1986). It has also been suggested that the collagen matrix of the demineralized graft acts as a substrate for attachment, proliferation and differentiation of new osteoprogenitor cells (Sampath and Reddi, 1983).

However, some difficulties have been encountered in the placement and retention of particulate FDDBA grafts especially in accessible and freely bleeding sites when the material may be flushed out. In an effort to overcome these difficulties and improve the biological and physical handling properties, these bone grafts have been combined with microfibrillar collagen (Blumenthal *et al.*, 1986). The combined graft helped to bind and retain the particles, created a space between the particles and acted as a scaffold for cell and blood vessel ingrowth. In addition, it was claimed that the collagen material became bound to the root surface and prevented epithelial downgrowth. The material consists of a combination of human freeze-dried bone powder with human tendon collagen. Following rehydration it can be layered into defect and expands to fill it. Clinical studies and experimental studies with dogs have been carried out with this material (Blumenthal *et al.*, 1986). Clinical re-entry was performed 5 months after the procedure and found a mean 61% bone in-fill. Histological studies showed evidence of bone formation, periodontal regeneration and prevention of epithelial migration. The material has also been used successfully in humans (Blumenthal, 1994).

The possibility of disease transfer with bone allografts obtained from human cadaver material is very unlikely if the material is procured and processed using established tissue banking protocols which incorporate medical and social screening, antibody testing, direct antigen tests, serological tests, bacterial culturing and follow-up studies (Mellonig, 1990; Friedlaender, 1987; American Association of Tissue Banks, 1984; Buck, Malinin and Brown, 1989; Martin, McDougal and Loskoski, 1985; Quinnan, Wells and Wittek, 1986; Resnick *et al.*, 1986; Buck *et al.*, 1990). The risk of disease transmission with FDDBA is 1 chance in 8 million. The HIV virus has been cultured from bone (Buck *et al.*, 1990) but is likely to be detected by the above tests and inactivated in the event of being missed in the screening process by the sterilisation procedures used in the preparation of these materials.

It seems likely that most grafts act simply as a replacement for the blood clot which usually breaks down, or as an inert scaffold on which some bone formation takes place prior to the resorption of the graft.

The use of synthetic bone substitutes avoids the problems of finding autograft bone and any tiny risk of disease transfer with FDDBA. Four types of synthetic bone substitute are

available (see above) and all seem to produce better results than surgical debridement alone.

Porous hydroxyapatite has a uniform pore size, which facilitates vascular ingrowth and subsequent new bone formation (Mellonig, 1990). Controlled studies in humans shows that it produces more bone in-fill in intrabony lesions than surgical debridement alone (Kenny *et al.*, 1985; Yukna *et al.*, 1986). Kenny *et al.* (1986) also showed histological evidence of new bone formation on the surface of and within the pores of porous hydroxyapatite. He placed this material into intrabony lesions of teeth with advanced periodontitis in human subjects and removed the teeth and surrounding tissues for light and scanning electron-microscopical examination. Spreading osteoblasts and new bone were seen in contact with the particles.

In a 5-year follow-up study (Yukna, Mayer and Amos, 1989) non-porous hydroxyapatite has also been shown to be superior to surgical debridement in producing bony in-fill. It also showed that the condition remained stable for long periods following this treatment. Porous and non-porous hydroxyapatite and surgical debridement have been compared in the treatment of intrabony defects (Krejci *et al.*, 1987) and this study showed that non-porous hydroxyapatite produced the most consistent results.

HTR polymer is a non-resorbable, microporous biocompatible composite of polymethylmethacrylate (PMMA) and polyhydroxyethylmethacrylate (PHEMA). This material has been used in the fabrication of contact lenses, lens transplants and prosthetic heart valves over many years. The polymer does not produce an inflammatory or immune response in contact with bone or soft tissue (Yukna, 1990). PMMA beads of 550–880 μm diameter with pores of 50–300 μm form the core of this material. These are coated with liquid PHEMA without the addition of any catalysts or inducers. The composite beads are then coated with calcium hydroxide/calcium carbonate. Thus, the actual surface interface with bone is the calcium surface layer and both fibrous tissue and bone can form on and attach to this layer. The composite is provided in a fine granular form for use in periodontal intrabony defects.

Stahl *et al.* (1990) used this material in 5 volunteer patients with advanced periodontitis and they provided 11 intrabony defects. These were surgically debrided and implanted with HTR polymer and the lesions were followed for 4–26 weeks. After this time the teeth and blocks of tissue were removed for histological examination. The clinical observations showed a reduction in probing depth due both to gingival recession and a gain in clinical attachment level. The patients showed no untoward symptoms or signs during this period. Histological examination showed that the grafts became surrounded by connective tissue capsules and some limited bone deposition was present on the surface of some implanted particles. The 11 lesions showed varied responses and there were different responses both between patients and different sites in the same patient. In 7 sites there was a long junctional epithelium between the root surface and the graft, whilst in 4 sites there was limited evidence of new attachment.

Yukna (1990) investigated the effectiveness of HTR polymer in treating intrabony lesions in 21 adult patients with moderate to advanced chronic periodontitis. Some sites were treated by surgical debridement alone and some by debridement followed by implantation of HTR polymer. They were followed by clinical and radiographical measurements for 6 months after which surgical re-entry procedures were carried out. The re-entry procedures showed that the sites implanted with HTR polymer showed significantly better mean bony in-fill (60.8%) than those treated by debridement alone (32.2%). Clinical and radiological measurements also showed significantly better results for the polymer group. These studies show that HTR polymer synthetic alloplast does show some promise for repair of periodontal osseous defects.

Possible formation of new attachment following bone grafting procedures

The ability of new attachment to form between bone and the treated root surface during the healing of intrabony defects has been extensively studied in human subjects by Bowers *et al.* (1989a,b,c). This was investigated on human subjects with advanced periodontitis who had teeth destined for extraction. These teeth were subjected to the experimental procedures and were then removed 6 months later with a block of surrounding bone

for histological examination. The intrabony defects were exposed surgically and thoroughly debrided and the root surfaces were then scaled and root planed. Some intrabony defects were grafted with freeze-dried demineralised bone allograft (FDDBA). Some teeth were left exposed in the mouth and others had their root surfaces submerged. This was done by cutting off the crown level with the highest level of the alveolar bone and coronally advancing the buccal flap to completely cover the root face (Bowers *et al.*, 1989a).

They found that on the teeth with osseous defects receiving debridement only no new attachment formed on the exposed teeth. All of these lesions healed by the formation of a long junctional epithelium which extended down the treated root surface. However, new attachment apparatus, consisting of new bone, new cementum and new periodontal ligament, did form on the submerged root surfaces (Bowers *et al.*, 1989a). They also found that grafting the intrabony defect with FDDBA did significantly increase the amount of new attachment apparatus which formed on submerged roots (Bowers *et al.*, 1989b). However, the formation of some new attachment apparatus was also seen on exposed teeth with defects that were additionally grafted with FDDBA (Bowers *et al.*, 1989c). New cellular cementum formed equally well on treated old cementum or dentine. No evidence of extensive root resorption, ankylosis or pulp death were seen on any of the exposed teeth or submerged roots. Thus, some new attachment apparatus may form in intrabony lesions grafted with FDDBA and possibly could also occur with other graft materials.

Summary of treatments of intrabony defects

In summary it can be said that new bone formation can regularly occur in surgically treated intrabony defects. The studies reported above indicate that surgical debridement of the lesion alone can result in up to 30% bony in-fill, whilst the additional use of autogenous bone grafts, freeze-dried bone allografts, demineralised freeze-dried bone allografts and synthetic bone substitutes produce varying responses but usually result in greater levels of bony in-fill up to a maximum of 60–70%. The extent of gain in new attachment is very variable with bone grafts but can sometimes occur presumably by the material acting as a barrier to epithelial downgrowth (*see below*). It is possible that some of the grafting materials, e.g. FDDBA, may also contain growth factors which may promote connective tissue, bone and cementum regeneration (*see above*). It is also possible that in the future synthetic bone allografts such as HTR-polymer may act as vehicles for selective growth promoting factors as the precise functions of these become known.

Guided tissue regeneration (GTR)

The capacity of the various periodontal tissues to regenerate has been discussed previously. Alveolar bone and cementum have good powers of regeneration provided that the necessary cell types and cell signals are present. The same is true for periodontal ligament, but for this to form a functional attachment the collagen fibres must become enclosed by newly formed bone on one surface and cementum on the other. This requires the regeneration of the three tissues to be finely integrated. Also, for any new attachment to form, junctional epithelium, which proliferates over exposed connective tissues, must be excluded from the wound. This last prerequisite forms the basis for the guided tissue regeneration technique (GTR) developed by Nyman *et al.* (1982a,b).

It was shown first in monkeys that periodontal ligament cells can proliferate over planed root surfaces if epithelial cells, bone cells and gingival connective tissue cells are excluded from the healing wound by the placement of a membrane (Nyman *et al.*, 1982b; Gottlow *et al.*, 1984). Similar results were reported in clinical studies on human teeth with advanced and intra-bony defects (Nyman, 1982a, 1983; Gottlow *et al.*, 1986). Some new attachment in the form of cementum with embedded collagen fibres and bone or bone-like tissue were formed using this technique and this has been demonstrated histologically both on monkey teeth (Nyman *et al.*, 1982b; Gottlow *et al.*, 1984) and extracted human teeth (Nyman, 1982a, 1983). It has also been observed by clinical observation on retained human teeth (Gottlow *et al.*, 1986). The basis of the

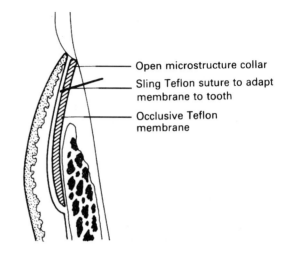

Open microstructure collar

Sling Teflon suture to adapt membrane to tooth

Occlusive Teflon membrane

Figure 17.3 Diagram to show the guided tissue regeneration technique described by Nyman (1983). After exposure of the area by raising a flap, all granulation tissue is removed and the root surface carefully planed. A Teflon membrane is then adjusted to cover the root surface from apical to the bone margin to just below the CEJ. It is interposed between these structures and the flap so that epithelium migrating apically-over the connective tissue surface is prevented from contacting the root

technique is the exclusion of epithelium by the membrane to allow time for periodontal ligament cells to migrate coronally.

The technique is carried out as follows. The area is first exposed by raising a flap developed with an intercrevicular incision to preserve keratinized gingiva. Pocket-lining epithelium is then removed from its inner aspect. All granulation tissue is removed and the roots are thoroughly planed. A flexible Teflon membrane (Gore-tex) is carefully trimmed to cover the lesion. This consists of a narrow, open microstructure margin which is designed to allow connective tissue penetration to produce a seal at the coronal margin of the root, as well as an occlusive membrane (*Figure 17.3*). It is adapted to fit over the intra-bony defect and the root of the tooth, extending from 2–3 mm below the bone margin to just below the CEJ on the root. This prevents the oral epithelium and gingival connective tissue contacting the root surface during healing. It is held in place by a Teflon sling suture which passes through both edges of the membrane upper margin and around the tooth. The flap is then sutured back to just cover the membrane. The membrane is left in place for 4–6 weeks and then removed. A further marginal incision exposes the membrane which is very carefully separated from the delicate healing tissue which appears like a gelatinous red membrane. The flap is then sutured back.

It must be stressed that this technique is applicable only to the treatment of single teeth with two- or three-walled intrabony defects. At present it is at the development stage and undergoing careful clinical assessments. As explained in the following text GTR can be used to treat either intrabony or furcation defects.

The results of short-term clinical trials with this technique using expanded polytetrafluoroethylene (PTFE) membranes (Gore-tex) (Gottlow *et al.*, 1986; Schallhorn and McClain, 1988; Becker *et al.*, 1988; Pontoriero *et al.*, 1988, 1989; Cortellini *et al.*, 1990; Caffesse *et al.*, 1990) have shown that a gain in probing attachment may occur on teeth with a variety of intrabony and furcation defects. More recently it has been shown that these changes can be maintained over 4–5 years (Gottlow *et al.*, 1992). Experimental studies using prepared defects in dogs and monkeys also showed evidence of regenerative new cementum with embedded collagen fibres at test sites in intrabony lesions and class II and III furcation defects (Nyman *et al.*, 1982b; Aukhil *et al.*, 1983, 1986; Gottlow *et al.*, 1984, 1990; Caffesse *et al.*, 1988, 1990; Pontoriero *et al.*, 1992). This did not occur at control sites. However, the results were variable at sites with Class III furcation involvement and extensive intrabony lesions. Thus, success was found to be partly dependent on the size, shape and apical extent of the lesion. Furthermore, there are some reports which show that the results of GTR are unpredictable and on many occasions show results that have no advantage over conventional surgery (Warren and Karring, 1992; Proestakis *et al.*, 1992; Pritlove-Carson *et al.*, 1993).

Some trials with biodegradable polylactic acid or polyurethane membranes have so far failed to produce regeneration (Warren *et al.*, 1992). However, recently several human and animal studies (Linde *et al.*, 1995; Sander and Karring, 1995a,b; Christgou *et al.*, 1995) have shown that the placement of resorbable membranes in GTR procedures can result in the formation of similar amounts of new attachment to the placement of conventional

e-PTFE membranes in the treatment of both two and three-walled intrabony defects and Class II and Class III furcation defects. These resorbable membranes include materials like collagen, polyglactin-910, polylactid and polyurethane (Christgou *et al.*, 1995). Some of these are commercially available.

However the above studies show that the achievement of membrane stability and total coverage of the membrane are important in achieving success. In this regard it has been clearly shown that artificially buried defects heal considerably better than exposed defects as in the clinical situation (Sander and Karring, 1995a). One of the reasons for this is that exposed membranes become extensively contaminated and penetrated by bacteria from the oral and subgingival flora (Simion *et al.*, 1995). Furthermore it has been shown that the topical application of chlorhexidine (Simion *et al.*, ibid) and metronidazole gel (Sander *et al.*, 1994; Frandesen *et al.*, 1994) to GTR membranes during their application may reduce, but not completely prevent bacterial contamination of the membrane. This has been reported to result in improved clinical results (Sander *et al.*, ibid).

Pritlove-Carson *et al.* (1993) reported on a series of matched intrabony lesions in patients. One lesion was treated with GTR and one with conventional surgery. They found no difference between the test and control sites in respect of probing depth, probing attachment level or recession.

GTR in combination with bone grafts

In clinical studies using GTR, some of which were cited above, there were a number of variables in the GTR technique including the concurrent use of bone grafts, root surface conditioning and coronally positioned flaps (Gantes and Garrett, 1991; Schallhorn and McClain, 1988; Mellonig, 1991). Combinations of GTR with the use of bone grafts has been shown to have some advantages over either technique used alone (Schultz and Gager, 1990). Schallhorn and McClain (1988) reported on a clinical study combining osseous composite grafting, root conditioning and GTR. They found a significantly greater gain of mean probing attachment with the combination compared to GTR alone.

Bowers *et al.* (1989a,b,c) showed that periodontal regeneration could take place using human freeze-dried decalcified bone allograft (FDDBA) in infrabony defects (*see* previous section). They concluded that the combination of highly osteogenic material such as FDDBA with GTR might offer promise for increasing the predictability of periodontal regeneration procedures.

This combination approach was investigated by Anderegg *et al.* (1991). They compared the use of FDDBA and GTR with GTR alone on human molar furcation defects. At the 6-month re-entry there was a distinct difference in the horizontal and vertical bone repair favouring the use of the graft. Stahl and Froume (1991) investigated the use of this combination on human intrabony defects and found gains in clinical attachment and histological evidence of new cementum, bone and periodontal ligament formation. However, the amount of new histological attachment varied from 0–1.7 mm in the four specimens studied.

Recently, this combination has been investigated by Guillemin *et al.* (1993a,b) using two paired sites in each of 17 patients with advanced periodontitis, one of which was treated with FDDBA and GTR and the other with GTR alone. The results were compared for the extent of bony in-fill assessed at re-entry 6 months after the procedure and bone density assessed by computerized densitometric analysis. No statistically significant differences were found for either comparison between the two groups. The average bony in-fill was 58% for the GTR alone sites and 70% for the combination sites. In addition the combination sites showed greater mean gingival recession (0.9 mm) than GTR alone sites (0.4 mm).

These studies would seem to indicate that both GTR and the use of FDDBA bone graft alone can produce periodontal regeneration. Their combined use seems to produce good results which may be slightly better than either used alone. However, the controlled studies do not show statistically significant differences between using GTR alone or with FDDBA.

The reasons for the unpredictability of GTR and bone grafting techniques may result from the cellular events leading to the formation of these tissues. These are not as simple as originally conceived and some new views on connective tissue regeneration have a bearing on this.

New views on connective tissue regeneration

There have been very significant advances in this area recently (Hughes, 1993). The cellular events of periodontal regeneration are not a simple race of cells but involve the controlled integration of a number of cell signalling systems. The following factors seem with our present knowledge to be the most important in determining the outcome of periodontal regenerative procedures:

- Excluding epithelium.
- Producing the conditions for the migration of stem and progenitor cells from the bone marrow. This involves the integrated production of the appropriate signal molecules.
- Production of signal molecules for cementoblasts and cementum formation.
- Production of signal molecules for osteoblasts and bone formation.
- Production of signal molecules for synchronized periodontal ligament formation.

So far we have only limited means of controlling these factors and the fine control of these systems in tissue healing almost certainly determines the type of tissue formed. Therefore, it is unlikely that periodontal regenerative procedures like GTR and bone grafting will be fully predictable until we have a better understanding of these processes and some practical means of controlling them.

The possible use of growth factors and cell mediators to produce periodontal regeneration

The new information described above has already begun to affect clinical methods to achieve periodontal regeneration. Melcher (1976) focused on the need to stimulate the regeneration of cementum and periodontal ligament as well as bone in periodontal regeneration. He postulated that if cells of the periodontal ligament and alveolar bone populated the healing tissue coronal to the residual alveolar bone, regeneration of new periodontium would occur. Guided tissue regeneration seeks to produce these conditions by excluding epithelial downgrowth and thus proving an anatomical environment for the coronal migration of these cells. Bone grafts such as human freeze-dried, demineralized bone allograft (*see* bone graft section *above*) seek to provide a stimulus for bone regeneration including the provision of bone morphogenic proteins and bone-derived growth factors. It would seem likely that the stimulation of all cells capable of regenerating all the tissues of the periodontium or their precursors by chemical messager molecules would induce them to differentiate and migrate into the healing area. It would also seem likely that cellular messenger molecules trigger all the stages of the complex events leading to periodontal regeneration. Recently some work has appeared in the literature which has experimentally tested some of these events.

Platelet-derived growth factor (PDGF) is mitogenic and chemotactic for connective tissue cells (Ross *et al.*, 1986). In combination with insulin-like growth factor-1 (IGF-1) in a carboxymethylcellulose carrier it has been tested in dogs with naturally-occurring periodontitis during treatment with periodontal surgery (Lynch *et al.*, 1991). In these experiments these factors produced regeneration of the periodontium with formation of new cementum, bone and periodontal ligament. A similar response with the same factors was also produced on the healing wound in experimental periodontitis in monkeys (Rutherford *et al.*, 1993). In these experiments only the growth factors in the gelled carrier separated the gingival tissue from the alveolar bone and root surface and no attempt was made to prevent the contact of gingival connective tissue with the root surface or the carrier as would be the case with GTR. In fact the amount and spatial distribution of the new periodontium formed suggested that cells present in the gingival connective tissue were induced by the growth factors and contributed cells to the healing process.

Glucocorticoids are known to modulate the effects of other hormones and mediators of cell functions. In this regard they enhance the mitogenic activity of fibroblast growth factor (Hooley and Kieran, 1974) and IGF-1 (Conover *et al.*, 1986), but inhibit epidermal growth factor (Otto *et al.*, 1981). They could thus modulate the activities of growth factors in wound healing. In this regard a potent synthetic glucocorticoid, dexamethasone, has

been shown to act synergistically with cartilage-derived growth factor to produce mitogenesis in cultured mouse cells while having no effect on PDGF mitogenesis (Levenson *et al.*, 1985). In contrast, it has been shown that dexamethasone acts synergistically with PDGF to induce proliferation of periodontal ligament and gingival tissue fibroblasts *in vitro* (Rutherford *et al.*, 1992). Dexamethasone has also been shown selectively to stimulate the proliferation of osteoprogenitor cells (Bellows *et al.*, 1990) and to induce adult bone marrow cells to differentiate into osteoblasts (Kasuggai *et al.*, 1991). It may therefore play a role in osteogenesis.

The role of a combination of dexamethasone and PDGF in a collagen carrier matrix has been used to test its effect on wound healing following periodontal surgery on experimental periodontitis lesions in monkeys. Paired lesions with horizontal and vertical bone loss and 3–5 mm of attachment loss were used. One site received an application of PDGF and dexamethasone in the collagen-carrier and the other the collagen-carrier only. A collagen matrix (CM) was used as the vehicle because it might produce an environment which favoured connective tissue formation and also might act as a barrier to epithelial migration. The regeneration of new periodontium, consisting of new cementum, bone and inserting periodontal ligament fibres coronal to the pretreatment levels, was seen after 4 weeks in the PDGF/dexamethasone/CM sites but not in the sites treated with CM or debridement alone. The application of PDGF/dexamethasone/CM produced 5-fold more new cementum and ligament and 7-fold more supracrestal bone than the control treatments. This included filling of intrabony defects and increased height of alveolar bone. In these experiments, it is possible that epithelial downgrowth was prevented both by the collagen matrix acting as a barrier and as a result of the inhibition of epithelial growth factor by PDGF (Otto *et al.*, 1981).

Thus, there is now good evidence that specific growth factors and cell mediators may interact with competent cells in the healing periodontal wound when applied locally in a suitable vehicle. The gingival and periodontal ligament cells would seem to react by differentiating and migrating into the wound area more rapidly than the rate of epithelial downgrowth to form the tissues of new periodontium. These factors would seem to have great potential in promoting the formation of new attachment in human periodontitis lesions either alone in a suitable carrier or in combination with other methods such as GTR. However, with GTR it would probably be preferable to use a resorbable membrane, such as resorbable collagen, polygalactin, polylactid or polyurethane membranes, so that the healing process is not disturbed by membrane removal.

The diagnosis and treatment of furcation involvement

Furcation involvement is caused by bone loss between the roots of multirooted teeth, usually the molars and upper premolar teeth. There is variation in the width of the neck of these teeth and this dictates whether furcation involvement occurs as a relatively early or late complication. The problem produced is inaccessibility to plaque control and scaling. The furcation opens buccolingually in two-rooted lower molars, buccolingually and mesiodistally in three-rooted upper molars and mesiodistally in two-rooted upper premolars. It may occasionally affect other teeth where there are aberrations in the number and shape of roots. Mesiodistal furcation involvement or the combinations that can occur with three-rooted upper molars cause the greatest access problems. Difficult and sometimes insoluble problems occur when roots lie close together or are partially fused, making the furcation extremely narrow and often totally inaccessible.

Furcation involvement results in the extraction of more molars than single-rooted teeth and is the commonest complication of periodontitis; it often necessitates extraction because of the development of acute lateral abscesses (Hirschfeld and Wasserman, 1978).

Classification

Furcation defects are classified according to the degree of inter-radicular bone loss as class 1, 2 or 3. This is discussed on p. 99.

Diagnosis

Furcation defects can be diagnosed by probing or with radiographs. Probing horizontally from within buccal or lingual pockets of lower or upper molars, as well as mesial and distal pockets of upper molars or first premolars, can detect furcation involvement hidden within the pocket. The best radiographs for confirmatory diagnosis are vertical bitewings or long cone intra-orals. They may also show on OPGs. Bisected angle periapical views are not good for this purpose because the tube angulation has the effect of projecting marginal bone coronally. Upper molar trifurcations are more difficult to interpret on radiographs because of the superimposition of the large palatal root. Upper first premolar furcations do not appear on standard radiographs but may show up if the tube is partly angled in a mesiodistal direction to try to project the rays between the roots.

Treatment

The aim of treatment is either to expose the furcation for access for cleaning which is easier in a buccolingual than a mesiodistal direction, or to induce regeneration of new bone. Treatment procedures are outlined below.

Class 1 and 2 incomplete defects

Early involvement may be treated conservatively by scaling and maintenance. More definite involvement is usually treated by a gingivectomy, if the attached gingival zone is wide, or more usually an apically repositioned flap. Granulation tissue is curetted from the lesion and the root surfaces are thoroughly scaled and planed. Minor bone reshaping may be carried out to produce a streamlined, easily cleaned contour. If a gingivectomy is used the new gingival margin should be carefully shaped to ensure good access for cleaning after healing. Much better access is achieved with a flap and the lesion is exposed by repositioning the flap margin next to, or even slightly apical to the bone margin. Following healing the furcation can be cleaned with a single tufted brush.

Guided tissue regeneration

GTR techniques have been successfully used to treat Class 2 furcation involvement on mandibular molars (Pontoriero *et al.*, 1988). The technique is essentially the same as that described on pp. 200–202.

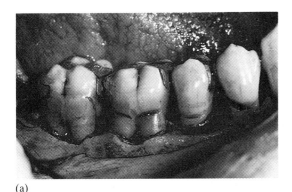

(a)

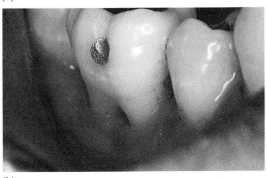

(b)

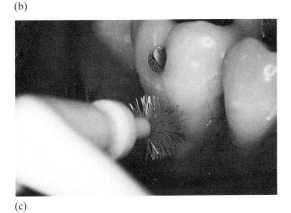

(c)

Figure 17.4 The treatment of Class 3 furcation involvement on the 6̄ of a 40 year old man. (*a*) Furcation area exposed by means of buccal and lingual inverse bevel flaps. The furcation space, the bone surface and the roots have been cleared of granulation tissue and deposits. The flap was then repositioned apically to expose the furcation area. (*b*) The postoperative result. (The picture was taken 6 months after surgery.) (*c*) The use of a spiral brush to clean the furcation

Over 90% of the sites treated showed complete resolution by in-filling of the defect with bone or bone-like tissue. The technique

may also be used to treat Class 3 defects but with less predictable results.

Class 3 complete defects

A number of options can be considered for complete, through-through furcation defects: simple exposure, tunnel preparation, root resection, tooth division, hemisection and extraction. The choice depends on the extent and pattern of bone loss and the root anatomy.

Simple exposure If the furcation is naturally wide enough for cleaning, it can be simply exposed by the apical positioning of inverse bevel flaps; this also gains access for curettage, scaling and root planing (*Figure 17.4a*). A periodontal dressing is placed over the wound and between the roots to ensure the exposure of the furcation (*Figure 17.4b*). After healing, cleaning is carried out with a spiral interproximal brush (*Figure 17.4c*).

Tunnel preparation This is applicable to lower molar bifurcation involvement. Exposure for curettage and scaling is gained by inverse bevel flaps buccally and lingually. The size of the furcation is then enlarged by bone contouring and sometimes by reshaping the inner root surfaces which is only necessary if the roots are close together. If possible this should be avoided because it can produce a high risk of root caries. The purpose of this contouring is to provide space for a spiral brush to pass freely through the furcation from the buccal to the lingual side. The flap is displaced apically to lie just below the bone margin. A periodontal pack is placed into the furcation so that the flap cannot ride up coronally. The area may need to be dressed for 2 weeks.

In some cases this procedure may be used for upper molar trifurcation involvement but the problem is more complicated. The palatal root will usually prevent complete access from the buccal side and additional mesial and distal approaches have to be made. These are particularly difficult for patient access using a spiral brush and demand a high degree of manual dexterity. Patients require careful instruction in the use of spiral interproximal brushes. They must replace the heads whenever the bristles show signs of wear. Vigorous use of these brushes and allowing the metal core to

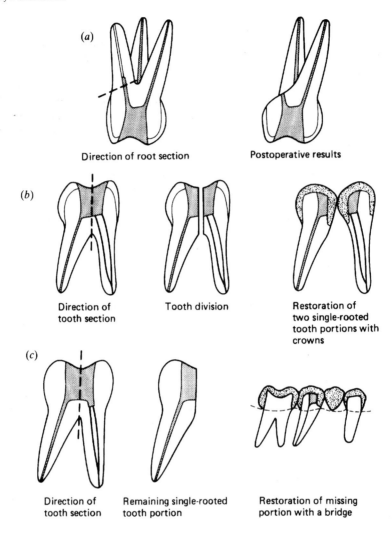

Figure 17.5 Diagrams to show three procedures for treating more advanced Class 3 furcation involvement: (*a*) root amputation; (*b*) tooth division; (*c*) hemisection. In all cases the tooth must first be root treated

contact the root will cause severe abrasion and must be avoided.

Root amputation, tooth division and hemisection (Figure 17.5) These procedures are indicated by extensive bone resorption around one of the roots of the affected tooth and are only possible if the remaining roots have sufficient support to ensure function. It must be remembered that the mobility of individual roots after separation will exceed the mobility of the whole tooth. These techniques all require endodontic treatment prior to the surgery. In some cases lack of access to narrow, curved and partially obliterated canals will preclude this. Very occasionally, in an emergency, e.g. when an unexpected problem is discovered during periodontal surgery, it may be necessary to amputate a root before endodontic treatment has been carried out. In this situation one must be sure that endodontic treatment is possible and that the tooth will be functional after the procedure. The exposed pulp at the amputation site is dressed with calcium hydroxide and arrangements are made for endodontic treatment after the surgery. In this situation it is necessary to prescribe a course of antibiotics.

Presurgical endodontics should ensure that all of the roots to remain are filled to the apex. A small cavity is made at the entrance of the canal of the root to be removed and packed with amalgam to produce a permanent seal at the point of amputation. The floor of the pulp chamber should also be packed with amalgam for a similar purpose. In the case of tooth division or hemisection the pulpal floor will be cut through and a permanent seal at this point is essential. The final restoration of these teeth will involve the provision of a crown(s) or a bridge.

Root amputation (*Figure 17.5a*) is particularly applicable to three-rooted upper molar teeth when it will involve the removal of either the mesiobuccal or distobuccal root. This will allow access to the furcation area for cleaning between the remaining two roots from a buccal approach. Care should be taken to balance the occlusion on these teeth before this procedure.

Buccal and palatal inverse bevel flaps are raised to gain access. Palatal pocketing can be treated by an inverse bevel gingivectomy. Granulation tissue is curetted away to reveal the shape of the furcation and its relation to the root to be amputated. Sectioning should start in the affected furcation and its path may be planned by passing a blunt probe through the space from buccal to palatal. The cut is made with a tapered diamond bur cooled by sterile water. A wide enough space should be made to elevate the root, taking care not to remove too much substance from the part of the tooth to be retained. The base of the crown should then be shaped so that it is cleanable from a buccal approach. The remaining roots are carefully scaled and planed and the buccal flap is placed apical to the furcation entrance between the two remaining roots. The position of the palatal gingival margin is determined by the position of the inverse bevel gingivectomy incision. A periodontal dressing is placed so that it passes between the margin of the flaps and the amputation site.

Tooth division (*Figure 17.5b*) is carried out less frequently than the other techniques. It is indicated for extensive furcation involvement of lower molars where bone loss around both roots is similar. Buccal and lingual inverse bevel flaps are raised and the furcation revealed by curettage. The tooth is then completely divided by extending a cut from the roof of the furcation through the crown. Each half of the tooth is reshaped into a single-rooted tooth and will be subsequently prepared to receive a crown. In this way a two-rooted molar is converted into two single-rooted teeth.

Hemisection (*Figure 17.5c*) is indicated for furcation involvement of lower molars where there is extensive bone resorption around one of the roots. It must be ensured that adequate restoration of the remaining half of the crown is possible before embarking on this procedure.

Buccal and lingual inverse bevel flaps are raised and the area is curetted. The sectioning process is begun at the roof of the furcation, extending upwards to divide the tooth. Tooth substance is preferentially removed from the half of the tooth to be sacrificed which is then removed with an elevator. The remaining root is scaled and planed. The remaining half of the crown is carefully contoured and smoothed and the flaps are repositioned to eliminate any pocketing. After healing the tooth will be crowned usually forming part of the bridge to replace the missing portion. Obviously a sufficient number of well-supported abutment teeth must be available.

Extraction Advanced furcation involvement with extensive bone resorption around two or more roots will necessitate extraction. Teeth with uncertain prognosis may be retained on a temporary basis providing the patient is aware of the uncertainty, the teeth are symptomless and there are no signs of infection or increasing mobility. However, the effect of retaining these teeth on the prognosis of adjacent teeth should be carefully considered.

Maintenance

All teeth with furcation involvement require frequent and regular maintenance. The importance of careful oral hygiene measures using spiral-tufted interproximal brushes must be stressed and taught to the patients. Successful long-term maintenance of teeth with furcation involvement can be achieved in many cases (Hirschfeld and Wasserman, 1978, Knowles *et al.*, 1980).

References

American Association of Tissue Banks (1984) *Standards for tissue banking.* Arlington, Va.: American Association of Tissue Banks

Anderegg, C.R., Martin, S.J., Gray, J.L. *et al.* (1991) Clinical evaluation of the use of decalcified freeze-dried bone allograft with guided tissue regeneration in the treatment of molar furcation invasions. *Journal of Periodontololgy* **62**, 264–268

Aukhil, I., Petterson, E. and Suggs, G. (1986) Guided tissue regeneration. An experimental procedure in beagle dogs. *Journal of Periodontology* **57**, 727–734

Aukhil, I., Simpson, D.M. and Schaberg, T. (1983) An experimental study of new attachment procedure in beagle dogs. *Journal of Periodontal Research* **18**, 643–654

Becker, W., Becker, B., Berg, L. *et al.* (1988) New attachment after treatment with root isolation procedures. Report for treated class II and class III furcations and vertical osseous defects. *International Journal of Clinical Periodontics and Restorative Dentistry* **3**, 9–23

Bellows, C.G., Heersche, J.N. and Aubin, J.E. (1990) Determination of the capacity for proliferation and differentiation of osteoprogenitor cells in the presence and absence of dexamethasone. *Developmental Biology* **140**, 132–138

Blumenthal, N.M. (1994) Future directions in periodontal regeneration therapy – a combined human collagen–bone multifunction implant. *Illinois Dental Journal* **34**, 35–38

Blumenthal, N.M., Sabet, T. and Barrington, E. (1986) Healing responses to grafting of combined collagen-decalcified bone in periodontal defects in dogs. *Journal of Periodontology* **57**, 84–90

Bowers, G.M., Chadroff, B., Carnevale, R. *et al.* (1989a) Histologic evaluation of new attachment apparatus formation in humans. Part I. *Journal of Periodontology* **60**, 664–674

Bowers, G.M., Chadroff, B., Carnevale, R. *et al.* (1989b) Histologic evaluation of new attachment apparatus formation in humans. Part II. *Journal of Periodontology* **60**, 675–682

Bowers, G.M., Chadroff, B., Carnevale, R. *et al.* (1989c) Histologic evaluation of new attachment apparatus formation in humans. Part III. *Journal of Periodontology* **60**, 683–693

Buck, B., Malinin, T. and Brown, M. (1989) Bone transplntation and human immunodeficiency virus. An estimate risk of acquired immunodeficiency syndrome (AIDS). *Clinical Orthopaedics and Releated Research* **240**, 129–136

Buck, B., Resnick, L., Shah, S. and Malinin, T. (1990) Human immunodeficiency virus cultured from bone. Implications for transplantation. *Clinical Orthopaedics and Related Research* **251** 249–253

Caton, J. and Nyman, S. (1980) Histometric evaluation of periodontal surgery. I. The modified Widman flap procedure. *Journal of Clinical Periodontology* **7**, 212–223

Caton, J., Nyman, S. and Zander, H. (1980) Histometric evaluation of periodontal surgery. II. Connective tissue attachment levels after four regenerative procedures. *Journal of Clinical Periodontology* **7**, 224–231

Caton, J. and Zander, H. (1975) Primate model for testing periodontal treatment procedures. I. Histologic investigation of localised periodontal pockets produced by orthodontic elastics. *Journal of Periodontology* **46**, 71–77

Christgou, M., Schmalz, G., Reich, E. and Wenzel, A. (1995) Clinical and radiographical split-mouth-study on resorbable versus non-resorbable GTR-membranes. *Journal of Clinical Periodontology* **22**, 306–315

Conover, C.A., Rosenfeld, R.G. and Hintz, R.L. (1986) Hormonal control of the replication of human fetal fibroblasts: the role of somatomedin C/insulin-like growth factor-1. *Journal of Cellular Physiology* **128**, 47–54

Cortellini, P., Pini Prato, G., Baldi, C. and Clauser, C. (1990) Guided tissue regeneration with different materials. *International Journal of Clinical Periodontics and Restorative Dentistry* **10**, 137–151

Caffesse, R.G., Dominguez, L.E., Nasjleti, C.E. *et al.* (1990) Furcation defects in dogs treated by guided tissue regeneration (GTR). *Journal of Periodontology* **61**, 45–50

Caffesse, R.G., Smith, B.A., Castelli, W.A. and Nasjleti, C.E. (1988) New attachment achieved by guided tissue regeneration in beagle dogs. *Journal of Periodontology* **59**, 589–594

Frandsen, E.V.G., Sander, L., Arnbjerg, D. and Theilade, E. (1994) Effects of local metronidazole application on periodontal healing following guided tissue regeneration. Microbiological findings. *Journal of Periodontology* **65**, 921–928

Friedlaender, G. (1987) Bone banking. *Clinical Orthopaedics and Related Research* **255**, 17–21

Gantes, B.G. and Garrett, S. (1991) Coronally displaced flaps in reconstructive periodontal therapy. *Dental Clinics of North America* **35**, 495–504

Gottlow, J., Nyman, S., Karring, T. and Lindhe, J. (1984) New attachment formation as the result of controlled tissue regeneration. *Journal of Clinical Periodontology* **11**, 494–503

Gottlow, J., Karring, T. and Nyman, S. (1990) Guided tissue regeneration following treatment of recession-like defects in the monkey. *Journal of Periodontology* **61**, 680–685

Gottlow, J., Nyman, S. and Karring, T. (1992) Maintenance of new attachment gained through guided tissue regeneration. *Journal of Clinical Periodontology* **19**, 315–317

Gottlow, J., Nyman, S., Lindhe, J. *et al.* (1986) New attachment formation in the human periodontium by guided tissue regeneration. *Journal of Clinical Periodontology* **13**, 604–616

Guillemin, M.R., Mellonig, J.T. and Brusvold, M.A. (1993a) Healing in periodontal defects treated by decalcified freeze-dried bone allografts in combination with ePTFE membranes. (I). Clinical and scanning electron microscope analysis. *Journal of Clinical Periodontology* **20**, 528–536

Guillemin, M.R., Mellonig, J.T., Brusvold, M.A. and Steffensen, B. (1993b) Healing in periodontal defects treated by decalcified freeze-dried bone allografts in combination with ePTFE membranes. Assessment by computerized densitometric analysis. *Journal of Clinical Periodontology* **20**, 520–521

Hauschka, P., Mavrakos, A., Lafrati, M.D. *et al.* (1986) Growth factor in bone matrix. Isolation of multiple types by affinity chromatography on heparin sepharose. *Journal of Biological Chemistry* **261**, 12665–12674

Hiatt, W. and Schallhorn, R. (1973) Intraoral transplants of cancellous bone and marrow in periodontal lesions. *Journal of Periodontology* **44**, 194–208

Hirschfeld, L. and Wasserman, B. (1978) A long-term survey of tooth loss in 600 treated periodontal patients. *Journal of Periodontology* **49**, 225–237

Hooley, R.W. and Kieran, J.A. (1974) Control of the initiation of DNA synthesis in 3T3 cells: serum factors. *Proceedings of the National Academy of Science (USA)* **71**, 2908–2911

Hughes, F.J. (1993) Surgical intervention: repair, guided tissue regeneration (growth factors; bone morphogenic proteins). Oral presentation at British Society of Periodontology Scientific Meeting at the Royal College of Surgery, June 5th 1993

Kasuggai, S., Todescan, R., Nagata, T. *et al.* (1991) Expression of bone matrix proteins associated with mineralized tissue formation by adult marrow cells *in vitro*: inductive effects of dexamethasone on osteoblast phenotype. *Journal of Cell Physiology* **147**, 111–120

Kenney, E.B., Lekovik, V., Han, T., Carranza, F.A. and Dimitrijevic, B. (1985) The use of porous hydroxyapatite implants in periodontal defects. I. Clinical results after 6 months. *Journal of Periodontology* **56**, 82–88

Kenney, E.B., Lekovik, V., Sa Ferreira, J.C., Han, T., Dimitrijevic, B. and Carranza, F.A. (1986) Bone formation within porous hydroxyapatite implants in human periodontal defects. *Journal of Periodontology* **57**, 76–83

Knowles, J.W., Burgett, F.G., Nissle, R.R. and Ramjford, S.P. (1979) Results of periodontal treatment related to pocket depth and attachment level: 8 years. *Journal of Periodontology* **50**, 225–233

Krejci, C., Bissada, N., Farah, C. and Greenwell, G. (1987) Clinical evaluation of porous and non-porous hydroxyapatites in the treatment of human periodontal defects. *Journal of Periodontology* **58**, 521–528

Levenson, R., Iwata, K., Klagsbrun, M. and Young, D.A. (1985) Growth factor- and dexamethasone-induced proteins in Swiss 3T3 cells. *Journal of Biological Chemistry* **260**, 8056–8063

Lindhe, J., Pontoriero, R., Berglundh, T. and Araujo, M. (1995) The effect of plaque management and bioresorbable occlusive devices in GTR treatment of degree III furcation defects. An experimental study in dogs. *Journal of Clinical Periodontology* **22**, 276–283

Lynch, S.E., Ruiz de Castilla, G., Williams, R.C. *et al.* (1991) The effects of short-term administration of a combination of platelet-derived and insulin-like growth factors on periodontal wound healing. *Journal of Periodontology* **62**, 458–467

Martin, L., McDougal, J. and Loskoski, S. (1985) Disinfection and inactivation of human T-lymphocyte virus type III/lymphadenopathy-associated virus. *Journal of Infective Disease* **152**, 400–403

Melcher, A.H. (1976) On the repair potential of periodontal tissues. *Journal of Periodontology* **47**, 256–260

Mellonig, J.T. (1991) Freeze-dried bone allografts in periodontal reconstructive surgery. *Dental Clinics of North America* **35**, 505–518

Mellonig, J.T. (1990) Regenerating bone in clinical periodontics. *Journal of the American Dental Association* **121**, 499–502

Mellonig, J., Bowers, G. and Bailey, R. (1981) Comparison of bone graft materials. I. New bone formation with autografts and allografts determined by strontium-85. *Journal of Periodontology* **52**, 291–296

Mellonig, J.T., Bowers, G.M., Bright, R.W. and Lawrence, J.J. (1976) Clinical evaluation of freeze-dried bone allograft in human periodontal osseous defects. *Journal of Periodontology* **47**, 125–131

Nyman, S., Lindhe, J. and Karring, T. (1990) Re-attachment – new attachment. In: Lindhe, J. (ed.) *Textbook of Clinical Periodontology*, 2nd ed. Copenhagen: Munksgaard, pp. 450–473

Nyman, S., Gottlow, J., Karring, T. and Lindhe, J. (1982a) The regenerative potential of the periodontal ligament. An experimental study in the monkey. *Journal of Clinical Periodontology* **9**, 257–265

Nyman, S., Lindhe, J. and Karring, T. (1983) Reattachment-new attachment. In: Lindhe, J. (ed.) *Textbook of Clinical Periodontology*. Copenhagen: Munksgaard, pp. 409–429

Nyman, S., Lindhe, J., Karring, T. and Rylander, H. (1982b) New attachment following surgical treatment of human periodontal disease. *Journal of Clinical Periodontology* **9**, 290–296

Otto, A.M., Natoli, C., Richmond, K.M.V. *et al.* (1981) Glucocorticoids inhibit the stimulatory effects of epidermal growth factor on the initiation of DNA synthesis. *Journal of Cell Physiology* **107**, 155–163

Pontoriero, R., Lindhe, J., Nyman, S., Karring, T., Rosenberg, E. and Savani, F. (1988) Guided tissue regeneration in degree II furcation involved mandibular molars. *Journal of Clinical Periodontology* **15**, 247–254

Pontoriero, R., Lindhe, J., Nyman, S. *et al.* (1989) Guided tissue regeneration in the treatment of furcation defects in mandibular molars. A clinical study of class III defects. *Journal of Clinical Periodontology* **16**, 170–174

Pontoriero, R., Nyman, S., Ericsson, I. and Lindhe, J. (1992) Guided tissue regeneration in surgically-produced furcation defects. An experimental study in the beagle dog. *Journal of Clinical Periodontology* **19**, 159–163

Pritlove-Carson, S., Palmer, R.M. and Floyd, P.D. (1993) Controlled trial of guided tissue regeneration in the treatment of periodontitis. *Journal of Dental Research* **72**, 717. Abstract 248

Proestakis, G., Bratthal, G., Söderholm, G. *et al.* (1992) Guided tissue regeneration in the treatment of infrabony defects on maxillary premolars. A pilot study. *Journal of Clinical Periodontology* **19**, 766–773

Quattlebaum, J., Mellonig, J. and Hansel, N. (1988) Antigenicity of freeze-dried cortical bone allograft in human periodontal osseous defects. *Journal of Periodontology* **59**, 394–397

Quinnan, G., Wells, J. and Wittek, M. (1986) Inactivation of human T-cell lymphotropic virus, Type III by heat, chemicals and irradiation. *Transfusion* **26**, 481–483

Quintero, G., Mellonig, J. and Gambill, V. (1982c) A six-month clinical evaluation of decalcified freeze-dried bone allograft in human periodontal defects. *Journal of Periodontology* **53**, 726–730

Resnick, L., Veren, K., Salahuddin, S., Tondreau, S. and Markham, P. (1986) Stability and inactivation of HTLV-III/LAV under clinical and laboratory environments. *Journal of the American Medical Association* **255**, 1887–1891

Rosenberg, M. (1971) Free osseous tissue autographs as a predictable procedure. *Journal of Periodontology* **42**, 195–209

Ross, R., Raines, E.W. and Bowen-Pope, D. (1986) The biology of platelet-derived growth factor. *Cell* **46**, 155–169

Rummelhart, J., Mellonig, J., Gray, J. and Towle, H. (1989) Comparison of freeze-dried bone allograft in human periodontal osseous defects. *Journal of Periodontology* **60**, 655–663

Rutherford, R.B., Niekrash, C.E., Kennedy, J.E. and Charette, M.F. (1992a) Platelet-derived and insulin-like growth factors stimulate the development of periodontal attachment in monkeys. *Journal of Periodontal Research* **27**, 285–290

Rutherford, R.B., Ryan, M.E., Kennedy, J.E. *et al.* (1993) Platelet-derived growth factor and dexamethasone combined with collagen matrix induce the regeneration of the periodontium in monkeys. *Journal of Clinical Periodontology* **20**, 537–544

Rutherford, R.B., Trail-Smith, M.D., Ryan, M.E. and Charette, M.F. (1992) Synergic effects of dexamethasone on platelet-derived growth factor mitogenesis *in vitro*. *Archives of Oral Biology* **37**, 139–145

Sampath, T.K., Coughlin, J.E. Whetstone, R.M. *et al.* (1990) Bovine osteogenic protein is composed of dimers of OP-1 and BMP-2A, two members of the transforming growth factor-B superfamily. *Journal of Biological Chemistry* **265**, 13198–13205

Sampath, T.K. and Reddi, A.H. (1983) Homology of bone inductive proteins from human, monkey, bovine and rat extracellular matrix. *Proceedings of the National Academy of Sciences (USA)* **80**, 6591–6595

Sander, L. and Karring, T. (1995a) New attachment and bone formation in periodontal defects following treatment of submerged roots with guided tissue regeneration. *Journal of Clinical Periodontology* **22**, 295–299

Sander, L. and Karring, T. (1995b) Healing of periodontal lesions in monkeys folowing the guided tissue regeneration procedure. A histological study. *Journal of Clinical Periodontology* **22**, 332–337

Sander, L., Frandsen, E.V.G., Arnbjerg, D., Warrer, K. and Karring, T. (1994) Effect of local metronidazole application on periodontal healing following guided tissue regeneration. Clinical findings. *Journal of Periodontology* **65**, 914–920

Sanders, J., Sepe, W., Bowers, G., Koch, R., Williams, J., Lekas, J. *et al.* (1983) Clinical evaluation of freeze-dried bone allograft in periodontal osseous defects—III. Composite freeze-dried bone allograft with and without autogenous bone grafts. *Journal of Periodontology* **54**, 1–8

Schallhorn, R.G. and McClain, P.K. (1988) Combined osseous grafting, root conditioning and guided tissue regeneration. *International Journal of Clinical Periodontics and Restorative Dentistry* **4**, 9–31

Schultz, A.J. and Gager, A.H. (1990) Guided tissue regeneration using an absorbable membrane (polygalactin 910) and osseous grafting. *International Journal of Periodontics and Restorative Dentistry* **10**, 9–17

Simion, M., Trisi, P., Maglione, M. and Piettelli, A. (1995) Bacterial penetration *in vitro* through GTAM membrane with and without topical chlorhexidine application. A light and scanning electron microscopic study. *Journal of Clinical Periodontology* **22**, 321–331

Stahl, S.S., Froum, S.J. and Tarnow, D. (1990) Human clinical and histologic responses to the placement of HTR polymer particles in 11 intrabony lesions. *Journal of Periodontology* **61**, 269–274

Stahl, S.S. and Froume, S. (1991) Histologic healing responses in human vertical lesions following the osseous allografts and barrier membranes. *Journal of Clinical Periodontology* **18**, 149–152

Turner, D. and Mellonig, J. (1981) Antigenicity of freeze-dried bone allograft in periodontal osseous defects. *Journal of Periodontal Research* **16**, 89–99

Urist, M.R. (1965) Bone formation by autoinduction. *Science* **150**, 893–899

Urist, M.R. and Strates, B. (1971) Bone morphogenic protein. *Journal of Dental Research* **60**, 1392–1406

Warren, K. and Karring, T. (1992) Guided tissue regeneration combined with osseous grafting in suprabony periodontal lesions. An experimental study in the dog. *Journal of Clinical Periodontology* **19**, 373–380

Warren, K., Karring, T., Nyman, S. and Gogoleweski, S. (1992) Guided tissue regeneration using biodegradable membranes of polyglactic acid or polyurethane. *Journal of Clinical Periodontology* **19**, 633–640

Yukna, R.A. (1990) HTR-polymer grafts in human

periodontal osseous defects. I. 6-months clinical results. *Journal of Periodontology* **61**, 633–642

Yukna, R.A., Cassingham, R., Caudrill, R. *et al.* (1986) Six months evaluation of calcitite (hydroxyapatite ceramic) in periodontal osseous defects. *International Journal of Periodontics and Restorative Dentistry* **6**, 34–45

Yukna, R.A., Mayer, E. and Amos, S. (1989) 5-year evaluation of Durapatite ceramic alloplastic implants in periodontal osseous defects. *Journal of Periodontology* **60**, 544–541

18

Mucogingival problems and their treatment

As described in Chapter 1 the attached gingiva or 'functional mucosa' extends from the gingival groove to the mucogingival junction where it meets the alveolar mucosa. At the mucogingival junction the mucoperiosteum splits so that the alveolar mucosa is separated from the periosteum by a loose highly vascular connective tissue. The width of the attached gingiva can vary from zero to about 9 mm, widest in the incisor regions and narrowest over canines and premolars. Its boundaries are defined on the buccal side by the insertion of the buccinator, the lip muscles and the frena, as well as by the morphology of the underlying bone. On the lingual side it is bounded by the insertion of the mylohyoid muscle, the insertions of lingual frena and the bone morphology.

Reduction in width of the attached gingiva is a consequence of gingival recession produced by atrophic changes, as described in Chapter 8, and/or as the result of progressive chronic periodontal disease.

In the past it had been assumed that some width of attached gingiva is necessary to maintain gingival health by separating the stable gingival margin from the mobile alveolar mucosa. It was also assumed that the depth of the vestibular sulcus was a significant factor in gingival health. As a result of this concept, a number of surgical 'vestibular extension' procedures were devised to achieve what were considered to be adequate anatomical dimensions. There was, however, no scientific evidence for these assumptions. Fortunately for the patient, notions of a normal vestibular depth were discarded, and ideas about the necessary width of attached gingiva questioned. Lang and Löe (1972) reported that a narrow band of 1–2 mm attached gingiva was necessary for gingival health, but other studies indicated that this is not the case. Miyasota et al. (1977), Wennstrom et al. (1982) and Salkin et al. (1987) have shown that it is possible to maintain a healthy and stable gingival margin with little or no attached gingiva, providing the individual maintains a high standard of oral hygiene. Wennstrom (1987) confirmed these results in a 5-year study. Addy et al. (1987) examined the relationship between frenal attachment, lip coverage and vestibular depth, and plaque and gingival bleeding scores in 1015 schoolchildren aged 11.5–12.5 years. They found that:

1. The position of the anterior maxillary frena appeared to affect plaque retention and gingival bleeding while the position of the mandibular labial frenum seemed to be unimportant.
2. Plaque and bleeding scores in the anterior area of the mandible seemed to decrease with an increase in vestibular depth, and
3. Decreased upper lip coverage at rest (lack of lip-seal) was related to increased plaque and bleeding scores in both jaws.

These various findings point to the fact that variations in the width of attached gingiva are significant only when oral hygiene is poor, and even then, as Addy et al. (1987) conclude, that significance is small, and alone does not justify surgical interference.

However, this study on children with gingival disease is not necessarily relevant to adults with various stages of periodontal disease. The precise form of treatment necessary depends on the anatomical and pathological variables involved in the lesion and in some cases the views of the patient.

Mucogingival problems can arise from the effects of:

• Chronic periodontitis
• Frenal pull
• Gingival recession

The effects of chronic periodontitis

1. Periodontal pocketing extending below the mucogingival junction where the apical limit of the pocket is:
   (a) level with some point between the mucogingival junction and the vestibular fold (*Figure 18.1*) so that after disease has been resolved there is enough healthy mucosa to cover the alveolar margin and produce a zone of attached mucosa and a vestibular sulcus. In this situation an apically repositioned flap may be indicated.
   (b) apical to the level of the vestibular sulcus so that any attempt at surgery to cover the alveolar margin would obliterate the gingival sulcus. In this case the apically displaced flap procedure could be used, plus a free gingival graft if tissue destruction is great.
2. Generalized gingival recession exposing root surfaces and reducing the zone of attached gingiva. This can be treated conservatively or surgically. Several surgical procedures could be considered including the free gingival graft combined with the coronally repositioned flap or the free connective tissue graft.

The effects of frenal pull

A frenum or muscle attachment which is inserted into an unhealthy gingival margin, which either:

(a) interferes with effective plaque removal (*Figure 18.2*) and/or
(b) pulls on the wall of the pocket and thereby aggravates the lesion (*Figure 18.2*). These

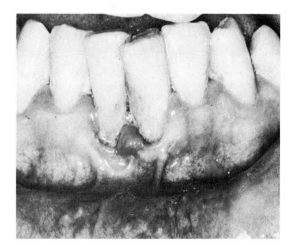

Figure 18.1 A combination of periodontal pocketing and gingival recession as a result of progressive chronic periodontitis. The pockets extend below the mucogingival junction and the gingival margin is subject to pull from muscle and frenal attachments

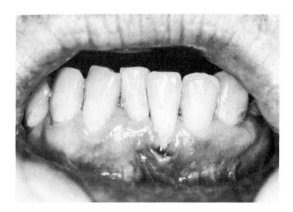

Figure 18.2 Gingival recession associated with soft-tissue attachment

lesions appear rather dramatic especially when related muscles are tensed by pulling (gently!) on the lip or cheek. Sometimes thorough scaling, root planing and efficient home care can keep the situation stable for several years. However, if gingival inflammation persists and/or there is evidence that the lesion is progressing surgical corrective treatment is indicated.

The first situation can be corrected by a simple frenectomy; the second may require a free gingival graft.

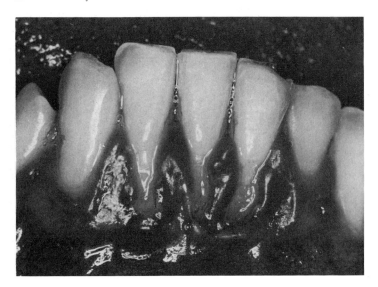

Figure 18.3 Destruction of gingival tissue caused by poor oral hygiene and the physical trauma of a very deep overbite, with the upper incisors impinging on the lower gingiva

Localized gingival recession

This may affect single or multiple teeth and may be caused by:

(a) an underlying local bony dehiscence(s) with associated toothbrushing trauma, or
(b) direct gingival trauma from the occlusion such as from a deep overbite associated with an Angle's Class 2, division II occlusion (*Figure 18.3*)

The first may be treated conservatively or surgically; surgical procedures include pedicle grafts and free gingival grafts and their variants (*see below*).

The second requires orthodontic treatment for the occlusal cause plus corrective surgery where possible. This is dependent on the precise nature of the defect.

Treatment of pocketing below the mucogingival junction

A number of surgical procedures have been developed to correct mucogingival problems of this type. All have the common aims of:

(a) the removal of disease, and
(b) the production of a periodontal anatomy which allows effective plaque control, and therefore prevent disease recurrence.

Deep pocketing of this type may be treated by the apically repositioned flap or the apically

displaced flap as appropriate. The former is described on pp. 188–191.

The apically displaced flap (*Figure 18.4*)

The apically displaced flap technique can be used where the base of the pocket lies apical to the MGJ and a zone of keratinized gingiva is either absent or very narrow and the vestibular depth shallow. For pocket elimination, the flap has to be moved apical by an amount equal to the depth of the pocket so that the flap margin coincides with the

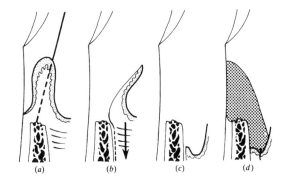

Figure 18.4 The apically displaced flap technique: (*a*) an inverse bevel incision is made (where there is considerable tissue destruction and distortion a horizontal incision can be made); (*b*) the flap is dissected from the underlying periosteum; (*c*) the tissue is displaced apical to the alveolar crest; (*d*) tissue sutured to underlying muscle and held in place by periodontal dressing. Healing is by secondary intention

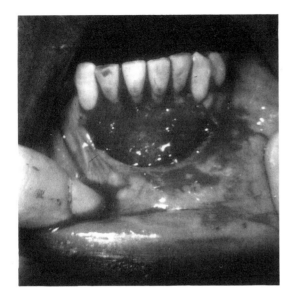

Figure 18.5 Apically displaced flap. A split-thickness flap has been dissected up, leaving periosteum on the bone surface

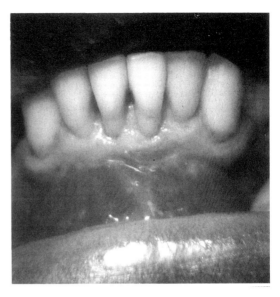

Figure 18.6 Apically displaced flap. Final result one year after procedure. There is pocket elimination with a functional zone of attached gingiva and a good vestibular depth

alveolar crest. However, where all or most of the attached gingiva has been destroyed, the flap has to be moved so that its margin is apical to the bone margin.

Procedure

If there is a usable zone of keratinized gingiva then this is preserved by making an inverse bevel incision along the gingival margin (*Figure 18.4a*). However, if very little keratinized gingiva remains and this is grossly misshapen than it is best discarded. In this case there is little point in making a scalloped gingival incision. A straight incision can be made and the inflamed and frequently misshapen marginal tissue discarded. Vertical releasing incisions are made delineating the area of tissue to be moved apically and the flap is lifted by sharp dissection through the loose connective tissue of the alveolar mucosa plus any associated muscles (*Figure 18.4b*), thus leaving the periosteum on the bone (*Figure 18.5*).

The flap is moved apical to the alveolar crest (*Figure 18.4c*) into a position which will allow the production, by secondary intention healing, of a zone of attached gingiva free of frenal and muscle attachments. After curettage and root planing of the exposed root surfaces, the flap is fixed by sutures at the releasing incisions and, if necessary, by a suture in the midline fixing the flap to the underlying mentalis muscle. The exposed alveolar margin, which is covered by periosteum, will heal by secondary intention.

A periodontal dressing is essential (*Figure 18.4d*). It is placed for 1 week and then removed; the wound is irrigated with a warm saline solution and the dressing is replaced for a further week. The surface of the wound becomes covered by stratified squamous epithelium over this period but the healing period is much longer than that for flap procedures which cover the bone surface. The formation of mature connective tissue and well-keratinized attached gingiva can take up to 6 weeks. During this period the patient needs to be kept on a chlorhexidine mouthwash and should receive professional cleaning every 2 weeks.

The final result of this procedure is good and should produce a functional zone of attached gingiva free from muscle and frenal pull and a good vestibular depth (*Figure 18.6*).

The treatment of the effects of frenal pull

This may be treated either by a frenectomy or a free gingival graft. The former is described below whilst the latter is included in the section on the treatment of gingival recession.

Frenectomy

A frenectomy is indicated where the attachment of a frenum or muscle attachment is so close to the gingival margin that it interferes with efficient plaque removal and contributes to persistent gingival inflammation. This problem is most frequently found on the labial surface between the upper central incisors, but can also occur in relation to the upper canines and premolars. In the lower jaw the frena are found labial to the lower incisors and rarely on the lingual aspect.

Procedure

1. After local anaesthesia the lip is extended and the frenum gripped with mosquito forceps. Incisions are made with a No. 15 Swann-Morton blade on either side of the forceps through the base of the frenum. The incisions should meet at the point of the instrument. The incision on the alveolar side is made close to the alveolar bone, leaving the periosteum in place.
2. The triangle of frenal tissue should come away easily if the incisions have been made correctly.
3. The edges of the lip wound are gently undermined so that they can be approximated without tension and sutured. It is not necessary to suture the alveolar wound.
4. Swabs are placed firmly over the wound to control bleeding and a periodontal dressing is applied. Retention of the dressing in this situation is often poor and the patient must be advised that if the dressing falls off it is not a calamity provided that the wound is kept clean with warm saline mouthwashes and a twice-daily rinse with 0.2% chlorhexidine solution.
5. After one week the sutures and any dressing are removed. Usually healing is rapid and uneventful.

The treatment of gingival recession

Localized gingival recession

Localized recession of the gingival margin with considerable exposure of the root is usually associated with the presence of an underlying bony dehiscence. It is most commonly seen on the buccal surface of teeth with buccally placed roots, associated with teeth with bulbous roots or in areas where the surface bone is naturally thin. Common teeth involved are lower incisors and upper canines, premolars or first molars. Recession progresses into the attached gingival zone, decreasing this as it deepens. If it progresses into the alveolar mucosa, below the mucogingival junction, the gingival margin is no longer protected from the pull of the muscles via frenal and mucosal attachments and it may be pulled away from the root surface during facial muscle activity. This relationship also interferes with plaque removal because the gingival margin at this point is no longer accessible to clean unless the lip is physically pulled back for access. Plaque and calculus therefore collect at the base of the lesion producing localized gingivitis. Inflammation persists unless there is frequent professional cleaning and lip movement produces further tension on the gingival margin so that progressive destruction is almost inevitable.

Localized or generalized gingival recession may be managed conservatively or surgically and these are described below.

Conservative management of gingival recession

Gingival recession which is not accompanied by disease, i.e. inflammation or pocketing, does not require intervention unless it presents a serious cosmetic problem. The patient must be reassured that recession, especially that produced by over enthusiastic toothbrushing, is of little significance, does not prejudice the life of the tooth and rarely justifies intervention; it simply signals that a less harmful cleaning technique is needed.

Where there is inflammation and/or pocketing, i.e. the recession is involved in a progressive periodontal lesion, or where labial recession produces a significant cosmetic problem, intervention may be indicated.

If the recession is isolated and reflects an underlying dehiscence, a laterally repositioned graft can be an effective method of correction. If the recession is associated with a muscle attachment and a related inadequate zone of attached gingiva a free gingival graft may be needed. These surgical techniques and some other alternatives are described in the section below.

Gingival recession occasionally produces root sensitivity to cold and sweet; this sensitivity often deters the patient from brushing properly so that plaque accumulates on the root surface. This actually aggravates the root sensitivity and the patient needs to be reassured that proper cleaning is necessary. Initially it may be necessary to use warm water for brushing but in many cases adequate plaque control reduces the sensitivity. If sensitivity to cold and sweet persists, one of the toothpastes especially formulated to treat the problem (Sensodyne, Emoform etc.) can be recommended. As stated earlier, sodium fluoride can be very effective as a desensitizing agent and it may be used as Lukomsky's paste (equal parts by weight of sodium fluoride, kaolin and glycerine) which is applied to the dried root on two or three occasions. An amine fluoride in a gel (Duraphat) applied to the dried root surface is also effective and convenient to use. Another useful medicament is 1% hydrocortisone solution applied several times to dried root. Topical guanethidine (1%) has also been recommended for rapid relief from dental hypersensitivity (Hannington-Kitt and Dunne, 1993).

One occasionally encounters intractable root sensitivity which does not respond to any topical applications. Usually this points to pulp pathology, produced either by a large restoration or by a microscopic lateral pulp canal; in this situation endodontics is needed. It must be stressed that surgical intervention is required in very few cases of recession. The chief criterion for such treatment is the presence of progressive disease which is definitely associated with the recession and which persists despite conservative measures.

Surgical treatment of gingival recession

The type of surgical treatment possible depends on the nature of the lesion(s) and these are classified below:

Classification of gingival recession

The classification of gingival recession into type defects is based upon the relationships between the base of the defect, the mucogingival junction and the height of the interdental papillae. This also gives a very reliable guide to the degree of reconstruction possible. These defects have been classified by Miller (1985a) and this is shown below along with a summary of the clinical criteria for each group and the possible results of treatment.

Classification	*Clinical Criteria*	*Possible Treatment Result*
Class I	Full height papillae Recession within attached gingiva	100% coverage possible
Class II	Full height papillae Recession at/ beyond MGJ	100% coverage possible
Class III	Reduced papilla height Recession at/ beyond MGJ	Coverage only to level related to papilla height
Class IV	Gross flattened loss of papillae	Not possible to cover

As already stated above there are two approaches to the treatment of gingival recession:

1. Accept and maintain

If the degree of recession is acceptable to the patient then a decision can be taken to try to maintain the condition. (The appropriate treatment for this has been described above.) Study models should be taken and the condition should be reviewed at regular maintenance visits to determine whether it is stable. If the gingival recession is found to be progressing and the recession is still acceptable to the patient but is close to or beyond the mucogingival junction then a free gingival graft can be carried out to increase the zone of attached gingiva and maintain the situation.

2. Repair and eliminate recession

If the recession is unacceptable to the patient and in one of the categories where successful repair is possible than an appropriate surgical technique to repair the defect can be discussed with the patient describing the probable outcome. The aim of these techniques is to cover the exposed root surface to the greatest degree possible and to increase and/or maintain a functional zone of attached gingiva.

The possible techniques to consider are listed below:

Pedicle grafts

- coronal repositioned flap
- lateral repositioned flap
- double papilla flap

Free grafts

- full thickness, thick epithelial
- connective tissue
- connective tissue with double papilla

Other regenerative techniques

- GTR with PTFE membranes
- GTR with resorbable membranes

In reparative techniques there is still debate about the need for root surface instrumentation or conditioning.

Root surface instrumentation

Miller (1992) states that root preparation will cause a reduction in inflammation which may result in a loss of papilla height by gingival shrinkage. This may affect the potential coverage of the exposed root surface. The reduction in vascularity also may affect the nutrient supply to the graft. However, any plaque, calculus and stain must be removed from the root surface prior to surgery and patients undergoing these procedures must have immaculate oral hygiene.

Root surface preparation

There is still considerable debate about the need to prepare the surface, and also, if this is deemed necessary, about which method of preparation should be used. A number of clinical researchers have reported good results using citric acid at pH 1 for between 2–3 minutes (Register and Burdick, 1975, 1976; Crigger *et al.*, 1978; Garrett *et al.*, 1978; Nyman *et al.*, 1981; Miller, 1982). This can be applied with a brush or a cotton bud, and may either be burnished into the root surface or left alone. Tetracycline has also been used as a solution in a similar manner to citric acid and beneficial results have been reported on its use (Wicksjö

et al., 1986; Demirel *et al.*, 1991; Terranova *et al.*, 1986). Terranove *et al.* (1986) showed that biochemical manipulation of the dentine surface could affect the cells attaching to it and their growth. They found that treatment of the dentine surface with tetracycline increased the binding of fibronectin to its surface. They also found that the absorbed fibronectin stimulated the attachment of fibroblasts to its surface and stimulated their growth. Furthermore, they also showed that the absorbed fibronectin suppressed the attachment of epithelial cells to the dentine surface and their growth.

Pedicle grafts

Laterally repositioned flap

The laterally repositioned flap is an effective procedure for treating an isolated area of gingival recession where a suitable donor site of keratinized tissue is present. The procedure was first introduced by Grupe and Warren (1956) and has been modified in small detail by several other clinicians. The exposed root is covered by mobilizing a pedicle graft from a suitable adjacent area which is then slid laterally to cover the defect. It is suitable to treat single tooth narrow areas of gingival recession with adequate interdental bone height and an adjacent donor area with an adequate zone of keratinized attached gingiva. This is a one-stage procedure whereby a pedicle flap is elevated by split-thickness dissection from an adjacent area of keratinized tissue. The blood supply that nourishes the flap over the avascular root surface is supplied by the wide base of the pedicle flap and from the periosteum over the bone surrounding the denuded roots. The flap is secured into position over the denuded root with interrupted silk sutures. The colour blend and root coverage are excellent in well-chosen cases. However, it is generally not suitable for treating isolated wide areas of recession or multiple recessions.

Procedure (Figure 18.7)

The area should receive preparatory periodontal treatment to remove all plaque and calculus from the root surface and resolve any gingival inflammation in the surrounding area and the rest of the mouth.

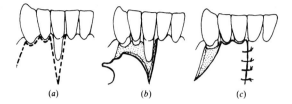

Figure 18.7 Diagram to illustrate laterally repositioned flap technique: (*a*) incisions are made around the defect and along the gingival margin, then a releasing incision is made approximately two teeth away from the defect; (*b*) a part full-thickness and part split-thickness flap is dissected from the underlying bone and (*c*) moved laterally to cover the defect

Preparation of the recipient area

Incisions are made down the margins of the defect to remove epithelium from its edges (*Figure 18.7a*). These incisions meet apically at the base of the defect where the incision is carried into the vestibule. More tissue should be removed from the margin of the defect which is to receive the leading edge of the sliding pedicle graft. This is to allow bone to be uncovered at this margin so that the sutured edge of the flap will lie over bone rather than root surface. This is very important to the success of this procedure and it dictates that the interproximal bone in this area must be at its normal height, i.e. there should be no interdental bone resorption. All the detached tissue should be carefully removed from around the exposed root surface and the root is carefully planed clean and smooth. Some clinicians have recommended root conditioning with citric acid for this procedure. Also if the recipient tooth has a bulky, outstanding root this lessens the chances of success. Planing back of these prominent roots with a Kirkland no. 7 curette has also been advocated and this would normally be followed by root conditioning.

Preparation of the pedicle graft

A gingival crevicular incision is then made around the next two teeth and a releasing incision is made from the gingival incision into the vestibule (*Figure 18.7a*). This should produce a flap which is twice as wide as the gingival defect. A part split thickness and part full thickness flap is then carefully developed. The full thickness mucoperiosteal flap is raised

from the tooth which will provide the part of the flap covering the exposed root so that the root is directly covered by periosteum. The part of the flap related to the adjacent tooth which when raised will expose the donor area bone should be developed as a split-thickness flap. This allows the exposed donor area of bone to retain its periosteal covering for protection and additional blood supply. This part of the flap is dissected up to separate the gingival epithelium and connective tissue from the underlying periosteum over the bone (*Figure 18.7b*). Great care should be taken with this stage of the procedure as perforation of the flap will mean inevitable failure. However, if this technique is attempted in an area potentially involving important nerves such as in the lower premolar area then a total full thickness flap should be raised to avoid nerve damage. The dissection of the flap is carried into the alveolar mucosa so that the flap can be moved laterally without any tension.

Repositioning of pedicle graft

The flap is moved across the root surface so that its leading margin approximates the receiving edge of gingival tissue making sure that the resulting suture line will lie over bone (*Figure 18.7c*). These margins are brought together and sutured using 4/0 or 5/0 silk sutures. Care must be taken that the flap fits tightly around the neck of the affected tooth. Three or four sutures may be needed to close the defect tightly and one of these is placed in the vestibule so that no residual eyelet defect is produced. An interdental suture is also placed in each interproximal space covered by the flap. A denuded area of periosteum-covered bone is left distal to the flap (or mesially to the flap if it was moved distally).

A moist sterile gauze is pressed firmly over the flap to fix it in position and minimize any underlying blood clot. A periodontal dressing such as Coe-Pack is placed over the wound area.

Postoperative care

The usual postoperative instructions are given with emphasis on the need to avoid vigorous lip movements. This procedure produces very little swelling or discomfort and healing is usually uneventful.

The dressing and sutures are removed after one week, by which time the suture line should be united and the denuded area covered by healing tissue.

Rarely does the wound need to be covered for more than a week. The patient is instructed to keep the area clean with a twice-daily chlorhexidine mouthwash and frequent warm saline washes. Irritation of the healing graft must be avoided. Careful toothbrushing with a soft brush can be started when the pack and sutures are removed but this should gently clean the tooth surface down to but not on to the gingiva.

Two weeks after surgery the suture line should be fading and the denuded area should be covered with epithelium. One month after surgery the wound is fully healed but it is still unwise to probe the gingival crevice over the defect. Probing is best left for about six months and should be carried out with great care.

Mode of healing

The exact form of healing that takes place after the laterally repositioned flap procedure is still debated. There are two possibilities:

1. Crevicular epithelium grows down the inner surface of the flap against the root surface to form a long epithelial attachment and the gingival fibre bundles keep the flap closely adapted to the root. It is also feasible that hemidesmosomes connect the epithelial downgrowth to the root surface so that a firm attachment is formed.
2. Epithelial downgrowth does not take place and a fibrous tissue connection forms between the flap and the root surface. This could imply the deposition of new cementum on to the root surface so that Sharpey's fibres can be formed. The differentiation of cementoblasts and formation of cementum seem unlikely without the concomitant formation of crestal bone and so far no evidence of such repair has been produced.

Whichever form of healing actually does take place, at a clinical level the graft can remain stable for many years providing that the gingival margin is free of plaque and therefore free of inflammation. Slight recession of the graft may take place but rarely recurrence of pocketing or of a new defect.

Modification of laterally repositioned flap

The standard laterally repositioned flap can sometimes result in some gingival recession in the donor area and a modification which spares the marginal gingiva at the donor site has been recently devised. This is only possible if a sufficiently wide zone of attached gingiva is present in the donor area to produce the desired zone of keratinized tissue at the recipient site. It has the advantage of leaving the interdental papillae *in situ* at the recipient site which makes it easier to secure the pedicle graft at the required height. It also leaves a much smaller exposed area at the donor site than the conventional technique.

Procedure

Recipient site

Horizontal incisions are made across the base of the two interdental papillae of the recipient tooth so that these are retained in their original positions. These will form a butt joint against which the repositioned sliding flap will lie. Two vertical incisions are then made down to the vestibule on either side of the recession area to expose bone around its margin (*Figures 18.8a* and *18.9a*). This tissue is cut off by a further horizontal incision at its base and the tissue is removed. The root surface is carefully scaled and planed and may be conditioned if desired.

Donor site

A slightly sloping horizontal incision is then made from the tip of the distal vertical recipient site incision and is carried below the interdental papillae and marginal gingiva of the donor site teeth. A further slightly sloping vertical incision is then made distally down into the vestibule to delineate the donor flap (*Figures 18.8a* and *18.9a*).

This flap is carefully dissected up as a split-thickness flap, leaving the periosteum in place. This flap is then fully mobilized and slid across to cover the defect where it fits into a butt joint with the recipient site papillae (*Figures 18.8b* and *18.9b*). The flap is sutured into position with resorbable 5/0 gut sutures. Two sutures join it to the retained papillae at the recipient site and a further two or three join the vertical flap margin to the mesial edge of

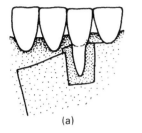 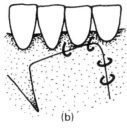

Figure 18.8 Modified laterally repositioned flap.
(*a*) Horizontal incisions below papillae of recipient teeth
and below gingival margins of donor teeth. Bone is
exposed around root of recipient tooth and a sloping
vertical incision is made to delineate flap; (*b*) Flap slid
over defect and sutured in place.

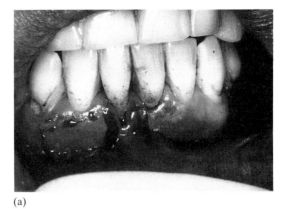

(a)

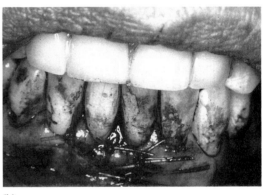

(b)

Figure 18.9 Clinical pictures of modified laterally
repositioned flap. (a) Incisions; (b) Sutured into new
position. (By courtesy of Mr C A Waterman)

the recipient site. Only a small area of donor
site periosteum is left uncovered with this
procedure.

The area is covered with either a conventional pack such as Coe-Pack or a Surgicel
cyanoacrylate pack. With this latter method,
Surgicel is placed over the area, and held in
place using cyanoacrylate glue (Superglue).
This can also be covered with Vaseline with
tetracycline powder mixed into it if required
(Miller, 1982, 1985b, 1992). Coe-Pack is
replaced after a week and replaced for a
further week if necessary. The latter pack is
left until it drops off, usually after 3 weeks.

Healing of both the donor and recipient
sites is usually uneventful.

Double papilla flap

This technique was introduced by Cohen and
Ross (1968) and is a variant of the laterally
repositioned flap. The basic technique is
similar except that the donor tissue is
mobilized from the adjacent papillae rather
than from an adjacent tooth. There is less
exposure of donor site bone with this procedure and less tension is placed on the donor
tissue. The interdental septum at the papillary
area is of greater thickness than the facial or
lingual alveolar plates and are less likely to be
damaged when the overlying tissues are
disturbed. A disadvantage of this technique is
that the proximal papillae must be of sufficient
bulk both mesio-distally and cervico-apically
to cover the defect. Small papillae imply small
interdental septa and under these conditions

this procedure would both fail to cover the
defect as well as possibly causing damage to
the underlying bony septa.

Procedure (Figure 18.10)

This procedure is suitable for a recession defect
on a tooth with bulky mesial and distal papillae. The exposed root surface is scaled and root
planed. A V-shaped incision is made around the
margin of the recessed gingiva to expose
connective tissue at its edge (*Figure 18.10a*).
The distal tissue is bevelled to expose a wider
zone of connective tissue to accept the mesial
portion of the graft. Mesial and distal vertical
incisions are made and carried into the
vestibule to mobilize the two papillae (*Figure
18.10a*). The two papillary flaps are carefully
raised and repositioned to cover the labial
surface of the exposed root so that the join line
coincides with the distal margin of the defect.

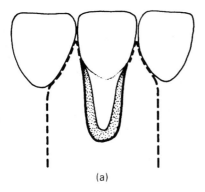 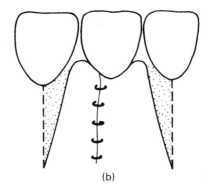

(a)   (b)

Figure 18.10 Double papilla flap. (*a*) Incisions (i) around root to expose bone with wider zone distally to provide base for suture line; (ii) delineating flap margins. (*b*) Papillae transposed to cover defect and sutured over bone exposed distal to defect

The flaps are sutured together in this position with resorbable 5/0 medium gut sutures (*Figure 18.10b*). This correct positioning is very important since placement of sutures at the midline of the exposed root will lead to inadequate coadaptation of tissue. This will result in the creation of a dehiscence at the suture line and failure of the procedure. The most apical suture is passed through the periosteum to stabilize the position of the graft. In addition, either mesial and distal sutures or a sling suture around the tooth can be placed to stabilize the graft further. A dressing such as Coe-Pack may be carefully placed over the area for a week.

Coronally repositioned flap

This procedure is usually in conjunction with the free gingival graft to treat the combined problem of gingival recession and lack of attached gingiva. These procedures are usually used where there are multiple sites of recession in the area to be treated.

Procedure

The free gingival graft is first carried out to increase the attached gingival zone (see full description in following section). After complete healing, a full-thickness mucoperiosteal flap is raised and extended to the base of the vestibule. It is then moved upwards in a coronal direction to cover the exposed roots of the teeth and maintained in this position by interdental suturing and the placement of a periodontal dressing. In the combined procedure the free gingival graft is used to provide new keratinized attached gingiva and the coronally repositioned flap to carry this up over the root surface.

Free grafts

Full thickness, thick epithelial flap

The free gingival graft was introduced by Nabors (1963). It is designed to increase the width of keratinized gingiva. Unlike the pedicle graft, this procedure takes keratinized palatal epithelium and connective tissue from its original site and relocates it to a remote donor site. The graft is placed over a freshly prepared bed of connective tissue and sutured in place. The underlying connective tissue bed nourishes the graft until it builds its own blood supply. This forms as the result of blood vessels growing into it from the underlying connective tissue base (*see below*).

As this graft retains none of its own blood supply and is totally dependent on the bed of recipient vessels, it was originally developed to increase the zone of attached gingiva and not specifically to cover denuded root. New attached gingiva is produced by grafting keratinized palatal mucosa and its inductive connective tissue over a recipient bed previously covered by non-keratinized alveolar mucosa. However, several modifications have improved this procedure's root coverage capabilities. Maynard (1977) developed two procedures: firstly the placement of a free gingival graft to create a band of keratinized gingiva and secondly a coronally repositioned flap (*see above*) to pull the tissue coronally over the exposed root(s). Holbrook and Oshsenbein (1983) used thick, stretched, free gingival grafts with intricate suturing to improve the graft's adaptation to the recipient bed and limit the amount of dead space, which could hinder vascularization. Miller (1982, 1985b) emphasized root planing and citric acid treatment of the exposed roots.

All of these modifications have improved the capability of free grafts to survive over avascular root surfaces. The coverage of wide or multiple areas of recession are best treated by the double procedure of Maynard (1977) (*see below*) whilst the free graft alone, using the modifications of Holbrook and Ochsenbein (1983) and Miller (1982, 1985b) can be used to cover single narrow root surface defects (*Figure 18.12a*).

Procedures

The procedure differs in several details according to whether the aim is only to increase the zone of attached gingiva, leaving the existing gingiva undisturbed (Procedure 1) or whether the aim is additionally to cover area(s) of root exposed by gingival recession (Procedure 2).

Suitable donor and recipient sites are chosen and local analgesia given.

Preparation of recipient site

The following technique has been proposed by Miller (1982, 1985b).

For Procedure 1, an incision is made along the mucogingival junction (*Figure 18.11a,c*). For Procedure 2 techniques, an incision made along the gingiva of the recipient site to allow butt joining of the graft to adjacent tissue (*Figure 18.11b,c*). The apical margin of the flap is raised and dissected through the connective tissue as a split thickness flap to delineate the connective tissue bed of the recipient site (*Figure 18.11d*). This extends into the area previously covered by non-keratinized alveolar mucosa. Bulow Dry Foil is then placed over the bed to act as a template for the graft and trimmed to size.

Root preparation

This is only necessary for type 2 procedures and the method outlined is that proposed by Miller (1985b). If the exposed root surface is buccally prominent it is planed back to reduce the possibility of recurrence and to reduce localized pressures on the graft. This is done either using a Kirkland No. 12 curette or a Gracey curette. A butt joint is made at the cement enamel junction of the tooth. The root surface is then conditioned using pH 1 citric acid using cotton buds or a burnishing technique. It is left until there is a frosted finish on the root surface after profuse rinsing.

Preparation of donor site

The template is placed on the palate and the graft outlined. It is delineated with a No. 15 Swann-Morton blade, making an incision about 3 mm deep so that the graft includes an adequate thickness of connective tissue. In fact it is this connective-tissue layer which is the functional part of the graft. A split-thickness graft is carefully dissected from the underlying deeper connective tissue with the No. 15 blade. The graft should be at least 2–3 mm thick and any adipose tissue on the inner side can be left for root coverage. However, if root coverage is not being attempted than it should be 1–2 mm with no adipose tissue.

Placement of graft

The graft should be placed *in situ* (*Figures 18.11e* and *18.12b*) and trimmed quickly, if necessary, to help to maintain its vitality. The flap raised at the recipient site can be cut off at this point as it is no longer needed, and the graft can be sutured in place.

Three types of suture have been described for use with this procedure (Miller, 1982, 1985; Jahnke *et al.*, 1993). These are (*Figure 18.11f,g*):

1. Papillary sutures positioned interdentally (*Figure 18.11f*)
2. Apical stretching sutures (*Figure 18.11f*)
3. Vertical stabilizing sutures (*Figure 18.11g*)

The vertical stabilizing sutures (*Figure 18.11g*) criss-cross over the graft without going through it. The suture passes from the palatal aspect of the tooth through the right interdental space. It then passes diagonally across the surface of the graft to its base at the opposite corner. It then penetrates through the

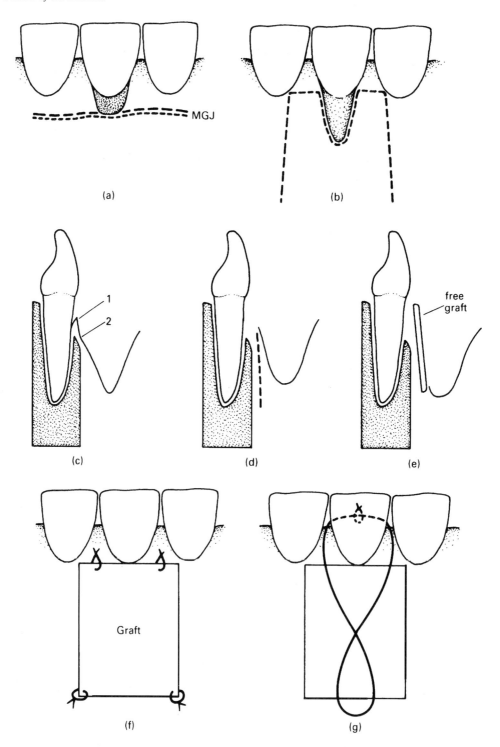

Figure 18.11 Free gingival graft. (*a*) Incision for procedure 1 at mucogingival junction. (*b*) Incisions for procedure 2 to cover exposed roots. Horizontal incision across base of papillae which are left *in situ*. The incision carries around the recession area. Two vertical incisions delineate flap. (*c*) Incision for procedure 1(1) and 2(2) in other plane. (*d*) Dissection of split-thickness flap to leave tissue over bone to nourish free graft. (*e*) Free graft in position. (*f*) Papillary and apical stretching sutures. (*g*) Vertical stabilizing sutures

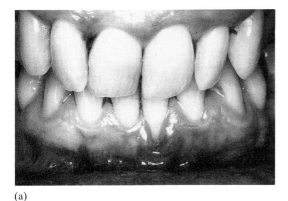

(a)

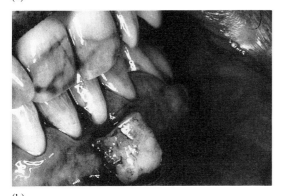

(b)

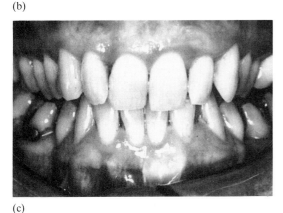

(c)

Figure 18.12 Free gingival graft to treat localized gingival recession. (*a*) Preoperative picture showing recession of ⌐1 extending to mucogingival graft; (*b*) Free graft placed into position before suturing; (*c*) Postoperative result after 1 year showing coverage of root and increase in attached gingival zone. (By courtesy of Mr C A Waterman)

periosteum at the base of the graft and then crosses diagonally in the opposite direction to the left interdental space. It finally passes through this to meet the starting end to be tied off palatally.

These sutures allow the graft to be approximated closely to the root surface, whilst still allowing flow of nutrient. Resorbable catgut sutures are used to avoid trauma to the healing area. To protect the graft, Surgicel is placed over the area, and held in place using cyanoacrylate glue (Superglue). This is then covered with Vaseline into which tetracycline powder has been mixed (Miller, 1982, 1985b, 1992). This is left until it drops off, usually after 3 weeks and cleanliness is maintained using chlorhexidine mouthwashes. The patient may be placed on tetracycline for 2 weeks.

The palate can be similarly covered, or an acrylic stent may be used, although there is good healing after only one week.

The end-result can look extremely good (*Figure 18.12c*), and this is a very predictable procedure with good long-term results. However, in some cases, it can look bulky or of a different colour.

Healing of the graft

Vascularization of the gingival graft takes place from the underlying connective-tissue bed. This can commence as early as the first 2–4 days, before which nutrients to the graft are supplied by tissue fluid. Capillary buds grow from the underlying connective tissue into the graft and these vessels anastomose and mature to form a new vasculature which is complete by about the 14th day. Because nutrition to the graft is minimal during the first 2–3 days the surface layers of the epithelium degenerate, necrose and are desquamated. A layer of new epithelium is present after 4–5 days, rete pegs are formed at 7–14 days and keratinization takes about 28 days. The maturation process takes place under the inductive influence of the palatal connective tissue.

Factors affecting success

1. Incorrect choice of site for procedure used, i.e. wrong class of gingival recession.
2. The graft may be too thick. If such a graft becomes vascularized the tablet of tissue stands away from the rest of the tissue.
3. If the graft is too thin it may perforate and necrose.
4. If the underlying blood clot is too thick the graft may be discarded.

Connective-tissue graft

This type of graft has a number of advantages over the free epithelial graft (Edel, 1974; Langer and Langer, 1985; Jahnke *et al.*, 1993). These are:

1. There is a closed palatal wound.
2. The aesthetic result is claimed to be better.
3. There is a better potential blood supply from the periosteum beneath and the split thickness flap above.

This procedure was introduced by Langer and Langer (1985) as a method of gaining root coverage in cases with severe recession involving either isolated or multiple teeth. The subepithelial connective tissue graft is a combination of a pedicle graft and a free autogenous connective-tissue graft performed simultaneously. In this procedure, the connective tissue receives a blood supply from the periosteum beneath and the split thickness flap above and this increases its chances of survival over the avascular root surface.

Procedure

Preparation of recipient site

A horizontal incision is made around the teeth to be treated and the area is bounded by two vertical relieving incisions which extend well beyond the mucogingival junction to create a wide base for the flap. The horizontal incision passes along the base of each included interdental papilla and then into the gingival crevice buccally to each tooth (*Figures 18.13* and *18.14*). Great care must be taken not to lift the papillae. The incisions are carefully deepened and the flap is carefully dissected from the underlying periosteum and deep connective tissue as a split thickness flap. The edge of the flap is first raised and held under tension with fine tissue forceps to allow careful sharp dissection with a No. 15 blade. Great care must be taken not to perforate the flap as this will compromise its blood supply, which is an important source of nutrient to the connective-tissue graft. The flap is freed apically so that there will be very little tension when it is ultimately pulled coronally. The size of the connective-tissue graft is determined by the size of the recipient base and its height and length are measured. The graft must be large enough to cover the exposed roots and

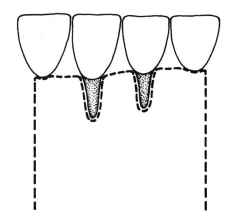

Figure 18.13 Incisions for connective-tissue graft at recipient site. The incision passes across the base of the papillae to leave these *in situ* for suturing

connective-tissue bed in all directions. The connective-tissue bed is the second important source of blood supply to the overlying graft.

Root preparation

Root planing of the exposed roots is carefully carried out. Additional preparation with citric acid or tetracycline may also be carried out as described in the last section. Opinion is divided as to whether this is necessary or beneficial.

Preparation of donor site

The donor site is prepared palatally by making two parallel horizontal bevelled incisions which are made 3 mm from the gingival margin using a No. 15 blade (*Figure 18.15a*). It is made from the canine to the first molar area since the connective tissue is thicker and better vascularized in this area and the rugae are of no concern because the graft is taken internally. A split thickness flap is raised with or without mesial and distal vertical relieving incisions. A wedge of connective tissue of about 1.5 mm thickness along with its thin border of epithelium is carefully dissected out (*Figure 18.15b*). Care should be taken to avoid the palatine vessels but staying anterior to the first molar should avoid this problem. The length of the flap and the depth of the dissection depend on the size of the recipient area to be covered. This procedure leaves the outer epithelialized flap to be replaced for primary intention wound closure.

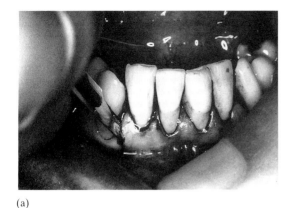

(a)

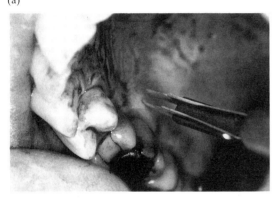

(b)

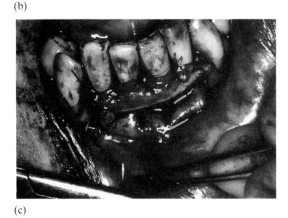

(c)

Figure 18.14 Connective tissue graft. (*a*) Incisions: the papillae are left *in situ* for suturing; (*b*) A special scalpel handle with two blades 1.5 mm apart for taking optimum thickness connective tissue graft from palate; (*c*) The connective tissue graft in position over root surfaces and prepared bed. (By courtesy of Mr C.A. Waterman)

A special scalpel handle (*Figure 18.14b*) has been devised to accept two blades 1.5 mm apart for use in obtaining a suitable connective-tissue graft. This was designed by Harris

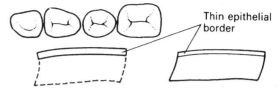

Figure 18.15 (*a*) Incisions for connective-tissue graft from palate. Two parallel incisions 1.5 mm apart from canine to first molar are made. Connective-tissue graft is then dissected out. (*b*) Resultant graft with thin epithelialized upper margin

(1992) for use in the double papilla graft/connective-tissue graft (*see below*) but can be used in this procedure also if available.

It is advisable to suture the palatal flap back into position immediately after removing the donor tissue as this will reduce the size of the blood clot which will form. A method of suturing which produces compression will also further this aim. Horizontal mattress sutures are used and they begin by passing through the mesial interproximal space on the buccal surface. They then penetrate the palatal mucosa apical and distal to the base of the graft and then exit the palate mesially. They finally cross to the distal interproximal space to be tied on the buccal surface. These sutures compress the palatal flap and approximate its edges. This should bring about rapid haemostasis. A dressing is optional and usually not necessary. The patient reports much less discomfort and bleeding problems than with the free gingival graft because of the full coverage.

Graft placement

The connective-tissue graft is carefully positioned over the denuded roots with its epithelialized border coronally (*Figure 18.14c*). It is stretched slightly to extend mesially and distally to cover the full length of the prepared bed and should extend down apically over the full depth of the prepared bed. Some authorities advocate suturing the graft to the papillae separately using interrupted chrome gut interdental sutures and an atraumatic needle. Alternatively, the graft and the overlying flap may be secured into place together (*see below*). This second method does, however, depend on completely covering the connective-tissue graft right up to its thin epithelial border. This thin border of epithelium is left on the graft because it helps to colour blend it with the adjacent tissues. It must be placed coronally to the cement-enamel junction.

Replacement of the recipient overlying flap

The recipient flap is repositioned coronally to cover as much of the connective-tissue graft as possible. It is sutured in place using resorbable gut sutures either separately by interdental gut sutures or in combination with securing the graft. In this alternative form of suturing the gut sutures pass through the flap, the graft and finally the papilla. The graft is protected by using a surgical cyanoacrylate and Vaseline covering (*see previous section*). The patient is instructed to use chlorhexidine mouthwashes and may be put on tetracycline for 2 weeks. The area is left until the pack comes off naturally, usually after 2–3 weeks.

Connective-tissue graft with double papilla flap

In both the above techniques when used separately, the graft over the root surface relies on the collateral circulation bringing nutrient from nearby areas. In this modification, proposed by Harris (1992), the graft is covered over the root surface with tissue brought together by a double papilla type flap. The graft gets its blood supply both from the underlying periosteum, mesial, distal and apical to the exposed root, and from the covering double papilla pedicle flaps.

Procedure

Preparation of recipient site

The recipient site incisions are the same as those previously described for a double papilla graft coverage of a recession defect (*see previous section*). The tips of the papillae are left *in situ* (*Figures 18.16a* and *18.17a*) to allow the graft to be sutured to them. For this combined procedure split thickness flaps are raised from both papillae.

Root preparation

The root surface is planed thoroughly to reduce any labial bulbosity of the affected tooth. It is then conditioned with tetracycline using a 250 mg tetracycline capsule dissolved in 2 ml saline.

Preparation of donor site

The procedure is the same as that described for the connective tissue graft (*see previous section*). A special scalpel handle (*Figure 18.14b*) has been devised to obtain an optimum thickness connective tissue graft with this procedure (Harris, 1992). It accepts two blades 1.5 mm apart which give an ideal incision in order to remove the graft.

Placement of the graft

The graft is tried in and its size slightly modified if necessary. It is sutured into position using 3/0 or 4/0 catgut in 3 parts.

1. Suture the connective-tissue graft to the remaining interdental papillae (*Figure 18.16b*).
2. To bring the flaps together as a double papilla (*Figures 18.16c* and *18.17b*).
3. A sling suture to hold the flap over the graft (*Figure 18.16d*)

The area is dressed using Surgicel and cyanoacrylate and this is covered with Vaseline and tetracycline. This last covering is made by mixing the contents of one 250 mg capsule of tetracycline into the Vaseline. Dietary restrictions are imposed and the patient is instructed to use a chlorhexidine mouthwash until normal oral hygiene can be carried out.

Resolution

The pack is left in position until it comes off naturally, usually after 2–3 weeks. Following this the resolution back to health and normal oral hygiene is usually quick and uneventful.

Histological result of grafting procedures over exposed root surfaces

At best all the grafting techniques which cover exposed root surfaces may result in a connective-tissue attachment to the root surface. However, most probably they will usually give rise to a long junction epithelium firmly

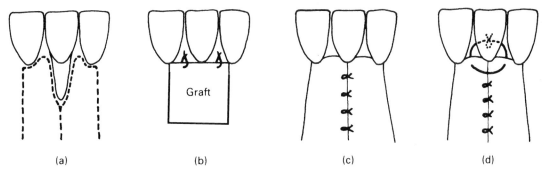

Figure 18.16 Connective-tissue graft with double papilla flap. (*a*) Incisions: the tips of both papillae are left for suturing of graft. (*b*) Connective-tissue graft sutured to papillae. (*c*) Double papillae flaps brought together and sutured over graft. (*d*) A sling suture tied lingually to hold flap tightly over graft

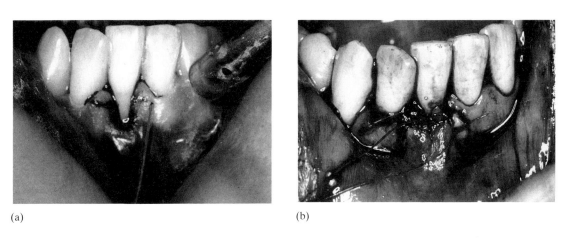

Figure 18.17 Connective tissue graft with double papilla flap. (*a*) Incisions: the tips of the papillae are left *in situ* for suturing; (*b*) Double papilla flap coronally repositioned to cover graft and sutured into position. (By courtesy of Mr C A Waterman)

adherent to the root surface. This relationship can be stable, but it is not as resistant to either inflammation or to trauma as would be the case if complete regeneration including bone had occurred.

Guided tissue regeneration

To have any chance of regenerating bone, cementum and periodontal attachment in these areas some form of guided tissue regenerative (GTR) technique needs to be performed. Standard GTR using Gore-tex membranes always require a secondary procedure to remove the PTFE membrane. This has the disadvantage of disturbing any newly formed osteoid material. Also flaps replaced over

Gore-tex membranes may shrink and therefore coverage of any osteoid which might form may be difficult with this two-stage technique.

In addition, space maintenance is a problem as PTFE membranes easily collapse, eradicating any space between the membrane and the root surface into which healing tissue from the periodontal ligament may grow (Nyman *et al.*, 1982). To avoid this disadvantage, two techniques have evolved to help maintain this space (Tinti *et al.*, 1992, 1993; Pini Prato *et al.*, 1992).

Two-stage GTR with PTFE membranes

A full thickness mucoperiosteal flap is developed from a crevicular horizontal incision,

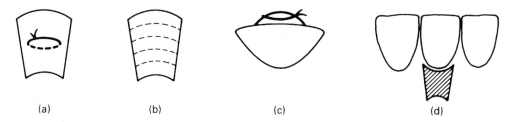

Figure 18.18 PTFE (Gore-tex) membrane for guided tissue regeneration on localized recession. (*a*) Membrane tented with suture; (*b*) Membrane with incorporated metal wires for tenting; (*c*) and (*d*) Tented membrane in position over exposed root

sparing the interdental papillae and vertical relieving incisions. It is raised until freely mobile to allow subsequent coronal repositioning. A single tooth Gore-tex membrane is modified so that it can be tented out to give a space between the membrane and the root to allow tissue ingrowth. This is accomplished by either placing a suture to tent it inwards (*Figure 18.18a*) or by tying it to a suitably bent gold bar or pre-cast gold framework. Recently, Gore-tex membrane with an incorporated metal framework has been manufactured to allow the membrane to be tented to the correct shape (*Figure 18.18b*). This membrane is then placed and secured by a sling suture to cover the exposed root surface, leaving a gap for tissue ingrowth (*Figure 18.18c,d*). The flap is then coronally repositioned to cover the membrane and sutured into place with PTFE sutures.

After 4 weeks, a marginal flap is gently lifted to allow the membrane to be removed. This should leave a definite soft tissue attachment against the root of the tooth. The flap is

sutured back after membrane removal and the sutures are removed one week later. The healing is usually uneventful thereafter.

It is unlikely that new hard tissues form after this procedure as downgrowth of gingival epithelium is not fully prevented as a result of the tenting of the membrane. The resultant relation to the root is therefore most probably an adherent long junctional epithelium.

Resorbable membranes

Resorbable membranes do not need to be removed as they are degraded by body tissues. They may also provide the suitable conditions for bone regrowth (Brady *et al.*, 1973; Gottlow *et al.*, 1992; Laurell *et al.*, 1992). The advantage of these techniques is that they are one-stage procedures. Furthermore, because of this there is no interference with the healing tissue inherent in the two-stage GTR procedure. The procedure is also considerably easier than grafting procedures because it only involves a

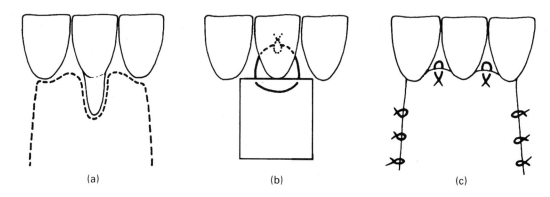

Figure 18.19 Guided tissue regeneration for gingival recession using resorbable membranes. (*a*) Incisions sparing tips of papillae; (*b*) Membrane held in position with sling suture; (*c*) Flap coronally positioned over membrane. It is sutured to papillae and vertically

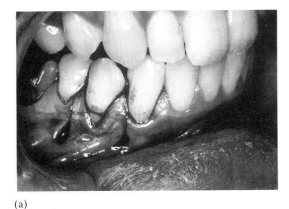

(a)

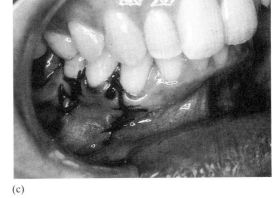

(c)

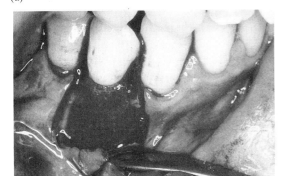

(b)

Figure 18.20 Guided tissue regeneration using resorbable membrane to cover localized gingival recession. (*a*) Incisions: sparing tips of papillae. Full-thickness mucoperiosteal flap; (*b*) Guidor resorbable membrane in position over root surface and surrounding bone. It adapts itself well to the shape of the root and adjacent bone. (*c*) Flap coronally repositioned and sutured over membrane. (By courtesy of Mr C A Waterman)

single surgical site and a full thickness mucoperiosteal flap is raised. It may have the potential to allow bone regeneration in areas of buccal osseous defects such as those associated with localized gingival recession (Waterman, personal communication).

Procedure

The procedure involves coronally repositioning a full thickness flap over the membrane. A flap is outlined (*Figures 18.19a* and *18.20a*) with an inverse bevel incision which allows partial removal over papillae tips the remainder of which are left *in situ* to facilitate suturing. Vertical relieving incisions are made down to the vestibule to allow a full-thickness mucoperiosteal flap to be fully mobilized. The exposed root surface is planed using Kirkland 12 or Gracey curettes. The margin of a flap is just raised on the lingual side to accommodate the resorbable retaining tie submucosally. The membrane can be tried in and then tied in place with resorbable sutures using a sling suture technique to suspend the membrane from the

lingual surface of the tooth (*Figure 18.19b*). A suitable membrane for this procedure is the Guidor membrane which has two layers with spaces on the underside to aid healing tissue/ osteoid ingrowth. It may be necessary to raise the apical edge of the retained interdental papilla in order to touch the edge of the membrane beneath. The membrane adapts itself well to the shape of the root and surrounding bone (*Figure 18.20b*). The flap is sutured coronally using interdental sutures through the papilla, and interrupted sutures for the relieving incisions (*Figures 18.19c* and *18.20c*). No packing is applied or the space below the membrane would be eliminated, and there would be no ingrowth of healing tissue. Tetracycline is prescribed for 2 weeks, and the external sutures are removed after 3–4 weeks. Chlorhexidine mouthwashes are used to maintain cleanliness until brushing can recommence at 6 weeks. Two-weekly professional cleaning should be carefully undertaken during this period.

The histology of the attachment to the root surface has not yet been fully assessed following this technique.

References

Addy, M., Dummer, P.M.H., Hunter, M.L. *et al.* (1987) A study of the association of fraenal attachment, lip coverage and vestibular depth with plaque and gingivitis. *Journal of Periodontology* **58**, 752–757

Brady, J.M., Cutright, D.E. and Miller, R.A. (1973) Resorption rate, route of elimination and ultra structure of the implant site of polylactic acid in the abdominal wall of the rat. *Journal of Biomedical Materials Research* **7**, 155–166

Cohen, D.W. and Ross, S.E. (1968) The double papilla repositioned flap in periodontal therapy. *Journal of Periodontology* **39**, 65–70

Crigger, M., Bogle, G., Nilveus, R. *et al.* (1978) The effect of topical citric acid application on the healing of experimental furcation defects in dogs. *Journal of Periodontal Research* **13**, 538–549

Demirel, K., Baer, P.N. and McNamara, T.F. (1991) Topical application of doxycycline on periodontally involved root surfaces in vitro: comparative analysis of substantivity on cementum and dentin. *Journal of Periodontology* **62**, 312–316

Edel, A. (1974) Clinical evaluation of free connective tissue grafts used to increase the width of keratinized gingiva. *Journal of Clinical Periodontology* **1**, 185–196

Garrett, J.S., Crigger, M. and Egelberg, J. (1978) The effects of citric acid on diseased root surfaces. *Journal of Periodontal Research* **13**, 155–163

Gottlow, J., Lundgren, D., Nyman, S. *et al.* (1992) New attachment formation in the monkey using Guidor, a bioabsorable GTR device. *Journal of Dental Research* **71**, 1535. Abstract

Grupe, H.E. and Warren, R.F. (1956) Repair of gingival defects by a sliding flap operation. *Journal of Periodontology* **27**, 92–95

Hannington-Kitt, J.G. and Dunne, S.M. (1993) Topical guanethidine relieves dental hypersensitivity and pain. *Journal of the Royal Society of Medicine* **86**, 514–515

Harris, R.J. (1992) The connective tissue and partial thickness double pedicle graft: A predictable method of obtaining root coverage. *Journal of Periodontology* **63**, 477–486

Holbrook, T. and Ochsenbein, C. (1983) Complete coverage of denuded root surface with a one stage gingival graft. *International Journal of Periodontics and Restorative Dentistry* **3**, 8–27

Jahnke, P.V., Sandifer, J.B., Gher, M.E. *et al.* (1993) Thick free gingival and connective tissue autografts for root coverage. *Journal of Periodontology* **64**, 315–322

Lang, N.P. and Löe, H. (1972) The relationship between the width of keratinised gingiva and gingival health. *Journal of Periodonology* **43**, 623–627

Langer, B. and Langer, L. (1985) Subepithelial connective tissue graft technique for root coverage. *Journal of Periodontology* **60**, 715–720

Laurell, L., Gottlow, J., Nyman, S. *et al.* (1992) Gingival response to Guidor, a bioabsorbable device in GTR therapy. *Journal of Dental Research* **71**, 1536. Abstract

Maynard, J.G. Jnr (1977) Coronal positioning of a previously placed autogenous gingival graft. *Journal of Periodontology* **48**, 151–155

Miller, P.D. (1982) Root coverage using a free soft tissue autograft following citric acid application. I Technique. *International Journal of Periodontics Restorative Dentistry* **2**, 65–70

Miller, P.D. (1985a) A classification of marginal tissue recession. *International Journal of Periodontics Restorative Dentistry* **5**, 9–13

Miller, P.D. (1985b) Root coverage using the free soft tissue autograft following citric acid application. Part III. A successful and predictable procedure in areas of deep wide recession. *International Journal of Periodontics and Restorative Dentistry* **5**, 15–37

Miller, P.D. (1992) Personal communication

Miyasoto, M., Crigger, M. and Egelberg, J. (1977) Gingival condition in areas of minimal and appreciable width of keratinised gingiva. *Journal of Clinical Periodontology* **4**, 200–209

Nabors, J. (1966) Free gingival grafts. *Periodontics* **4**, 243–245

Nyman, S., Lindhe, J. and Karring, T. (1981) Healing following surgical treatment and root demineralisation in monkeys with periodontal disease. *Journal of Clinical Periodontology* **8**, 249–258

Nyman, S., Gottlow, J., Karring, T. and Lindhe, J. (1982) The regenerative potential of the periodontal ligament. *Journal of Clinical Periodontology* **9**, 257–265

Pini Prato, G., Tinti, C., Vincenzi, G. *et al.* (1992) Guided tissue regeneration versus mucogingival surgery in the treatment of human buccal gingival recession. *Journal of Periodontology* **63**, 919–928

Register, A.A. and Burdick, F.A. (1975) Accelerated re-attachment with cementogenesis to dentin, demineralized in situ. I optimum range. *Journal of Periodontology* **46**, 646–655

Register, A.A. and Burdick, F.A. (1976) Accelerated reattachment with cementogenesis to dentin, demineralised in situ. II Defect repair. *Journal of Periodontal Research* **47**, 263–267

Salkin, L.M., Freedman, A.L., Stein, M.D. and Bassiouny, M.A. (1987) A longitudinal study of mucogingival defects. *Journal of Periodontology* **58**, 164–166

Terranove, V.P., Franzetti, L.C., Hic, S. *et al.* (1986) A biochemical approach to periodontal regeneration. Tetracycline treatment of dentin promotes fibroblast adhesion and growth. *Journal of Periodontal Research* **21**, 330–337

Tinti, C., Giampaolo, V. and Cocchetto, R. (1993) Guided tissue regeneration in mucogingival surgery. *Journal of Periodontology* **64**, 1184–1191

Tinti, C., Vincenzi, G., Cortellini, P. *et al.* (1992) Guided tissue regeneration in the treatment of human facial recession. *Journal of Periodontology* **63**, 554–560

Waterman, C. (1994) The treatment of buccal recession defects using a bioabsorbable membrane (Personal communication of paper in preparation)

Wennstrom, J.L. (1987) Lack of association between the width of attached gingiva and the development of soft tissue recession. A 5 year longitudinal study. *Journal of Clinical Periodontology* **14**, 181–184

Wennstrom, J., Lindhe, J. and Nyman, S. (1982) The role of keratinised gingiva in plaque associated gingivitis in dogs. *Journal of Clinical Periodontology* **9**, 75–85

Wicksjö, U.M.E., Baker, P.J., Christersson, L.A. *et al.* (1986) A biochemical approach to periodontal regeneration: tetracycline treatment conditions dentin surfaces. *Journal of Periodontal Research* **21**, 322–369

19

The periodontal abscess

A periodontal or lateral (as opposed to apical) abscess is a localized area of inflammation in which the formation of pus has taken place in the periodontal tissues. It is produced by endogenous pyogenic microorganisms, possibly toxic factors in the plaque and/or some reduction in host resistance caused by local or systemic factors.

A number of factors appear to provoke the formation of an abscess:

1. Obstruction of the opening to a deep pocket, frequently one which is tortuous, e.g. associated with a furcation defect.
2. Gingival injury with a foreign body, e.g. toothbrush bristle or woodstick, etc. which carries bacteria into the tissues. Careless subgingival scaling may also carry microorganisms into damaged tissue, as can powerful irrigation of a pocket.
3. Incomplete removal of plaque and subgingival calculus from the depths of a pocket. Frequently after scaling there is tightening of the gingival cuff which occludes a pocket containing bacteria.
4. Infection of tissues damaged by excessive occlusal stress which may be produced by:
   (a) A blow on a tooth
   (b) Excessive orthodontic pressure
   (c) Bruxism (see p. 268).
5. As a consequence of pulp disease:
   (a) Where a periapical lesion spreads up the lateral surface of a tooth.
   (b) Where lateral pulp canals link with the periodontal ligament. This is especially common in the furcation. Accessory pulp canals are extremely common and may not be evident on the radiograph. The furcation abscess produced by pulp pathology is frequently misdiagnosed as a primary periodontal lesion.
   (c) Perforation of the lateral wall of a tooth during endodontics.
6. Altered host response as in diabetes. Diabetes has been frequently diagnosed following the appearance of multiple periodontal abscesses.

Clinical features

The onset of symptoms can be sudden with pain on biting and a deep throbbing pain. The involved tooth may feel high and mobile. The overlying gingiva becomes red, swollen and tender but at first there is no fluctuation or discharge of pus. There may be enlargement of the associated lymph glands.

The next stage is characterized by the presence of pus. This may discharge into a periodontal pocket when the symptoms reduce, or the pus may track through the bone to form an abscess under the alveolar mucoperiosteum. Once the pus enters the soft tissue the severe pain diminishes and the abscess appears as a red, shiny and very tender swelling over the alveolus. The abscess usually points and discharges but if this does not happen the inflammation may spread into the surrounding connective tissue to produce a cellulitis. This occurs most commonly if the

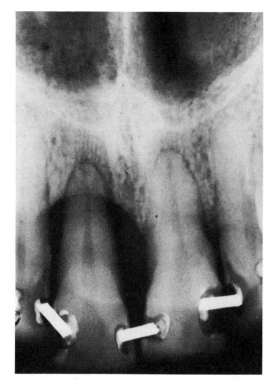

Figure 19.1 Radiographic appearance of a periodontal abscess which is on the palatal aspect of the central incisor

1. The position of the abscess swelling. If this is over the root apex it is likely to be periapical.
2. The presence of periodontal disease with pocketing and bone destruction. If the periodontal condition is generally quite good and pocketing is absent or shallow the abscess is unlikely to be periodontal.
3. If the involved tooth is heavily filled it is likely that pulp pathology is present, and a history of sensitivity to hot and cold tends to confirm this. If the tooth is non-vital the abscess could be either periapical or periodontal, or both as a combined abscess. Pulp vitality tests can be extremely misleading but if the tooth gives a normal reading this points to periodontal infection. If the tooth is caries free and unfilled the abscess is likely to be periodontal.
4. Radiographs taken in the earliest stages provide little useful information but once the lesion is established its position can be identified (*Figure 19.1*). However, a periodontal abscess on the facial or lingual aspect of the tooth may not be clearly discernible on the radiograph. A radiograph taken with a gutta-percha point inserted gently into the suspected pocket can help to define the origin of the abscess.

patient's resistance is low. If the abscess is in the upper jaw, depending upon the tooth involved, the lip, cheek, side of the nose or the infra-orbital area and lower eyelid may swell. Infection in the vicinity of the infra-orbital foramen is particularly dangerous. If the abscess is in the lower jaw, the lower lip, chin, cheek, angle of the mandible and neck may swell. If infection involves the lower third molar there may also be trismus and difficulty in swallowing. At this stage the patient is obviously unwell, in pain and distressed and his temperature may be elevated.

Differential diagnosis

These clinical features can be produced by both periapical and periodontal abscesses and a differential diagnosis must be made because the treatments for the two forms of abscess are different. Sometimes a differential diagnosis may not be easy. A number of features must be taken into account:

Treatment of the abscess

Treatment depends upon the stage of abscess development, the amount of bone loss and whether pulp pathology is also involved. The initial aims of treatment are the relief of pain and control of infection. Once this has been achieved the residual lesion must be treated; otherwise recurrent abscess formation is inevitable.

In the first stage infection can be controlled by an antibiotic, e.g. penicillin V 250 mg four times a day for 5 days (or erythromycin in the same dosage if the patient is sensitive to penicillin). It helps to relieve the occlusion by grinding the opposing tooth.

Once the abscess is fluctuant and pointing drainage is essential. The abscess is incised under local anaesthesia but the injection must be made well away from the inflamed area. Regional anaesthesia or even general anaesthesia may be needed if the inflamed area is large. This is supplemented by regular hot salt water mouthwashes. The drainage incision should be horizontal and made through the most fluctuant site. The margins of the wound may be spread to facilitate drainage. If adequate drainage is established an antibiotic may not be needed. Relieving the occlusion by grinding the opposing tooth should allow the patient to eat on the other side of the mouth.

If the infection has spread to produce a cellulitis an intramuscular injection of Triplopen or erythromycin should bring this under control and drainage can then be established.

Once the acute condition is under control, treatment of the residual condition can be started. If there is considerable bone loss, extraction may be necessary. If the tooth is to be conserved a flap can be raised and the bone defect which is associated with the abscess curetted. Frequently the abscess has perforated the facial or lingual plate of bone, leaving a bridge of marginal bone. If this bridge of bone is narrow it may be cut away and the fragments of bone used as a graft in the bone defect. If the bridge is wide it is conserved in the hope that the perforation will repair. On the first occasion of abscess formation the prognosis can be good but if recurrent abscesses have been present the prognosis may be doubtful.

The combined periodontal-periapical lesion

The combined lesion can develop in a number of ways:

1. Where an apical abscess has spread laterally to create a periodontal lesion or united with a pre-existing lateral lesion.
2. Where pulp infection has spread via accessory canals into the periodontal tissues. This is most frequent in the furcation where accessory canals are common.
3. Where a periodontal lesion extends close to the tooth apex and causes secondary pulpal infection.

At one time the presence of a combined periapical-periodontal lesion justified extraction, especially occurring in a furcation. Today, endodontics has achieved a high level of success and predictability and the prognosis for a tooth involved in a combined lesion can be good.

Treatment

Once acute inflammation has been controlled and the occlusion adjusted, root-canal treatment should be initiated. A lateral compression technique is necessary to occlude accessory canals and when endodontics has been satisfactorily completed periodontal surgery can be carried out.

If a multirooted tooth is involved and (i) bone destruction about one root is much more advanced than that about the other root(s), or (ii) the furcation defect is of such labyrinthine complexity that it cannot be kept clean, or (iii) the divergent roots of neighbouring teeth, usually the buccal roots of upper molars, are very close together or actually touch, then root resection is indicated (*see* Chapter 17).

20

Early onset periodontitis

A variety of names have been given to a form of periodontal disease characterized by deep pockets and advanced alveolar bone loss in the young, in children, adolescents and young adults, without any associated systemic disease. Gottlieb (1923, 1928) designated the condition(s) diffuse atrophy of alveolar bone, and subsequently other names were devised: deep cementopathia, paradontosis, periodontosis, juvenile periodontitis, prepubertal periodontitis, rapidly progressive periodontitis. Page and Baab (1985) suggested that all forms of the disease be designated early onset periodontitis (EOP).

At a population level there is direct correlation between oral hygiene status, the degree of gingival inflammation and the severity of periodontal destruction. However, at an individual level there is a great deal of variation in the way in which the tissues respond to plaque irritation. Some individuals with poor oral hygiene suffer little periodontal destruction while others with little plaque have advanced periodontal destruction. Two hypotheses have been proposed to account for this variation:

1. Certain plaque bacteria have a greater potential for tissue destruction than others and when they are present disease will occur.
2. Host factors determine the tissue response to plaque.

Of course both of these factors could be important in both adult periodontitis and EOP.

Early onset periodontitis can be practically divided into 3 groups:

- Prepubertal periodontitis
  Severe gingivitis and destructive periodontitis in primary dentition.
- Rapidly progressive periodontitis
  Generalized rapid attachment loss in permanent dentition.
- Juvenile periodontitis
  Localized:
  Severe localized attachment loss in permanent first molars and incisors.
  Generalized:
  Involvement of these teeth and a few or many other teeth.

Prepubertal periodontitis

This is an extremely rare form of periodontal disease characterized by rapid periodontal destruction of the primary dentition (Page et al., 1983a). The gingivae are grossly inflamed and the patient commonly has other bacterial infections. In some cases the condition may affect the permanent dentition as well. In many instances there is a familial pattern to the disease and most if not all cases are probably genetically mediated. A number of inherited conditions described in Chapter 6 also produce these effects including hypophosphatasia, Papillon–Lefèvre syndrome, cyclic neutropenia, familial neutropenias, Chediak–Higashi syndrome.

Rapidly progressive periodontitis

Rapidly progressive periodontitis (RPP) is characterized by severe generalized periodontal destruction and may affect any or all of the permanent dentition of patients between the ages of 20 and 35 (Page *et al.*, 1983b). The clinical features and subgingival flora resemble active chronic periodontitis with *Porphyromonas gingivalis*, *Prevotella intermedia*, *Eikenella corrodens* and *Actinobacillus actinomycetemcomitans*, all being reported to be present. There is a lack of epidemiological evidence for this condition as a separate entity although there is evidence of some cases having a familial tendency. On present available evidence, it is difficult to justify the classification of this condition as a separate disease entity as it could well represent a rapidly progressive chronic periodontitis in a susceptible individual.

It is also important to distinguish this condition from post-juvenile periodontitis (*see below*) and to remember that some conditions such as Down's syndrome (*see* Chapter 6) have a high susceptibility to severe rapidly progressive periodontitis in the permanent dentition.

Juvenile periodontitis

Usually multiple names for a disease entity indicate an ill-defined knowledge of the precise aetiology and pathogenesis; indeed it is possible for similar clinical manifestations to be produced by different causal factors and pathological processes. In this text the term juvenile periodontitis (Butler, 1969) is used because it refers to the general population affected and does not imply any particular cause or disease process. Baer (1971) described juvenile periodontitis as a well-defined clinical entity different from adult periodontitis in that it appears to start around puberty, seems more common in girls, appears to occur in families, and is rapidly progressive.

Two forms of the disease were described, local and general. In the localized form the tissue destruction is restricted to the first molars and incisors, and is characterized by a symmetrical distribution; in the generalized form many or all the teeth are involved. Gradations between these two extremes are often seen. The variability of these forms was recently demonstrated by Yosof (1990) in a study of 47 Malaysian children (22 boys and 25 girls) with the condition. He divided the children into four groups according to the distribution of the bone loss:

Type 1 Bone destruction limited to first molars and incisors (14.9%).

Type 2 Bone destruction involving first molars and incisors and some other teeth (25.5%).

Type 3 Generalized destruction but worse around the first molars and incisors (14.9%).

Type 4 Generalized involvement of more than 14 teeth (44.7%).

Juvenile periodontitis (JP) has distinctive clinical and bacteriological features which justify its classification as a separate disease entity.

The main epidemiological and clinical features of this disease are as follows:

Prevalence

The disease occurs in approximately 1 in 1000 adolescents and seems to have a racial predisposition, occurring most frequently in people of West African origin. Recent epidemiological studies using precise diagnostic criteria have reported an incidence of between 0.1 and 0.4% (Saxen, 1980a,b; Saxby, 1984; Kronauer *et al.*, 1986; Bial and Mellonig, 1987). These studies all confirm that the incidence varies amongst different ethnic groups and a study in Britain (Saxby, 1984) showed an incidence of 0.02% for Caucasians, 0.8% for Negroes and 0.2% for Asians. In a recent study of the radiographs of 1038 children aged 10–12 years, Neely (1992) found a prevalence rate of 4.6 per thousand. In an examination of 2500 children in Chile Lopez *et al.* (1991) found a JP prevalence of 0.32%, and in Iraq Albander (1993) recorded a prevalence of 1.8%. The disease seems more prevalent in Africa as exemplified by Nigerian studies (Hartley and Floyd, 1988). A racial tendency receives further support from a study of mixed American naval recruits (Melvin *et al.*, 1991) which examined 5013 individuals, 3158 men and 1855 women and found 38 cases (0.78%) with JP; 2.9% of Black recruits, 0.09% of Caucasians and 0.8% of Oriental and Hispanic origin. However, too many variables, e.g. oral hygiene, nutritional status, socio-economic factors, enter the picture to allow valid comparison, and in the Chilean study the authors state that JP was found most commonly in people from low socio-economic groups.

Age

The patient is usually an adolescent at the time of examination but may be much younger; the onset of the disease may be several years before the time of examination. Sjobin *et al.* (1993) carried out a retrospective study of early radiographs of 118 young patients aged 13–19 with JP, taken when they were 5–12 years old, and compared these with early radiographs of 168 13–19 year olds without JP. They found that some of the individuals with JP had bone loss around primary teeth.

A similar clinical picture to JP, but with obvious signs of gingival inflammation, has been found in individuals in their 20s and has been called post juvenile periodontitis. It appears to result from the evolution of JP.

Sex

Many studies have found that the condition appears more commonly in females than males at a ratio of about 3:1 (Baer, 1971; Manson and Lehner, 1974). In Iraqi children Albander (1993) recorded a ratio of 3.5:1, and the ratio of girls to boys in the Lopez *et al.* (1991) study was 7:1. Perhaps we should enter the same qualifications as for the prevalence studies. It was suggested that some of the findings reflect the way in which the data have been collected. In those studies based upon patients presenting at periodontal clinics, the adolescent girl who is usually more concerned about her appearance and well-being than the adolescent boy will figure more frequently. Also, the patient is more likely to be accompanied by the mother from whom the enquiries about the family are made. Fathers are often invisible, and prevalence in males may be underestimated simply because they are not examined. When the data is obtained from an epidemiological survey, as in the study of Melvin *et al.* (1991) an almost equal (1.1:1) sex prevalence is found. As Hart *et al.* (1992) point out, there is no female preponderance after correction for 'ascertainment basis'. Thus the method of

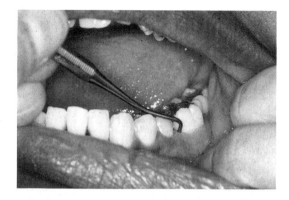

Figure 20.1 Juvenile periodontitis. A periodontal probe measuring a 10 mm pocket mesial to the ⌐6 of an 18-year-old girl. Note the lack of clinical inflammation, plaque and calculus

collecting data must be scrutinized before conclusions can be drawn.

Clinical manifestations

The gingivae usually show few if any signs of clinical inflammation and little or no supra-gingival plaque and calculus. Subgingival calculus deposits are usually absent from root surfaces and because of the absence of clinical inflammation and gingival bleeding the condition may escape detection until it becomes advanced when mobility and drifting of teeth, usually incisors, occur. An acute periodontal abscess may develop at this stage and the associated pain and swelling bring the patient to the dentist for examination. As stated, the condition is frequently localized to the incisors and first molars but may affect other teeth.

In regularly attending patients the disease should be diagnosed much earlier and at this stage treatment is more successful. The early clinical signs are periodontal pocketing and attachment loss, often on the mesial surface of the first molar (*Figure 20.1*). Attachment loss may increase rapidly. Baer (1971) estimated that 50–75% of the attachment of affected teeth may be lost in 4–5 years.

Bone destruction

The pattern of bone destruction and distribution of the lesions represent two of the intriguing aspects of the disease. In the classic case

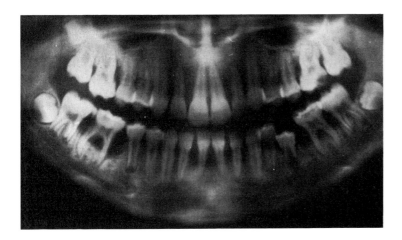

Figure 20.2 Juvenile periodontitis. Classic first molar-incisor involvement in a 12-year-old boy. The orthopantogram shows advanced bone loss around the upper and lower first molars and incisors

advanced bone destruction is localized to the incisors and first molars in a symmetrical or mirror-image distribution (*Figure 20.2*). Deep angular or crescentic bone defects around these teeth, particularly the affected molars, are characteristic and the areas of bone resorption are sharply demarcated from the neighbouring bone which on the radiograph appears completely healthy. Because the alveolar bone is thinner around incisors then these teeth often lose all the interdental bone and this appears on the radiographs as marked horizontal bone loss. Other teeth, in particular second premolars and second molars, may be involved.

With regular attenders, the first radiographical signs are likely to be seen on routine bitewing radiographs usually on the mesial surface of the first molar. Any early signs of bone loss on these teeth should be taken seriously and should lead to a detailed examination of the patient. These radiographs should always be checked for any signs of bone loss since they clearly show the alveolar crest. They are probably the only means of early diagnosis of JP since children and adolescents are unlikely to have a detailed periodontal examination.

In a proportion of cases apparently random, asymmetrical involvement occurs. On rare occasions the condition may spread with time to other teeth so that the bone around almost every tooth is involved.

Familial tendency

Many researchers have described a familial tendency in this disease. Benjamin and Baer (1967) described its occurrence in twins, siblings, cousins and other family connections. This has suggested a genetic transmission, and because of the apparently greater frequency in females an X-linked dominant inheritance has been suggested (Melnick *et al.*, 1976; Spektor *et al.*, 1985). However, re-interpretation of this evidence (Hart *et al.*, 1992) this supports the notion of autosomal transmission. In this connection some studies have suggested that it is an autosomal recessive condition (Saxen, 1980c; Long *et al.*, 1987) and still others that it is autosomal dominant (Roulston *et al.*, 1985; Boughman *et al.*, 1986). Boughman *et al.* (1986) reported one child with JP and dentinogenesis imperfecta (a genetically transmitted autosomal dominant fault) which both showed genetic markers on chromosome 4, whilst the same group also discovered a family in which five generations displayed JP and dentinogenesis imperfecta always occurring together (Roulston *et al.*, 1985). In yet another study by one of these groups (Boughman *et al.*, 1988), genetic-model testing was used on 28 families with a history of JP. They showed that an autosomal recessive mode of inheritance was most applicable to the data.

The various genetic studies showed that if a patient has JP there is a 50% chance that the disease will develop in a brother or sister (Saxen, 1980c; Spektor *et al.*, 1985; Van Dyke *et al.*, 1985).

It has also been shown that JP occurs frequently in blood group B (Kaslick *et al.*, 1971). Tissue typing has also been used to determine a possible predisposition to JP. The major histocompatibility complex, MHC (*see*

Chapter 3) has at least six human leucocyte antigen (HLA) types and the composition of these is genetically determined and varies in different individuals. Available information indicates a great variation in HLA profiles amongst JP patients (Saxen, 1980c; Saxen and Koskimies, 1984), although there is an increased frequency of antigens A9, A28 and B15 in these patients (Reinholdt *et al.*, 1977). Thus although there is much evidence to support the genetic inheritance of JP, its mode of inheritance is still unclear. It is also not known how the genes are expressed.

General health

There seems to be no relationship with any systemic condition, although a somewhat similar dental picture is found in the rare Papillon–Lefèvre syndrome but with a generalized distribution and also involving the deciduous dentition.

The role of cementum

Gottlieb (1928) first suggested that the underlying cause of periodontosis was a defect in cementum formation. This concept has been re-examined more recently (Lindstog and Blomlöf, 1983; Blomlöf *et al.*, 1986). They carried out a comparative histological study on teeth from patients with JP, adult chronic periodontitis and healthy controls. They found that the cementum on the teeth from JP subjects had extensive areas of hypoplasia in both the exposed and intra-alveolar root surfaces. This suggests that the defect is related to impaired cementum formation rather than the pathology of the pocket. This defect in cementum formation could be hereditary and could be an important aetiological factor.

Bacteriology

The subgingival microflora of JP is scanty when compared with that associated with adult periodontitis and its composition is very difficult. Examination with dark ground microscopy shows that it is dominated by coccoid and straight non-motile rods (Liljenberg and Lindhe, 1980). The dominant cultivatable microflora consists of Gram negative capnophilic and facultative rods and these make up about two-thirds of the isolates (Newman and Socransky, 1977). The principal bacteria present are *Actinobacillus actinomycetemcomitans*, *Capnocytophaga* species and *Eikenella corrodens*. Some motile anaerobic rods, mainly *Campylobacter (Wolinella) recta*, may also be present in some cases (Slots, 1976; Zambon *et al.*, 1983a). Using selective media for *Actinobacillus*, *A. actinomycetemcomitans* can be isolated from nearly all JP patients (Slots *et al.*, 1980; Zambon *et al.*, 1983a). Mandell (1984) found 100-fold higher numbers of *A. actinomycetemcomitans* and 50-fold higher numbers of *Eikenella corrodens* in active versus non-active sites.

The bacteria associated with JP may invade the periodontal connective tissue in this condition (Gillett and Johnson, 1982) and *A. actinomycetemcomitans* is the principal invading species (Saglie *et al.*, 1982).

Several bacteria associated with JP produce substances capable of damaging the host defences and tissues and these will be described in association with each bacteria. By far the most important bacteria associated with this condition is *A. actinomycetemcomitans* and this has been the subject of most of the research on this subject. This is therefore the first bacteria described below.

Actinobacillus actinomycetemcomitans

Numerous studies have shown the association between *A. actinomycetemcomitans* and JP and have suggested that it plays an important role in its pathogenesis (Haffajee *et al.*, 1984; Zambon, 1985). *A. actinomycetemcomitans* is found in low numbers in the subgingival flora of healthy and adult chronic periodontitis sites whereas in JP it is found in 97% of affected sites and forms up to 70% of the total flora at these sites (Zambon, 1985). Furthermore resolution of JP coincides with a reduction or elimination of this bacteria from the subgingival flora and recurrence of disease is associated with a recolonization of the site with this bacteria (Slots and Rosling, 1983).

However, there is now no doubt that a significant number of young healthy subjects also harbour *A. actinomycetemcomitans* in their oral flora. The global distribution of *A. actinomycetemcomitans* varies considerably and in normal periodontally healthy individuals its prevalence is about 13% in Finland

(Alanuusua and Asikainen, 1988), 20–25% in urban USA (Slots *et al.*, 1980) and 60% in Panama (Eisenmann *et al.*, 1983). Interestingly, this bacterial distribution seems to mirror the relative occurrence of JP in these 3 countries which was lowest in Finland, intermediate in the USA and highest in Panama (Lindhe and Slots, 1989). Possibly if there is a higher infection rate with this bacteria in the population then there is a higher risk that susceptible individuals may acquire the bacteria and develop JP (Slots and Schonfeld, 1991). This may to some extent explain the higher prevalence of JP in Black subjects in the USA and UK. It is possible that the high level of *A. actinomycetemcomitans* infection in these subjects represents a carriage of the bacteria from African populations with high prevalence of JP (Franklin, 1978). Tracing *A. actinomycetemcomitans* transmission in racial and family groups is being aided by the development of sensitive microbial genetic methods to trace genotypes of this bacteria in various populations (Di Rienzo and Slots, 1990; Zambon, Gregory and Smutko, 1990).

Similarly, familial distribution of *A. actinomycetemcomitans* may be due to transmission of bacteria between family members and this could be particularly relevant in families with one or more members susceptible to JP. Convincing evidence of intrafamilial transmission was produced by Zambon *et al.* (1983a) who found that each infected subject in the family harboured the same biotype and serotype of the bacteria. This was also shown with genetic methods using restriction fragment length polymorphism (RFLP) typing of strains (Di Rienzo and Slots, 1990). They showed at least one common RFLP type in each infected family member.

More than one serotype or genotype of *A. actinomycetemcomitans* can colonize the oral cavity of an individual. Asikainen *et al.* (1991) recovered 2 serotypes from 1 of 13 infected Finnish subjects and Chung *et al.* (1989) found 2 serotypes in 3 of 12 infected Korean patients. In addition, Di Rienzo and Slots (1990) found 2 and 3 RFLP types in two black families. Both the intrafamily transmission of strains of *A. actinomycetemcomitans* and the presence of uninfected members in affected families (Zambon *et al.*, 1983a) shows that close contact between individuals is necessary for transmission to occur. The apparently poor

transmissibility of this organism may in part explain the low prevalence of JP.

However, as many as 25% of the adolescents in the USA harbour periodontal strains of *A. actinomycetemcomitans* but only 0.1% of this group develop JP. This could either be because host factors determine disease development or because only certain strains of *A. actinomycetemcomitans* alone or in combination with other bacteria have pathogenic potential (Slots and Schonfeld, 1991).

Three serotypes of *A. actinomycetemcomitans* can be distinguished and in a study in the USA (Zambon, Slots and Genco, 1983c), serotype b has been detected in twice as many JP affected sites as serotypes a and c. In Finland (Asikainen *et al.*, 1991) serotype b has been found in periodontitis patients and serotype c in healthy individuals.

Using restriction fragment length polymorphism (RFLP) typing of *A. actinomycetemcomitans* different patterns were observed and these did not correspond to serotypes of the bacteria (Di Rienzo and Slots, 1990). One of these RFLP types named RFLP B seemed particularly virulent and was present in the flora of 3 subjects who converted from health to JP. This genotype was not recovered from any healthy sites.

It has also been suggested (Preus, Olsen and Namork, 1987) that genetic material acquired by phage infection could influence the virulence of *A. actinomycetemcomitans*. They found that phage infected bacteria were present in 12 sites which had experienced bone loss within the preceding year in 5 JP patients whilst 9 non-progressing sites infected with the bacteria had non phage infected strains.

A. actinomycetemcomitans strains also vary in their ability to produce the leucotoxin (*see below*) against human PMNs and monocytes. It has been found that sites with JP lesions are usually infected with strongly leucotoxin-producing strains whilst the healthy sites are generally infected with non-leucotoxin producing strains (Zambon *et al.*, 1983b; Tsai and Taichman, 1986).

A. actinomycetemcomitans produces a variety of factors which could increase its virulence and potentially damage the tissues of the host. These are:

- A leucotoxin which can destroy PMNs and monocytes

- Chemotactic inhibition factors
- Surface-associated material (SAM) which stimulates bone resorption
- A lipopolysaccharide (LPS) which can also cause bone resorption
- Proteases that degrade immunoglobulins
- Collagenase which may degrade connective tissue collagen
- Extracellular outer membrane vesicles
- Factors affecting the immune response
- Factors damaging host cells.

Leucotoxin

It was first shown by Baehni *et al.* (1979) that *A. actinomycetemcomitans* strain Y4 isolated from a patient with JP was cytotoxic to PMNs. It was later shown that some strains of *A. actinomycetemcomitans* associated with JP produce a leucotoxin which can kill PMNs and monocytes (Taichmann *et al.*, 1980; McArthur *et al.*, 1981; Zambon *et al.*, 1983b; Ohta and Kato, 1991). The purified leucotoxin has a mass of 115 000 Daltons and its amino-acid sequence and sequence of its coding gene has major similarities with similar toxins from other bacteria, notably *Escherichia coli* haemolysin, *Pasturella haemolytica* leucotoxin and *Pseudomonas aeruginosa* leucotoxin (Ohta and Kato, 1991). It appears to be mainly present in the outer cell membrane and in the extracellular outer membrane vesicles (Lai *et al.*, 1981; Ohta and Kato, 1991). *A. actinomycetemcomitans* strains vary in their ability to produce the leucotoxin (*see above*) and the strains can be classified into leucotoxin-producing strains (Y4 (ATCC 43718), ATCC 29522 and 29524) and non-leucotoxin-producing strains (627, 652) (Ohta and Kato, 1991). Zambon *et al.* (1983a) found a high prevalence of leucotoxin activity in serotype b and low or none in the other two serotypes. However, Chung *et al.* (1989) found variation in leucotoxic activity between all 3 strains. This is partly explained by the work of Kolodrubetz *et al.* (1989) who cloned the leucotoxin gene and showed that copies of it were present in both the leucotoxin-producing and the non-leucotoxin gene and concluded that this was probably responsible for the strain differences in leucotoxin production. There have been two recent studies of its mechanism of leucotoxicity (Iwase *et al.*, 1990; Sakurada, 1990). These showed that it had a membranolytic activity

producing pores in the target cell (Iwase *et al.*, 1990) and that phospholipid was the receptor on the cell for the toxin whose activity resulted in a rapid influx of Ca^{2+} into the cell (Sakurada, 1990). These results indicate that its mechanism of action is very similar to that of *Escherichia coli* haemolysin and *Pseudomonas aeruginosa* leucotoxin (Ohta and Kato, 1991).

Chemotactic inhibition factors

A. actinomycetemcomitans produces factors which inhibit the chemotaxis of PMNs (Van Dyke *et al.*, 1980, 1982). These factor(s) could reduce the number of PMNs in the local lesion available to phagocytose and kill these bacteria.

Surface-associated material (SAM)

A. actinomycetemcomitans produces surface-associated material (SAM) composed of a bacterial capsule and other molecules loosely bound to the outer surface of the external membrane. SAM from several putative periodontal pathogens can induce bone resorption *in vitro* (*see* Chapter 5). All of these are much more potent bone resorbing agents than lipopolysaccharide (*see below*). The SAM from *A. actinomycetemcomitans* is extremely active at inducing bone resorption *in vitro* at low concentrations (Wilson *et al.*, 1985; Kamin *et al.*, 1986). It does this by different mechanisms to the SAMs from other bacteria (Wilson *et al.*, 1988) which do so by stimulating osteoclasts to produce bone resorption inducing cytokines such as interleukin (IL)-1 and tumour necrosis factor (TNF) or prostaglandins (*see* Chapter 5). The SAM from *A. actinomycetemcomitans* is composed of several proteins and peptides. A 64 KDa protein is the factor which produces the bone resorption but the precise mechanism of its action has not yet been established. There is some evidence that it could directly stimulate the proliferation and differentiation of osteoclasts or act indirectly to do this by stimulating osteoblasts to produce signals other than the cytokines or prostaglandins mentioned above (Kamin *et al.*, 1986). In addition, the SAM contains a peptide component which stimulates fibroblasts to produce IL-6 (Reddi *et al.*, 1994, 1995). This may significantly contribute to bone resorption because IL-6 stimulates the proliferation of osteoclast precursors (Roodman, 1992).

JP patients produce high levels of serum antibodies to SAM from *A. actinomycetemcomitans* and serum from these patients can block the bone resorbing activity of this SAM (Meghji *et al.*, 1992). However, it has not yet been clearly established what role these enzymes play *in vivo* in protecting against these defects.

Lipopolysaccharide (LPS)

LPS is a major integral component of the outer membrane of Gram negative bacteria. The LPS of *A. actinomycetemcomitans* has a broad spectrum of immunological and endotoxic activities including stimulating *in vitro* bone resorption, the production of IL-1, an IL-1 inhibitor and prostaglandin (PG) E_2 from macrophages and polyclonal activation of B-lymphocytes (Iino and Hopps, 1984; Nishihara *et al.*, 1988; Garrison *et al.*, 1988; Koga *et al.*, 1991). It seems likely that the bone resorptive activities of this LPS are the result of PGE_2 and IL-1 from osteoblasts and other cells (Koga *et al.*, 1991). However, it is a much less potent bone resorbing agent than SAM from this bacteria (*see above*). Patients with JP have high serum antibody levels to this LPS (Ebersole *et al.*, 1983).

Proteases that degrade immunoglobulins

A. actinomycetemcomitans produces protease enzymes which degrade immunoglobulins (Killian, 1981). This could reduce the local effectiveness of antibodies produced against this bacteria.

Collagenase

A. actinomycetemcomitans produces a collagenolytic proteinase which can attack collagen (Robertson *et al.*, 1982). This could contribute to degradation of collagen and connective tissue breakdown in the periodontal tissues.

Extracellular outer membrane vesicles

A. actinomycetemcomitans produces numerous extracellular outer membrane vesicles which are shed from the surface of the bacteria (Holt, Tanner and Socransky, 1980). These vesicles contain the leucotoxin (*see above*) and LPS (Lai *et al.*, 1981; Nowotney *et al.*, 1982; Tervahartiala *et al.*, 1989; Koga *et al.*, 1991). Their small size could easily permit them to cross epithelial barriers such as the pocket epithelium (Maryland and Grenier, 1989).

Factors affecting the immune response

A. actinomycetemcomitans produces a potent polyclonal B-lymphocyte activating factor (Bick *et al.*, 1981) which may contribute to the pathogenesis of the condition by inducing B-lymphocytes to produce antibodies with determinants unrelated to the bacterial antigens. This may at least in part be due to its LPS present in outer membrane vesicles (*see above*).

Factors damaging host cells

A. actinomycetemcomitans produces an epitheliotoxin which can damage epithelial cells and could facilitate bacterial penetration of the junctional and pocket epithelium (Birkedal-Hansen *et al.*, 1992). It also produces a fibroblast-inhibiting factor which may impair tissue repair (Stevens and Hammond, 1982).

Eikenella corrodens

The surface associated material (SAM) and LPS of *E. corrodens* stimulate bone resorption *in vitro* by releasing IL-1 and TNF from osteoblasts (Holt and Ebersole, 1991) and the SAM produces polyclonal B-lymphocyte activation (Bick *et al.*, 1981). *E. corrodens* also produces factors which inhibit PMN chemotaxis (Van Dyke *et al.*, 1982).

Capnocytophaga species

Capnocytophaga species produce proteases which can degrade types I and IV collagens, immunoglobulins and the glycosaminoglycan components of proteoglycans (Killian *et al.*, 1983; Seddon and Shah, 1989; Söderling *et al.*, 1991). They inhibit PMN chemotaxis (Van Dyke *et al.*, 1982) and their LPS produce weak bone resorption *in vitro* by the same mechanism as *E. corrodens*.

Host response

Local

The primary defence of the periodontal pocket is provided by PMNs and reduction in their function gives rise to severe disease. It has been shown that PMNs from the periodontal pockets of JP cases have reduced chemotactic activity and phagocytic function which could in part be related to the secretion of leucotoxin by *A. actinomycetemcomitans* (Murray and Patters, 1980).

The local lesion of JP in the connective tissue adjacent to the pocket and junctional epithelium is mainly populated by plasma cells and blast cells (Liljenberg and Lindhe, 1980). Gingival explant cultures have been shown to produce immunoglobulins against the associated bacteria and this shows that plasma cells in the local tissues are capable of local production of these immunoglobulins (Hall *et al.*, 1990).

General

The majority of patients with JP have peripheral blood PMNs with an impaired ability to react to chemotactic stimuli (Clark *et al.*, 1977; Van Dyke *et al.*, 1980). This appears to be caused by a cell-associated defect.

Patients with JP have increased levels of serum IgG, IgM and IgA. They also show an impaired blastogenic response to some Gram negative bacteria (Lehner *et al.*, 1974). More recently it has been shown that they have raised antibody titres to *A. actinomycetemcomitans* (Ebersole *et al.*, 1982; Ranney *et al.*, 1982) and over 90% develop neutralizing antibodies against its leucotoxin (Tsai *et al.*, 1981), its LPS (Ebersole *et al.*, 1983) and the bone resorbing activity of its SAM (Meghji *et al.*, 1992).

Aetiology

From these findings it appears that JP is a distinct bacterial disease from adult chronic periodontitis. It appears that the susceptibility to infection by certain Gram negative, facultative bacteria is mainly the result of impaired PMN function that may be inherited. The impaired lymphocytic blastogenic response to certain Gram negative bacteria may also play a part as may also the inherited cementum

hypoplasia. These impairments may be further compromised by infection with a suitable strain of *A. actinomycetemcomitans* and its production of leucotoxin and chemotactic inhibitor which could allow the bacteria to invade the tissues. Its production of SAM with its potential to stimulate bone resorption may also be a key factor.

The tendency of the disease to stabilize in early adult life may well be associated with the production of neutralizing antibodies against the leucotoxin, SAM and LPS.

None of these findings fully explain the condition. The bacterial theory may explain the classic incisor-first molar syndrome, as these teeth erupt first and are exposed to the oral flora for longer. However, it does not explain classic distributions where some teeth are spared, e.g. upper incisors involved and lower incisors spared or the cases with a random or asymmetrical distribution of lesions.

Post-juvenile periodontitis

Post-juvenile periodontitis is seen in patients of 20 or more years of age and shows some of the features of localized JP. The main differences are that the gingival condition and bacterial flora resemble chronic periodontitis. The gingival tissues show clinically obvious inflammation associated with supra- and subgingival plaque and calculus. It would seem that the marked attachment loss seen in this condition mainly resulted from the active phase of JP. It seems likely that when JP comes under control by the development of effective immunity the pockets become colonized by the usual indigenous bacteria associated with chronic periodontitis which produce clinically obvious inflammation. Further progression of the condition then becomes related to the same factors which operate in chronic periodontitis.

Diagnosis of juvenile periodontitis

The early diagnosis of JP depends on careful and regular periodontal examinations of children and young adolescents from the time of eruption of the permanent teeth. This would need to include careful periodontal probing around the first molars and incisors. It should, of course, be remembered that deep false pocketing is a feature around erupting teeth.

JP usually starts on the first molar and early signs of bone loss may be noticed on routine bite-wing radiographs. Full-mouth radiographs may be necessary for comprehensive diagnosis. As the condition has a familial tendency, siblings and offsprings of JP patients should always be carefully examined.

Treatment of juvenile periodontitis

Early diagnosis on this condition is very important because the chances of saving affected teeth are only good if treatment is given before significant attachment is lost.

JP is mainly associated with *A. actinomycetemcomitans* infection and elimination of this bacteria with antibiotics is the mainstay of the primary treatment of this disease. *A. actinomycetemcomitans* is susceptible to tetracycline, a bacteriostatic protein synthesis inhibiting antibiotic *in vitro*. Following systemic administration of tetracycline the serum and crevicular fluid concentrations are high enough to suppress the bacteria *in vivo*. A combination of systemic tetracycline and scaling and root planing has been shown to suppress *A. actinomycetemcomitans* much better than scaling alone (Slots and Rosling, 1983) and this has been shown to be an effective treatment for JP. This has therefore become the mainstay of the primary treatment of this disease. However, recently it has been shown that tetracycline often fails to eliminate *A. actinomycetemcomitans* completely from the subgingival flora (Mandell *et al.*, 1986). Topical application of tetracycline into the pocket produces much higher local concentrations but in spite of this only reduces the numbers of *A. actinomycetemcomitans* to a very limited extent (Nakagawa *et al.*, 1991) and this suggests that its *in vivo* susceptibility is much less than that *in vitro*.

A. actinomycetemcomitans is moderately susceptible to metronidazole but is 2–4 times more susceptible to its hydroxymetabolite (Pavicic *et al.*, 1991). The combination of metronidazole and amoxycillin has been found to be very effective in eliminating *A. actinomycetemcomitans* from the subgingival flora (van Winkelhoff *et al.*, 1989). Complete elimination of *A. actinomycetemcomitans* was found in 97% of all the patients treated with this combination and scaling and root planing (van Winkelhoff *et al.*, 1992) and 2 out of 4 patients

which were still positive for this bacteria were colonized by metronidazole resistant stains. After 2 years of follow-up, recolonization by *A. actinomycetemcomitans* was only found in 1 out of 48 patients (Pavicic *et al.*, 1995). The highly predictable therapy may be explained by the synergism found between metronidazole and amoxycillin (Pavicic *et al.*, 1991) and this also occurs between the hydroxymetabolite of metronidazole and amoxycillin. Thus on present evidence these would seem to be the antibiotics of choice for the elimination of *A. actinomycetemcomitans* from the subgingival flora (Pavicic *et al.*, 1992). However, in addition, Saxen and Asikainen (1993) compared the systemic administration of metronidazole and tetracycline as adjuvants in the treatment of juvenile periodontitis in 27 patients with juvenile periodontitis which were all positive for *A. actinomycetemcomitans* at the affected sites. At baseline they were divided into 3 groups. One group received metronidazole (200 mg tds for 10 days), one group received tetracycline (250 mg tds for 10 days) and the final control group received no antibiotics. All groups received full periodontal treatment consisting of scaling and root planing, maintenance and periodontal surgery when indicated. The clinical parameters were measured at 6 and 18 months after treatment and bacterial samples were also taken for *A. actinomycetemcomitans* culture at the same time intervals. The clinical condition markedly improved in all groups. *A. actinomycetemcomitans* was eliminated from all the test sites in the metronidazole group, 17 out of 26 sites in the tetracycline group and 19 out of 26 sites in the control group. They therefore concluded that metronidazole was more effective than tetracycline in eliminating *A. actinomycetemcomitans* from infected juvenile periodontitis pocket sites. Therefore, there is evidence that the adjuvant administration of metronidazole alone is effective treatment for the complete elimination of *A. actinomycetemcomitans* in juvenile periodontitis.

Thus, providing sufficient support is remaining on the affected teeth then the aim of the primary treatment is elimination of *A. actinomycetemcomitans* from the pockets by a combination of antibiotics, oral hygiene instruction and scaling and root planing. This should be followed by regular 3-monthly maintenance scaling to prevent recolonization. If *A. actomycetemcomitans* re-infects a site(s) then the patient should be re-treated with the appropriate antibiotic(s) based on the results of microbiological sensitivy tests. Regular microbiological monitoring of *Actinobacillus actinomycetemcomitans* in the subgingival flora should be carried out if such facilities are available. Practitioners should refer patients to a dental hospital if oral microbiological facilities are not available to them locally.

Where appropriate, periodontal surgery may be considered for the treatment of residual deep pockets. Where there is insufficient support remaining extractions and prosthetic replacement need to be considered. A plan for such treatment is set out below:

1. Samples of subgingival flora of affected sites should be taken for microbiological investigation and in particular to monitor *Actinobacillus actinomycetemcomitans* and its antibiotic sensitivity. A suitable collection and transport system using an appropriate medium must be worked out with the microbiology laboratory.
2. Oral hygiene instruction and counselling of the patient with emphasis laid on the special nature of the condition and therefore the special responsibility of the patient in maintaining a high level of home care.
3. Administration of either metronidazole 200 mg and amoxycillin 375 mg 3 times daily for 7 days, metronidazole 200 mg 3 times daily for 10 days, or tetracycline 250 mg four times daily for 14 days.
4. Scaling and root planing of affected sites. Subgingival calculus deposits are usually absent. However, debridement and root planing help to create conditions unfavourable to the microflora.
5. Extraction when necessary, with immediate replacement of anterior teeth, of teeth with a hopeless prognosis due to excessive bone loss and drifting.
6. Localized inverse bevel periodontal surgery. This should only be carried out if the patient's cooperation is good and is best done with preoperative and postoperative antibiotic administration. Any suprabony pockets in posterior teeth can be eliminated by apical positioning but, with anterior teeth, replaced flaps are necessary because of aesthetic considerations. A majority of teeth with this condition will have deep intrabony pocketing with associated angular bony defects. These lesions should be curetted with the aim of producing bony in-fill. Certain isolated intrabony lesions with suitable morphology can be treated with guided tissue regenerating and/or bone grafting techniques (*see* Chapter 14, pp. 194–204). The tissues heal rapidly after surgery and often show evidence of in-fill of bone defects. In some cases, advanced bone loss around one of the roots of a first molar may be treated by root amputation or hemisection.
7. Occlusal adjustment. Migration of incisors is a late characteristic of JP but orthodontic treatment of these cases is usually contraindicated. If teeth which are to remain have drifted into premature contact, these should be treated by selective grinding. In a few cases after successful periodontal treatment and after the condition has become fully stable, gentle orthodontic retraction of labially drifted upper incisors might be considered if they can be stabilized behind the lower lip or splinted in a stable position.
8. Prosthetics. Any necessary partial dentures must be carefully designed so that gingival irritation is avoided and abutment teeth loaded as near axially as possible. Chrome cobalt skeleton dentures are usually indicated and acrylic dentures should only be used in the immediate replacement phase.
9. Maintenance. The observation by Waerhaug (1977) that successfully treated cases can subsequently show signs of relapse indicates that long-term maintenance is essential. These patients should be recalled every 3 months for oral hygiene reinforcement and scaling. The affected sites should be monitored and if any deterioration occurs samples of subgingival flora be taken for microbiological investigation in order to monitor possible recurrence of *Actinobacillus actinomycetemcomitans*. If this bacteria is found by the microbiologists, its antibiotic sensitivity should be determined. Appropriate antibiotic treatment can then be given to eliminate this bacteria from the flora. For these reasons it is usually appropriate to refer these cases to a dental hospital where microbiological facilities are available.

Evaluation of treatment procedures for JP

Antibiotics and scaling and root planing

It has been shown by Christersson *et al.* (1985) that scaling and root planing alone may improve the clinical condition somewhat but fails to reduce significantly the number of *A. actinomycetemcomitans* in the subgingival flora. However, a number of studies have shown that a 2-week course of tetracycline or related drugs both brought about clinical improvement and significantly reduced the numbers of *A. actinomycetemcomitans* (Slots and Rosling, 1983; Christersson *et al.*, 1985). However, tetracycline often fails to eliminate *A. actinomycetemcomitans* from the subgingival flora (Mandell *et al.*, 1986). Penicillin and metronidazole used separately have been reported to be ineffective in treating JP (Mitchell, 1984; Kunihira *et al.*, 1985) but in contrast metronidazole and amoxycillin used in combination have been found to be very effective (van Winkelhoff *et al.*, 1989, 1992). In a 2-year follow-up study (Pavicic *et al.*, 1995) this combination of drugs with scaling and root planing (*see above*) has been shown to eliminate totally *A. actinomycetemcomitans* from the subgingival flora for 2 years. Recently, however, the administration of metronidazole alone has been shown to be effective in eliminating *A. actinomycetemcomitans* from the flora (Saxen and Asikainen, 1993).

Antibiotics and surgery

A combination of antibiotics and surgery seems to be very effective in controlling JP. A 2-week course of tetracycline plus replaced flap surgery (Lindhe and Liljenberg, 1984) controlled the progress of the disease in 16 study patients, although 2 patients had recurrence and needed re-treatment. After 5 years of follow-up there was improvement in all clinical measurements and evidence of bony in-fill of bone defects. Bacterial monitoring of this combination of treatment (Kornmann and Robertson, 1985) showed that sites with high levels of *Actinobacillus actinomycetemcomitans* showed a better response to surgery plus tetracycline than scaling plus tetracycline. It has also been shown that surgery plus tetracycline can completely eliminate *A. actinomycetemcomitans* from the subgingival flora

for up to 12 months (Mandell and Socransky, 1988). However, it has now been shown (Pavicic *et al.*, 1995) that this can be achieved for 2 years with metronidazole and amoxycillin plus scaling and root planing (*see above*). There are as yet no reported studies of these antibiotics in combination with surgery.

References

Alanuusua, S. and Asikainen, S. (1988) Detection and distribution of *Actinobacillus actinomycetemcomitans* in the primary dentition. *Journal of Periodontology* **59**, 504–507

Albander, J.M. (1993) Juvenile periodontitis – pattern of progression in relationship to clinical periodontal parameters. *Community Dentistry and Oral Epidemiology* **21**, 185–189

Asikainen, S., Lai, C-H., Alanuusua, S. and Slots, J. (1991) Distribution of *Actinobacillus actinomycetemcomitans* serotypes in periodontal health and disease. *Oral Microbiology and Immunology* **6**, 115–118

Astemborski, J.A., Boughman, J.A., Myrick, P.O. *et al.* (1989) Clinical and laboratory characteristics of early onset periodontitis. *Journal of Periodontology* **60**, 557–563

Baehni, P.C., Tsai, C-C., McArthur, W.P. *et al.* (1979) Interactions of inflammatory cells and oral microorganisms. VII. Detection of leukotoxic activity of a plaque-derived gram negative microorganisms. *Infection and Immunity* **24**, 233–243

Baer, P.N. (1971) The case for periodontitis as a clinical entity. *Journal of Periodontology* **42**, 516–519

Benjamin, S.D. and Baer, P.N. (1967) Familial patterns of advanced alveolar bone loss in adolescence (periodontitis). *Periodontics* **5**, 82–88

Bial, J.J. and Mellonig, J.T. (1987) Radiographical evidence of juvenile periodontitis (periodontosis). *Journal of Periodontology* **58**, 321–326

Bick, P.H., Betts-Carpenter, A., Holdman, L.V. *et al.* (1981) Polyclonal B-cell activation induced by extracts of gram negative bacteria isolated from periodontally diseases sites. *Infection and Immunity* **34**, 43–49

Birkedal-Hansen, H., Caulfield, P.W., Wannameumier, Y. and Pierce, R. (1992) A sensitive screening assay for epitheliotoxins produced by oral organisms. *Journal of Dental Research* **61**, 192 Abstract 125

Blomlöf, L., Hammerström, L. and Linskog, S. (1986) Occurrence and appearance of cementum hypoplasias in localized and generalized juvenile periodontitis. *Acta Odontologica Scandinavica* **44**, 313–320

Boughman, J.A., Beaty, T.H., Yang, P. *et al.* (1988) Problem of genetic model testing in early onset periodontitis. *Journal of Periodontology* **59**, 332–337

Boughman, J.A., Halloran, S.L. and Roulston, D. (1986) An autosomal dominant form of juvenile periodontitis (JP): its localization to chromosome No. 4 and linking to dentinogenesis imperfecta. *Journal of Craniofacial and Genetic Development Biology* **6**, 341–350

Butler, J.H. (1969) A familial pattern of juvenile periodontitis (periodontosis). *Journal of Periodontology* **40**, 115–118

Chung, H-J., Chung, C-P., Son, S-H. and Nisengard, R.J. (1989) *Actinobacillus actinomycetemcomitans* serotypes and leukotoxicity in Korean localized juvenile periodontitis. *Journal of Periodontology* **60**, 509–511

Clark, R.A., Page, R.C. and Wilde, G. (1977) Defective neutrophil chemotaxis in juvenile periodontitis. *Infection and Immunity* **18**, 694–700

Christersson, L., Slots, J., Rosling, B. and Genco, R.J. (1985) Microbiological and clinical effects of surgery treatment of localized juvenile periodontitis. *Journal of Clinical Periodontology* **12**, 465–476

Di Rienzo, J.M. and Slots, J. (1990) Genetic approach to the study of epidemiology and pathogenesis of *Actinobacillus actinomycetemcomitans* in localized juvenile periodontitis. *Archives of Oral Biology* **35**, 79S–84S

Ebersole, J.L., Taubman, M.A., Smith, D.C. and Socransky, S.S. (1982) Humoral immune responses and the diagnosis of human periodontal disease. *Journal of Periodontal Research* **17**, 478–480

Ebersole, J.L., Taubman, M.A., Smith, D.J. *et al.* (1983) Human immune responses to oral microorganisms. II. Serum antibody responses to antigens from *Actinobacillus actinomycetemcomitans* and correlation with localized juvenile periodontitis. *Journal of Clinical Immunology* **3**, 321–331

Eisenmann, A.A.C., Eisenmann, R., Sousa, O. and Slots, J. (1983) Microbiological study of localized juvenile periodontitis in Panama. *Journal of Periodontology* **54**, 712–713

Franklin, E.R. (1978) Periodontal diseases, a socioeconomic problem in Black Africa. *Odonto-Stomatologie Tropicale* **6**, 16–28

Garrison, S.W., Holt, S.C. and Nichols, F.C. (1988) Lipopolysaccharide-stimulated PGE_2 release from human monocytes. Comparison of lipopolysaccharide prepared from suspected periodontal pathogens. *Journal of Periodontology* **59**, 684–687

Gillett, R. and Johnson, N.W. (1982) Bacterial invasion of the periodontium in a case of juvenile periodontitis. *Journal of Clinical Periodontology* **9**, 93–100

Gottlieb, B. (1923) Die diffuse Atrophie des Alveolarknochens Weitere Beitrage zur Kenntnis des Alveolarschwandes und dwssen Wiedergutmachung durch Zementwachstum. *Zeitschrift für Stomatologie* **21**, 195–262

Gottlieb, B. (1928) The formation of the pocket: diffuse atrophy of alveolar bone. *Journal of the American Dental Association* **15**, 462–476

Haffajee, A.D., Socransky, S.S., Ebersole, J.L. and Smith, D.J. (1984) Clinical, microbiological and immunological features associated with treatment of active periodontal lesions. *Journal of Clinical Periodontology* **11**, 600–618

Hall, E.P., Falkler, W.A. and Suzuki, J.B. (1990) Production of immunoglobulins in gingival tissue explant cultures from juvenile periodontitis patients. *Journal of Periodontology* **61**, 603–608

Hart, T.C., Marazita, M.L., Schenkein, H.A. and Diehl, S.R. (1992) Reinterpretation of the evidence for X-linked dominant inheritance of juvenile periodontitis. *Journal of Periodontology* **63**, 169–173

Hartley, A.F. and Floyd, P.D. (1988) Prevalence of juvenile periodontitis in school children in Lagos, Nigeria. *Community Dentistry and Oral Epidemiology* **16**, 299–301

Holt, S.C. and Ebersole, J.L. (1991) The surface of selected periodontopathic bacteria: possible role in virulence. In: Hamada, S., Holt, S.C. and McGhee, J.R. (eds) *Periodontal Disease Pathogens and Host Immune Response*. Tokyo: Quintessence Publishing Co. Ltd. pp. 79–96

Holt, S.C., Tanner, A.C.R. and Socransky, S.S. (1980) Morphology and ultrastructure of oral strains of *Actinobacillus actinomycetemcomitans* and *Haemophilus aphrophilus*. *Infection and Immunity* **30**, 588–600

Iino, Y. and Hopps, R.M. (1984) The bone resorbing activities of lipopolysaccharides from the bacteria *Actinobacillus actinomycetemcomitans*, *Bacteroides gingivalis* and *Capnocytophaga ochracia* isolated from human mouths. *Archives of Oral Biology* **29**, 59–63

Iwase, M., Lalley, E.T., Berthold, P. *et al.* (1990) Effects of cations and osmotic protectants on cytolytic activity of *Actinobacillus actinomycetemcomitans* leukotoxin. *Infection and Immunity* **58**, 1783–1788

Kamin, S., Harvey, W., Wilson, M. and Scutt, A. (1986) Inhibition of fibroblast proliferation and collagen synthesis by capsular material from *Actinobacillus actinomycetemcomitans*. *Journal of Medical Microbiology* **22**, 245–249

Kaslick, R.S., Chasens, A.I., Tuckman, M.A. and Kaufman, B. (1971) Investigation of periodontosis with periodontitis: literature survey and findings based on ABO blood groups. *Journal of Periodonotology* **42**, 420–427

Killian, M. (1981) Degradation of immunoglobulins A1, A2, and G by suspected principal periodontal pathogens. *Infection and Immunity* **34**, 757–765

Killian, M., Thompson, B., Petersen, P.E. and Bleeg, H.S. (1983) Occurrence and nature of bacterial IgA proteases. *Annals of the New York Academy of Science* **409** 612–624

Koga, T., Nishihara, T., Amano, K. *et al.* (1991) Chemical and biochemical properties of cell-surface components of *Actinobacillus actinomycetemcomitans*. In: Hamada, S., Holt, S.C. and McGhee, J.R. (eds) *Periodontal Disease Pathogens and Host Immune Response*. Tokyo: Quintessence Publishing Co. Ltd. pp. 117–127

Kolodrubetz, D., Dailey, T., Ebersole, J. and Kraig, E. (1989) Cloning and expression of leukotoxin gene from *Actinobacillus actinomycetemcomitans*. *Infection and Immunity* **57**, 1465–1469

Kornmann, K.S. and Robertson, P.B. (1985) Clinical and microbiological evaluation of juvenile periodontitis. *Journal of Periodontology* **56**, 443–446

Kronauer, E., Borsa, G. and Lang, N.P. (1986) Prevalence of incipient juvenile periodontitis at age 16 in Switzerland. *Journal of Clinical Periodontology* **13**, 103–108

Kunihira, D., Caine, F. and Palicanis, K. (1985) A clinical trial of phenoxymethyl penicillin for adjunctive treatment of juvenile periodontitis. *Journal of Periodontology* **56**, 352–360

Lai, C-H., Listgarten, M.A. and Hammond, B.F. (1981) Comparative ultrastructure of leukotoxic and non-leukotoxic strain of *Actinobacillus actinomycetemcomitans. Journal of Periodontal Research* **16**, 379–389

Lehner, T., Wilton, J.M.A., Ivanyi, L. and Manson, J.D. (1974) Immunological aspects of juvenile periodontitis (periodontosis). *Journal of Periodontal Research* **9**, 261–272

Liljenberg, B. and Lindhe, J. (1980) Juvenile periodontitis. Some microbiological, histopathological and clinical characteristics of juvenile periodontitis. *Journal of Clinical Periodontology* **7**, 48–61

Lindhe, J. and Liljenberg, B. (1984) Treatment of localised juvenile periodontitis results after 5 years. *Journal of Clinical Periodontology* **11**, 399–410

Lindhe, J. and Slots, J. (1989) Periodontal disease in children and young adults. In: Lindhe, J. (ed.) *Textbook of Clinical Periodontology*. Copenhagen: Munksgaard. pp. 193–220

Lindstog, S. and Blomlöf, L. (1983) Cementum hypoplasia in teeth affected by juvenile periodontitis. *Journal of Clinical Periodontology* **10**, 443–451

Long, J.C., Nance, W.E. and Waring, P. (1987) Early onset periodontitis: a comparison and evaluation of two proposed modes of inheritance. *Genetics and Epidemiology* **4**, 13–24

Lopez, N.J., Rios, V., Pareja, M.A. and Fernandez, O. (1991) Prevalence of juvenile periodontitis in Chile. *Journal of Clinical Periodontology* **18**, 529–533

McArthur, W.P., Tsai, C-C., Baehni, P.C. *et al.* (1981) Leucotoxic effects of *Actinobacillus actinomycetemcomitans. Journal of Periodontal Research* **16**, 159–170

Mandell, R.L. (1984) A longitudinal microbiological investigation of *Actinobacillus actinomycetemcomitans* and *Eikenella corrodens* in juvenile periodontitis. *Infection and Immunity* **45**, 778–780

Mandell, R.L. and Socransky, S.S. (1988) Microbiological and clinical effects surgery plus doxycycline on juvenile periodontitis. *Journal of Periodontology* **59**, 373–379

Mandell, R.L., Tripodi, L.S., Savitt, E. *et al.* (1986) The effect of treatment on *Actinobacillus actinomycetemcomitans* in localised juvenile periodontitis. *Journal of Periodontology* **57**, 94–99

Manson, J.D. and Lehner, T. (1974) Clinical features of juvenile periodontitis (periodontosis). *Journal of Periodontology* **45**, 636–640

Maryland, D. and Grenier, D. (1989) Biological activities of outer membrane vesicles. *Canadian Journal of Microbiology* **35**, 607–613

Meghji, S., Wilson, M., Henderson, B. and Kinane, D. (1992) Antiproliferative and cytotoxic activity of surface-associated material from periodontopathic bacteria. *Archives of Oral Biology* **37**, 637–644

Melnick, M., Shields, E.D. and Bixler, D. (1976) Periodontitis: a phenotypic and genetic analysis. *Oral Surgery, Oral Medicine, Oral Pathology* **42**, 32–41

Melvin, W.L., Sandifer, J.B. and Grey, J.L. (1991) The prevalence and sex ratio of juvenile periodontitis in a young racially mixed population. *Journal of Periodontology* **62**, 330–334

Mitchell, D. (1984) Metronidazole: its use in clinical dentistry. *Journal of Clinical Periodontology* **11**, 145–158

Murray, P. and Patters, M. (1980) Gingival crevice neutrophil function in periodontal lesions. *Journal of Periodontal Research* **15**, 463–469

Nakagawa, T., Yamada, S., Oosuka, Y. *et al.* (1991) Clinical and microbiological study of local minocycline delivery (Periocline) following scaling and root planing in recurrent periodontal pockets. *Bulletin of Tokyo Dental College* **32**, 63–70

Neely, A.L. (1992) Prevalence of juvenile periodontitis in a circumpubertal population. *Journal of Clinical Periodontology* **19**, 367–372

Newman, M.G. and Socransky, S.S. (1977) Predominant cultivatable microbiota in periodontitis. *Journal of Periodontal Research* **12**, 120–128

Nishihara, T., Koga, T. and Hamada, S. (1987) Extracellular proteinous substances from *Haemophilus actinomycetemcomitans* induce mitogenic responses in murine lymphocytes. *Oral Microbiology and Immunology* **2**, 48–52

Nishihara, T., Koga, T. and Hamada, S. (1988) Suppression of murine macrophage interleukin-1 release by the polysaccharide portion of the lipopolysaccharide of *Haemophilus actinomycetemcomitans. Infection and Immunity* **56**, 619–625

Novak, M.J., Stamatelakys, C. and Adair, S.M. (1991) Resolution of early lesions of juvenile periodontitis with tetracycline therapy alone: long term observations in 4 cases. *Journal of Periodontology* **62**, 628–633

Nowotney, A., Behling, U.H., Hammond, B. *et al.* (1982) The release of toxic microvesicles by *Actinobacillus actinomycetemcomitans. Infection and Immunity* **37**, 151–154

Ohta, H. and Koga, K. (1991) Leucotoxic activity of *Actinobacillus actinomycetemcomitans*. In: Hamada, S., Holt, S.C. and McGhee, J.R. (eds) *Periodontal Disease Pathogens and Host Immune Response*. Tokyo: Quintessence Publishing Co. Ltd. pp. 143–154

Page, R.C., Altman, L.C., Ebersole, J.L. *et al.* (1983b) Rapidly progressive periodontitis, a distinct clinical condition. *Journal of Periodontology* **54**, 197–209

Page, R.C. and Baab, D.A. (1985) A new look at the etiology and pathogenesis of early onset periodontitis. *Journal of Periodontology* **56**, 748–751

Page, R.C., Bowen, T., Altman, L. *et al.* (1983a) Prepubertal periodontitis. 1. Definition of a clinical disease entity. *Journal of Periodontology* **54**, 257–271

Pavicic, M.J.A.M.P., van Winkelhoff, A.J. and de Graaff, J. (1991) Synergistic effects between amoxycillin, metronidazole and its hydroxymetabolite against

Actinobacillus actinomycetemcomitans. Antimicrobial Agents and Chemotherapy **35**, 961–966

Pavicic, M.J.A.M.P., van Winkelhoff, A.J. and de Graaff, J. (1992) Susceptibilities of *Actinobacillus actinomycetemcomitans* to a number of antimicrobial combinations. *Antimicrobial Agents and Chemotherapy* **36**, 2634–2638

Pavicic, M.J.A.M.P., van Winkelhoff, A.J., Douqué, N.H. *et al.* (1995) Microbiological and clinical effects of metronidazole and amoxycillin in *Actinobacillus actinomycetemcomitans* associated periodontitis: a 2 year evaluation. *Journal of Clinical Periodontology*, In press

Preus, H.R., Olsen, I. and Namork, E. (1987) The presence of phage-infected *Actinobacillus actinomycetemcomitans* in localised juvenile periodontitis. *Journal of Clinical Periodontology* **14**, 605–609

Ranney, R.R., Yanni, N.R., Burmeister, J.A. and Tew, J.G. (1982) Relationship between attachment loss and precipitating antibody to *Actinobacillus actinomycetemcomitans* in adolescents and young adults having severe periodontal destruction. *Journal of Periodontology* **53**, 1–7

Reddi, K., Meghji, S., White, P. *et al.* (1995) A 5–7 KDa protein from *A. actinomycetemcomitans* which directly stimulates fibroblasts IL-6 synthesis. *Bone.* In press

Reddi, K., Poole, S., Nair, S. *et al.* (1994) Comparison of the IL-6 inducing activity of periodontopathic bacterial surface-associated proteins. *Journal of Dental Research* **73**, 816. Abstract 237

Reinholdt, J., Bay, I. and Svjgaard, A. (1977) Association between HLA antigens and periodontal disease. *Journal of Dental Research* **56**, 1261–1263

Robertson, P.B., Lantz, M., Marucha, P.T. *et al.* (1982) Collagenolytic activity associated with *Bacteroides* species and *Actinobacillus actinomycetemcomitans*. *Journal of Periodontal Research* **17**, 275–283

Roodman, G.D. (1992) Interleukin-6: An osteotropic factor? *Journal of Bone and Mineralisation Research* **7**, 475–478

Roulston, D., Schwartz, S., Cogan, M.M. *et al.* (1985) Linkage analysis of dentinogenesis imperfecta and juvenile periodontitis: creating a 5 point map of 4q. *American Journal of Human Genetics* **37**, Abstract 206

Saglie, F.R., Carranza Jnr, F.A., Newman, M.G. *et al.* (1982) Identification of tissue-invading bacteria in human periodontal disease. *Journal of Periodontal Research* **17**, 452–455

Sakurada, S. (1990) Leucotoxic mechanism of *Actinobacillus (Haemophilus) actinomycetemcomitans* leukotoxin on human neutrophils. *Japanese Journal of Oral Biology* **32**, 103–114

Saxby, M. (1984) Prevalence of juvenile periodontitis in a British school population. *Community Dentistry and Oral Epidemiology* **12**, 185–187

Saxen, L. (1980a) Prevalence of juvenile periodontitis in Finland. *Journal of Clinical Periodontology* **7**, 177–186

Saxen, L. (1980b) Juvenile periodontitis. *Journal of Clinical Periodontology* **7**, 1–19

Saxen, L. (1980c) Heredity of juvenile periodontitis. *Journal of Clinical Periodontology* **7**, 276–288

Saxen, L. and Koskimies, S. (1984) Juvenile periodontitis – no linkage with HLA-antigens. *Journal of Periodontal Research* **19**, 441–444

Saxen, L. and Asikainen, S. (1993) Metronidazole in the treatment of juvenile periodontitis. *Journal of Clinical Periodontology* **20**, 166–171

Seddon, S.V. and Shah, H.N. (1989) The distribution of hydrolytic enzymes among Gram-negative bacteria associated with periodontitis. *Microbial Ecology in Health and Disease* **2**, 181–190

Sjobin, B., Mattson, L., Unell, L. and Egelberg, J. (1993) Marginal bone loss in the primary dentition of patients with juvenile periodontitis. *Journal of Clinical Periodontology* **20**, 32–36

Slots, J. (1976) The predominant cultivatable organisms in juvenile periodontitis. *Scandinavian Journal of Dental Research* **49**, 248–255

Slots, J., Reynolds, H.S. and Genco, R.J. (1980) *Actinobacillus actinomycetemcomitans* in human periodontal disease: a cross-sectional microbiological investigation. *Infection and Immunity* **29**, 1031–1020

Slots, J. and Rosling, B. (1983) Suppression of periodontopathic microflora in localized juvenile peridontitis by systemic tetracycline. *Journal of Clinical Periodontology* **10**, 465–486

Slots, J. and Schonfeld, S.E. (1991) *Actinobacillus actinomycetemcomitans* in localised juvenile periodontitis. In: Hamada, S., Holt, S.C. and McGhee, J.R. (eds) *Periodontal Disease Pathogens and Host Immune Response*. Tokyo: Quintessence Publishing Co. Ltd. pp. 53–64

Söderling, E., Mäkinen, P.L., Syed, S.A. and Mäkinen, K.K. (1991) Biochemical comparison of proteolytic enzymes present in rough- and smooth-surfaced *Capnocytophaga* isolated from the subgingival plaque of periodontitis patients. *Journal of Periodontal Research* **26**, 17–23

Spektor, M.D., Vandersteen, G.E. and Page, R.C. (1985) Clinical studies of one family manifesting rapidly progressing juvenile periodontitis and prepubertal periodontosis. *Journal of Periodontology* **56**, 93–101

Stevens, R.H. and Hammond, B.F. (1982) Inhibition of fibroblast proliferation by extracts of *Capnocytophaga spp.* and *Actinobacillus actinomycetemcomitans*. *Journal of Dental Research* **61**, 347 Abstract 1515

Taichmann, N.S., Dean, R.T. and Sanderson, C.J. (1980) Biochemical and morphological characterization of the killing of human monocytes by leukotoxin derived from *Actinobacillus actinomycetemcomitans*. *Infection and Immunity* **28**, 258–268

Tervahartiala, B., Uitto, V-J., Kari, K. and Laako, T. (1989) Outer membrane vesicles and leukotoxic activity of *Actinobacillus actinomycetemcomitans* from subjects with different periodontal status. *Scandinavian Journal of Dental Research* **97**, 33–42

Tsai, C-C., McArthur, W.P., Bachni, P.C. *et al.* (1981) Serum neutralizing activity against *Actinobacillus actinomycetemcomitans* leukotoxin in juvenile periodontitis. *Journal of Clinical Periodontology* **8**, 338–348

Tsai, C-C. and Taichmann, N.S. (1986) Dynamics of infection by leukotoxic strain of *Actinobacillus actinomycetemcomitans* in juvenile periodontitis. *Journal of Clinical Periodontology* **13**, 330–331

Van Dyke, T.E., Bartholomew, E., Genco, R.J. *et al.* (1982) Inhibition of neutrophil chemotaxis by soluble bacterial products. *Journal of Periodontology* **53**, 502–508

Van Dyke, T.E., Horoszewicz, H.O., Cianciola, L.J. and Genco, R.J. (1980) Neutrophil chemotactic dysfunction in human periodontitis. *Infection and Immunity* **27**, 124–132

Van Dyke, T.E., Schweinebraten, M., Cianciola, L.J. *et al.* (1985) Neutrophil chemotaxis in families with juvenile periodontitis. *Journal of Periodontal Research* **20**, 503–514

van Winkelhoff, A.J., Rodenberg, A.J., Goené, R.J. *et al.* (1989) Metronidazole plus amoxycillin in the treatment of *Actinobacillus actinomycetemcomitans* associated periodontitis. *Journal of Clinical Periodontology* **16**, 128–131

van Winkelhoff, A.J., Tijhof, C.J. and de Graaff, J. (1992) Microbiological and clinical results of metronidazole plus amoxycillin therapy in *Actinobacillus actinomycetemcomitans*-associated periodontitis. *Journal of Periodontology* **63**, 52–57

Waerhaug, J. (1977) Plaque control in the treatment of juvenile periodontitis. *Journal of Clinical Periodontology* **4**, 29–40

Wilson, M., Kamin, S. and Harvey, W. (1985) Bone resorbing activity of purified capsular material from *A. actinomycetemcomitans*. *Journal of Periodontal Research* **20**, 484–491

Wilson, M., Meghji, S. and Harvey, W. (1988) Effect of capsular material from *Haemophilus actinomycetemcomitans* on bone collagen synthesis *in vitro*. *Microbios* **54**, 181–185

Yosof, Z.A. (1990) Early-onset periodontitis: radiographic patterns of alveolar bone loss in 55 cases from a selected Malaysian population. *Journal of Periodontology* **61**, 751–754

Zambon, J.J. (1985) *Actinobacillus actinomycetemcomitans* in human periodontal disease. *Journal of Clinical Periodontology* **12**, 1–20

Zambon, J.J., Christersson, L.A. and Slots, J. (1983a) *Actinobacillus actinomycetemcomitans* in human periodontal disease. Prevalence in patient groups and distribution of biotypes and serotypes within families. *Journal of Periodontology* **54**, 707–711

Zambon, J.J., de Louca, C., Slots, J. and Genco, R.C. (1983b) Studies of leukotoxin from *Actinobacillus actinomycetemcomitans* using the promyelocytic HL-60 cell line. *Infection and Immunity* **40**, 205–212

Zambon, J.J., Gregory, G.J. and Smutko, J.S. (1990) Molecular genetic analysis of *Actinobacillus actinomycetemcomitans* epidemiology. *Journal of Periodontology* **61**, 75–80

Zambon, J.J., Slots, J. and Genco, R.C. (1983c) Serology of oral *Actinobacillus actinomycetemcomitans* and serotype distribution in human periodontal disease. *Infection and Immunity* **41**, 19–27

21

Acute and infectious lesions of the gingiva

Introduction

Acute lesions are by definition of sudden onset, limited duration and with well-defined clinical features; by contrast with chronic gingivitis which is frequently not obvious, acute gingival lesions are usually easier to diagnose.

There are some pathological conditions that can affect other parts of the oral mucosa, as well as the gingivae, which are impossible to classify because their aetiology is uncertain, e.g. erythema multiforme, or because they may be chronic with acute episodes, e.g. the fungal disease candidiasis. Syphilis, tuberculosis and other bacterial and viral infections may occasionally involve the gingiva but the lesions are widespread, involving many parts of the mouth as well as other parts of the body.

The gingival lesions to be described are:

- Traumatic lesions, both physical and chemical
- Viral infections
  - Acute herpetic gingivostomatitis
  - Herpangina
  - Hand, foot and mouth disease
  - Measles
  - Herpes varicella/zoster virus infections
  - Glandular fever
- Bacterial infections
  - Tuberculosis
  - Syphilis
- Fungal infections
  - Candidiasis
- Gingival abscess
- Aphthous ulceration
- Erythema multiforme
- Drug allergy and contact hypersensitivity.

Traumatic lesions

Physical injury can be mechanical or thermal. A carelessly wielded toothbrush or woodstick, a sharp piece of food such as a fish-bone, hot food and drink are the most common causes of injury. Occasionally the cause is rather more bizarre, a cigarette burn, a pencil pushed into the mouth, a hair-grip, a musical instrument – the range of human oral activity is extensive.

Chemical causes of damage include aspirin placed against the gum to alleviate toothache, escharotics such as silver nitrate, even hydrogen peroxide solution used too strong and too frequently. Careless use of a caustic by the dentist, e.g. phenol, trichloracetic acid, can cause considerable tissue damage.

Usually there is little doubt about the diagnosis. The patient is aware of the accident and may suffer immediate and fairly severe pain. The acute symptoms may last for a day or so and be followed by several days of soreness and sensitivity to further irritation.

A localized area of inflammation and ulceration may form. In the case of a burn there may be vesicle formation followed by ulceration. The wound is seen as a bright red area denuded of epithelium and with a ragged edge of necrotic tissue which can be felt by the tongue. The healing wound is quickly covered by epithelium unless secondary infection takes place as it might do in the debilitated individual. In this case pain persists, the wound may suppurate and this may be accompanied by lymph gland enlargement and malaise. Abscess formation may follow damage by a piece of woodstick or bone if the foreign object is not removed.

Treatment

Frequently the wound heals without any active intervention. The patient should and probably will avoid irritant foods or hot drinks. Rinsing with cold water or a very dilute saline solution might soothe. Strong antiseptics should be avoided. Troches containing a topical anaesthetic, e.g. benzocaine lozenge, can be recommended and some analgesic such as aspirin or paracetamol prescribed.

If the cause of the injury is still there, e.g. a fish-bone, it should be removed as gently as possible.

If there is secondary infection an antibiotic may need to be prescribed.

It can be helpful to protect the wound with a bland dressing such as carboxymethylcellulose gelatin paste (Orabase) which is spread gently over the wound several times a day.

Infections

Viral infections

Acute herpetic gingivostomatitis

Primary infection by the herpes simplex virus (HSV) type I usually occurs in children (1–10 years) but may affect older children or adults. The virus is transmitted by infected saliva or skin lesion contact. Infection in neonates can produce encephalitis or meningitis but in children or adults it produces either a febrile illness or subclinical infection. The incubation period is about 5 days. Symptoms appear abruptly with mild to severe fever. Temperature may be raised as high as 39.4°C. There is lymph gland enlargement and malaise, and the mouth and throat may be very painful. In young children there is irritability, profuse salivation and refusal to eat, even before the oral lesions become apparent. Small vesicles form on the gingivae, the tongue, buccal mucosa and lips, in fact anywhere in the mouth.

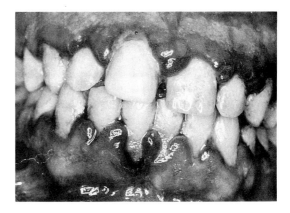

Figure 21.1 Acute herpetic gingivomatitis. The grey membrane of sloughing epithelium is in contrast to the underlying gingival inflammation

Usually the vesicles burst before they are seen and the resultant round or irregular ulcers form a grey membrane surrounded by bright red mucosa. There is an acute gingivitis with redness, swelling and bleeding. Symptoms subside in 10–21 days as the titre of protective antibodies rises (*Figure 21.1*).

A large proportion (30%) of patients who have had a primary herpetic infection early in life develop recurrent infection years later. The commonest recurrent lesion is on the lip (herpes labialis or cold sore). The lesion develops at the mucocutaneous junction of the upper lip and on the skin up to the nostril, although it can occur on the lower lip, and rarely on the gingiva or palate. An itching or burning sensation precedes the appearance of the lesion and a blister or cluster of blisters form which burst, crust and heal after about 10 days. The blisters occur as a result of reactivation of latent virus in the trigeminal ganglion. This can occur as a result of any infection which lowers the resistance or dries the skin, or as a result of excessive exposure to sunlight.

Laboratory diagnosis may be made by direct smear to show characteristic giant cells or by staining with specific fluorescent antisera to HSV. The virus can be isolated in tissue culture. A considerably raised antibody titre indicates recent infection.

Treatment

Treatment of the oral infection is largely symptomatic and supportive, i.e. bed rest, cool, soft food and plenty of fluid. In the infant, milk of magnesia or 55% Dequadin paint may be gently applied on cotton wool to the lesions. Benzocaine lozenges are useful in the older child or adult.

Aspirin or paracetamol will help to reduce pain and temperature. Phenergan is a useful sedative in the child.

In severe cases acyclovir (Zovirax) tablets (200 mg 5 times daily for 5 days) or suspension (5 ml of suspension 5 times daily for 5 days) may be prescribed. Acyclovir cream (apply 5 times daily for 5 days) may also be used as a preventive measure for herpes labialis.

Herpangina

This is an acute febrile illness caused by infection with Coxsackie A types 1–6, 8, 10, 16 or 22. It occurs in sporadic outbreaks mainly in children. The patient complains of a sore throat due partly to oral ulceration. Small ulcers appear mainly on the anterior faucial walls but also on the hard and soft palate, posterior pharyngeal wall, buccal mucosa and tongue. They heal in a few days and recovery is uneventful in 7–10 days.

Hand, foot and mouth disease

This is an acute febrile illness caused by infection with Coxsackie A type 16 or occasionally 5 or 6. It occurs in sporadic outbreaks affecting mainly young children. Maculopapular and vesicular lesions appear on the skin and oral mucosa. The skin lesions mainly affect the hands, arms and feet. The oral vesicles break down into small ulcers. Recovery is uneventful in 10–14 days.

Measles

Measles is a severe febrile illness affecting mainly children and protective vaccination is available against it. There is fever, malaise, cough, conjuctivitis, photophobia and lacrimation. There is a typical blotchy macular rash. Oral lesions known as Koplik's spots precede the skin lesions by a number of days. These are bluish-white specks surrounded by a bright red margin and they occur mainly on the buccal mucosa.

Recovery takes place in 2–3 weeks in otherwise healthy, fit and well-fed children but the infection can be serious in previously unexposed populations particularly when poor and malnourished.

Herpes varicella/zoster virus infections

Varicella or chickenpox is an acute febrile illness mainly of children. It produces a widespread maculo-papular or vesicular eruption on the skin. Small vesicles also form on the oral mucosa including the tongue and gingiva. Recovery is uneventful in 2–3 weeks.

Herpes zoster or shingles is caused by reactivation of latent varicella virus or reinfection of a person who has previously had chickenpox. It is commonest in middle-aged to older adults and affects sensory nerves producing a severe neuralgia. A vesicular eruption occurs on the skin or mucosa innervated by the affected sensory nerve. If the trigeminal nerve or sensory portion of the facial nerve is affected the vesicles can affect the skin of the face and oral mucosa.

Glandular fever

Glandular fever is caused by infection with the Epstein–Barr virus (EBV) which is a herpes-like virus. It is thought to be spread in infected saliva and is most common in children, adolescents and young adults. The infection may be prolonged and this particularly occurs in adults. It is characterized by fever, malaise, sore throat, headache, chills, cough and widespread lymphadenopathy. The liver and spleen may also be enlarged. There is oral involvement with a pharyngitis and oral lesions which take the form of palatal petechiae. There is also an acute gingivitis and stomatitis.

Good oral hygiene and regular professional cleaning are important to treat the gingivitis. Sometimes acute necrotizing ulcerative gingivitis (ANUG) may occur and require treatment.

Bacterial infections

The commonest acute gingival bacterial infection, ANUG, is described separately in Chapter 22. Other bacterial infections affecting the oral mucosa are described below.

Tuberculosis

Oral lesions are rare and are usually secondary to sputum infection from open pulmonary tuberculosis. Deep ulcers may occur on any part of the oral mucosa and a tuberculous gingivitis has been reported (Shafer *et al.*, 1983).

Syphilis

Secondary syphilis occurs about 6 weeks after primary infection and it produces a widespread skin rash and oral eruption. In the mouth ulcers known as mucous patches form and also irregular long winding ulcers known as snail track ulcers. These lesions are teeming with spirochaetes and are highly infectious.

Fungal infections

Candidiasis

The fungus *Candida albicans* is normally found in the mouth as a saprophyte until some changes in the balance of the oral flora or alteration in the local and systemic defence mechanisms occur, producing lowered resistance. Then the fungus proliferates and infects the tissues. It is the most common fungal infection of the mouth. Factors which predispose to infection are prolonged use of antibiotics, steroids, and immunosuppressive drugs. It is also associated with diabetes, leukaemia and conditions of the gastrointestinal tract which promote malabsorption and malnutrition. Vaginal candidiasis is common in pregnancy and the newborn infant may be infected from the vagina. It is also a very common feature of HIV infection and its presence in a severe form should alert one to the possibility of this infection.

Candidiasis occurs in many forms. Three forms tend to be confined to the mouth; fortunately these are usually transient and easy to treat.

1. Acute pseudomembranous candidiasis (thrush)

Thrush is found in infants, debilitated older adults and patients with HIV infection. Lesions occur in the gingivae, tongue, cheeks and throat. They are creamy white, elevated patches which can be wiped away to leave a

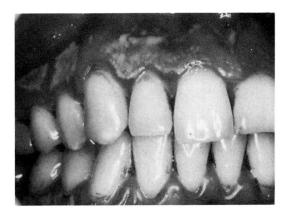

Figure 21.2 Thrush (acute pseudomembranous candidiasis). Creamy white particles are present on the attached gingiva over the right upper incisors and premolars. (By courtesy of Professor C. Scully)

raw red base (*Figure 21.2*). The patient complains of a sore dry mouth or throat.

Diagnosis can be made by demonstrating the yeasts in scrapings from the lesion.

Treatment

In infants a suspension of nystatin (100 000 I.U./ml) can be painted on the lesions two or three times a day. In adults amphotericin B lozenges BP (10 mg) or nystatin pastilles DPF (100 000 I.U.) are sucked 3 or 4 times a day. In severe cases miconazole oral gel DPF can be used.

2. Acute atrophic candidiasis

This form is usually associated with an upset in balance between tissues and oral flora which follows the prolonged use of steroids or antibiotics. The mucosa is thin, fiery red and painful. Nystatin or amphotericin B reduces the symptoms.

3. Chronic atrophic candidiasis (denture sore mouth)

This condition is produced by *Candida* infection of tissue which is being irritated by a denture, often one which is worn day and night. The most usual site is the palate where the tissue is bright red and spongy.

The condition is often accompanied by an angular cheilitis which is produced by overclosure following alveolar resorption under the

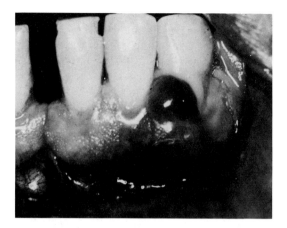

Figure 21.3 Gingival abscess caused by injury from a carelessly used dental woodstick

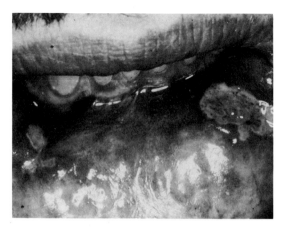

Figure 21.4 Aphthous ulceration. (By courtesy of Dr F. Nally and *Dental Update*)

denture. The corners of the mouth become folded and wet and subsequently infected by *Candida albicans*.

Treatment consists of: (i) leaving the denture out as much as possible; (ii) coating the lesions and the denture when worn with nystatin or amphotericin B; (iii) remodelling the dentures and remaking them when the infection is controlled.

Gingival abscess

The term 'gingival abscess' should be used for abscesses confined to the gingivae. It is often associated with physical damage to the gingival margin by a woodstick, fish-bone, etc. with subsequent infection of the wound but it can also arise within the wall of a gingival pocket where drainage has been impeded.

The abscess appears as a localized, shiny red swelling which is painful (*Figure 21.3*); associated teeth are sensitive to percussion. The abscess may discharge spontaneously or spread into the underlying tissue to form a periodontal abscess.

Treatment

If the cause of the abscess is still present it should be removed carefully. Drainage can be established by hot salt water mouthwashes used every 2 hours. If the lesion persists it can be curetted under local anaesthesia or incised if it is pointing. If persistent and severe a

systemic antibiotic may be needed. Any residual pocketing can be removed by thorough subgingival curettage or localized gingivectomy.

Aphthous ulceration

Recurrent mouth ulcers are the most common lesions of the oral mucosa. There are three types of ulcer: minor aphthous ulcers, major aphthous ulcers and herpetiform ulcers. Their common characteristics are that they are painful lesions which appear without any reason, last for several days or weeks, heal and then after a variable interval recur. The cause is as yet unknown but it is thought that the ulcers may be a manifestation of autoimmunity to a component of the oral mucosa. Several related factors have been suggested, such as emotional stress and hormonal change. In a number of patients the ulcers appear to be related to the menstrual cycle, the peak incidence being found in the postovulation period. There may be a relationship between ulceration and iron-deficiency anaemia, deficiency of folic acid and vitamin B_{12}.

Minor aphthous ulcers (Mikulicz's aphthae)

These are the most common type. One or several small ulcers occur on non-keratinized oral mucosa, especially the lips, cheeks, vestibule and margins of the tongue (*Figure*

21.4). They are shallow ulcers less than 10 mm in length with a surrounding zone of inflammation and slight swelling. They may be very painful or scarcely noticed by the patient unless traumatized. Sometimes tissue breakdown is heralded by localized paraesthesia. The ulcer(s) may last 4–14 days, heal without scarring and recur after weeks or months. They are found in the age group 10–40 years, slightly more frequently in females than males.

Major aphthous ulcers (periadenitis mucosa necrotica recurrens)

These are much less common than the minor variety. They are larger (up to 30 mm), last as long as 40 days and are much more painful. Sometimes they recur so rapidly that involvement seems continuous. They can be found anywhere on the oral mucosa. They start as a submucosal nodule which breaks down to form a deep crater-like ulcer with considerable tissue destruction which heals with a scar.

Herpetiform ulcers

Despite their name they are not related to herpes. They are most frequent in females and occur as a group of pin-head ulcers which may coalesce to form a large painful ulcer. They can occur on any part of the oral mucosa, including the tongue, palate and oropharynx in which case they cause dysphagia (discomfort or pain on swallowing).

Treatment

Treatment for all aphthous ulceration is symptomatic and depends on the frequency and severity of the ulceration. The patient needs to be reassured that the ulcer is not malignant. In the case of minor ulcers treatment may be unnecessary but if they are painful topical anaesthetics or applications of Bonjela can be useful. Where the ulcer is more painful and persistent the application of topical corticosteroid preparations, such as 0.1% triamcinolone (Adcortyl A in Orabase), may be beneficial. Tablets of hydrocortisone hemisuccinate (2.5 mg, Corlan) can be used four times a day, allowing the tablet to dissolve next to the ulcer.

Tetracycline mixture BP as a mouthwash is useful for herpetiform ulcers in adults.

Very rarely, systemic corticosteroids may be needed in severe cases but in these patients it is essential to have comprehensive blood tests and assessment of iron, folic acid and vitamin B_{12} levels.

If the patient has a problem keeping the mouth clean a 0.2% chlorhexidine mouthwash is useful and can speed up the rate of healing.

Erythema multiforme

This is a syndrome of multiple aetiology with a wide spectrum of clinical features. The oral and cutaneous lesions may occur separately or together. In about a third of cases the condition is recurrent.

The aetiology of the syndrome may involve several underlying mechanisms. Drug allergy can cause the condition, especially to long-acting sulphonamides, penicillin and barbiturates. Several cases have also been associated with *Mycoplasma pneumoniae* infection which causes primary atypical pneumonia. In many cases no cause can be found.

The major form of the disease produces systemic involvement whilst the minor form produces local manifestations only. The patient is usually a child or young adult. In the major form there is a skin eruption with conjunctivitis and lesions of the mouth and upper respiratory tract. The patient becomes progressively ill over 7–14 days with fever and malaise.

In the mouth there is diffuse inflammation of the oral mucosa and gingivae. There are widespread erosions on the mucosa and these have a red, velvety base and bleed freely. Some vesicles also form. The lips are severely involved with extensive crusting and they may crust together at night. Eating, talking and oral examination are painful.

On the skin there is an extensive erythematous and macular rash. Iris target lesions with a central bulla which breaks down to crust may be seen. The hands, feet and flexural surfaces are most involved.

There is a diffuse conjunctivitis which can become secondarily infected to produce corneal ulceration. The upper respiratory tract is often involved with epistaxis, dysphagia and tracheitis. Pneumonia, urinogenital involvement, nephritis and myocarditis can occur in severe cases.

In the minor form these are only local manifestations in the mouth or the skin or both and no fever or prostration.

The patient should be referred to a physician. In the minor form topical corticosteroids may be used in the mouth. In the major form systemic steroids and supportive treatment are necessary. If *Mycoplasma pneumoniae* infection is present a course of tetracycline is given.

Drug allergy and contact hypersensitivity

As the number and variety of drugs and chemicals used as food additives increase, oral manifestations of hypersensitivity become more common.

Adverse reactions are basically of two types:

1. Those following systemic administration of a drug or chemical.
2. Those following direct contact with the oral mucosa.

Drug allergy

These reactions can be provoked by penicillin, diazepam, local anaesthetics, codeine, tetracycline, barbiturates and many other drugs in common use.

Manifestations depend on the type of allergic response provoked, ranging from simple drying of the mouth to the most severe response, anaphylactic shock, which is potentially fatal. A severe reaction is angioneurotic oedema in which there is swelling of the face, eyelids, lips, tongue and even pharynx. A fairly common response, especially to penicillin, is urticaria, skin rash, pains in the joints and fever. In the mouth, patches of inflammation, vesicles and ulcers may appear.

Contact hypersensitivity

Reactions of the oral mucosa have been reported to chewing gum, mouthwashes, toothpaste, sweets, cosmetics, topical antibiotics, periodontal dressings, etc. Often flavouring agents, such as peppermint, menthol, cinnamon, eugenol, are implicated.

Symptoms start with a burning sensation of the oral mucosa and swelling and redness of the tongue, lips and gingivae. The epithelium may peel off to leave very sore ulcerated areas. The gingivae are characteristically bright red and sensitive and because the patient cannot clean the mouth it can become very dirty.

Management

The drug or chemical suspected must be immediately withdrawn. Antihistamines, such as Piriton, are useful where symptoms are mild but more severe reactions, e.g. angioneurotic oedema, may require injection of hydrocortisone hemisuccinate.

In anaphylactic shock intramuscular injection of 0.5 ml of 1:1000 adrenaline is necessary.

The mouth can be kept clean by frequent warm water or weak saline mouthwashes.

Reference

Shafer, W.G., Hine, M.K. and Levy, B.M. (1983) *A Textbook of Oral Pathology*, 4th edn. Philadelphia: Saunders

22

Acute necrotizing ulcerative gingivitis

This condition has many synonyms including acute ulcerative gingivitis (AUG), acute necrotizing gingivitis (ANG), Vincent's disease, trench mouth and fuso-spirochaetal gingivitis. Acute necrotizing ulcerative gingivitis (ANUG) is an acute necrotizing inflammatory disease produced by endogenous infection where systemic changes, as yet not precisely defined, predispose the gingiva to invasion by some bacteria in the oral flora, in particular spirochaetes and fusiform bacteria.

In Western countries, ANUG is usually seen in the 16–30 age group. Epidemiological studies from 1950–1960 reported a 5% incidence of this condition in young adults particularly in large groups living in cramped conditions such as military recruits and college students. However, the prevalence of the disease has reduced markedly over the past 20 years and this may reflect improved general health and nutrition and better standards of plaque control. More recently the disease has been seen in patients with HIV infection and AIDS (see Chapter 7) and this now needs to be considered in the diagnosis of this condition.

In some developing countries, such as those in Africa, ANUG is often seen in children and is often associated with malnutrition and infectious disease such as measles and herpes simplex infections (Osuji, 1990). Environmental factors are entirely responsible for this situation because it occurs in the poor malnourished children and not in those children with rich families who are of the same race and tribe. In a few of these affected children with severe malnutrition and recent infections the infection may spread from the gingiva to involve the oral and facial tissues producing a condition known as cancrum oris or noma. This may result in massive oro-facial necrosis and is life threatening. If the child recovers from the infection gross facial deformity results.

In a study of 58 Nigerian children with ANUG Osuji (1990) found 5 cases of cancrum oris. These children had all had a recent history of febrile illness. Predisposing factors for cancrum oris are severe malnutrition, infectious childhood diseases, HIV infection and any disease in which the immune system is compromised, as well as poor oral hygiene.

Clinical features of ANUG

In developed countries the condition is a disease of young adults and occurs equally in both sexes. It appears to be seasonal, occurring most frequently in autumn and winter months. The condition rarely occurs in a clean mouth and then only if there is a major predisposing factor.

The condition is very painful and plaque accumulates around the affected areas. Patients complain of gingival soreness, which is sometimes severe, and eating becomes difficult. There may be spontaneous gingival bleeding, an objectionable taste and a powerful halitosis.

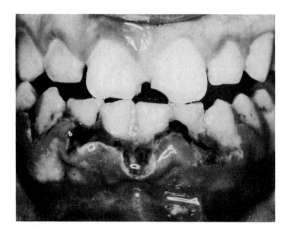

Figure 22.1 Acute ulcerative gingivitis (involving gingivae in the lower jaw). (By courtesy of Dr F. Nally and the Editor of *General Practitioner*)

ANUG is characterized by necrotic ulceration of the affected gingival margins (*Figure 22.1*). In the early stages of the disease the gingival papillae become red and swollen and the tips of the papillae become ulcerated. Necrotic ulceration of the papillae increases and the ulcers may spread laterally along the gingival margins. The ulcers are painful to touch and are covered by a yellowish-grey slough. They have a characteristic 'punched out' appearance (*Figure 22.1*) and if the 'false membrane' of sloughing tissue is removed a raw and bleeding surface is exposed.

The ulceration may be localized to one area or involve the whole mouth. Localized infections are most often seen around the lower anterior teeth. They may also be related to sites of bacterial stagnation such as a partially erupted lower third molar.

There are frequently no systemic symptoms, although cervical or submandibular lymphadenopathy is commonly present. In some severe cases there may be mild to moderate fever and malaise and more marked lymphadenopathy. In a study of 35 ANUG patients presenting at an urban USA dental school, Falker *et al.* (1987) found lymphadenopathy in 61% and fever in 39% of their cases.

Ulceration can also rarely occur on the contacting surface of the tongue or cheek, the palate and the fauces (Vincent's angina) but only when there is very severe debilitation. When ANUG occurs in association with HIV infection the lesion may spread more deeply and lead to exposure and infection of the underlying bone (Chapter 7).

Even without active intervention the acute symptoms will subside and the ulcers heal in 10–14 days. However, the normal gingival form does not return and the gingival margin becomes thickened by fibrous repair tissue and the papillae retain the concave shape of the healed ulcer. This saucer-shaped deformity of the gingiva is so characteristic of ANUG that an episode of previous infection can be diagnosed years later.

Once an episode of ANUG has occurred there is a tendency for recurrence and in a susceptible individual this can occur more than once a year. This can result in progressive destruction of the periodontal tissues with typical loss of the interdental papillae and the formation of characteristic gingival craters. The additional stagnation produced by this tissue deformity also encourages the progression of any underlying chronic periodontitis.

Predisposing factors

The main predisposing factors in most cases are poor oral hygiene, smoking and emotional stress. However, it can be precipitated by malnutrition, blood dyscrasias such as acute leukaemia, infections such as AIDS and glandular fever, malignant neoplasms and chemotherapy. Probably any condition in which the immune and defence systems are compromised would act in the same way.

The reduction in this condition in recent times probably reflects better standards of oral hygiene and improved health and nutrition. The name trench mouth derives from the high prevalence of ANUG in soldiers suffering the appalling conditions of trench warfare in the First World War. The disease occurred in groups living together in these grossly unhygienic conditions and under immense stress.

Microbiology

ANUG is a mixed bacterial infection caused by a group of anaerobes consisting of spirochaetes and fusiform bacteria which is often termed a fuso-spirochaetal complex. These bacteria include *Treponema vincentii, T. denticola, T. macrodentium, Fusobacteriun nucleatum, Prevotella intermedia* and *Porphyromonas gingivalis* (Loesche *et al.*, 1982). These bacteria are all found in large numbers in the slough and necrotic tissue at the surface of the ulcer and also invade a small distance into the underlying intact tissue at the base of the ulcer. Spirochaetes can be seen under electron microscopy to invade the greatest distance into the tissue. The aetiological role of these bacteria is suggested by the fact that ANUG resolves rapidly following short-term treatment with metronidazole.

Other bacterial species commonly found in the subgingival flora are also present on the surface of the lesion in lesser numbers.

There are many reports of ANUG in closely confined groups of young adults (*see above*). However, there is no evidence that the condition is transmissible. This view is supported by experiments in which the inoculation of microorganisms from affected to healthy animals did not result in development of ANUG except when the recipients were severely immunosuppressed. It is therefore thought that the reported group outbreaks of ANUG were due to common exposure to stressful conditions and poor oral hygiene rather than direct transmission of an infecting agent. This view is also supported by the fact that all of the bacteria infecting the tissues in ANUG are bacteria found in the subgingival flora of patients with chronic gingivitis and periodontitis who do not develop ANUG.

Histopathology

The histopathological changes of ANUG are largely non-specific. The surface epithelium and adjacent connective tissue on the surface of the lesion is necrotic. There is a dense acute inflammatory infiltration of the underlying tissues with large numbers of polymorphonuclear neutrophil leucocytes (PMNs) in the tissues. Bacteria can be seen invading this area, with the spirochaetes spreading deepest. Below this area is viable tissue infiltrated with plasma cells, lymphocytes and some macrophages.

Host responses

The exact way in which the predisposing factors trigger the infection is not clear.

However, the fact that ANUG occurs in AIDS and in severely immunosuppressed animals suggests that immunosuppression might be an important factor.

ANUG usually develops when there is poor oral hygiene and pre-existing gingivitis. It will, however, rarely occur in a clean mouth when a severe debilitating factor is present, e.g. acute leukaemia.

A number of studies (Macgregor, 1992) have indicated that smoking is an important predisposing factor in ANUG (*see also* Chapter 4). In a study of 35 ANUG patients in an urban dental school Falker *et al.* (1987) found that 83% of these patients were smokers. Smokers tend to have poorer levels of oral hygiene than non-smokers but this is not sufficient to explain the association. Smoking may cause vasoconstriction of gingival blood vessels and might in this way favour the colonization of an anaerobic bacterial flora.

Emotional stress as a predisposing factor in ANUG has been long recognized by clinicians. However, there are only a few well controlled studies which demonstrate the association between ANUG and stress. Stress may alter behaviour such as decreasing oral hygiene, reducing salivary flow and local blood flow and probably affects immune function. In spite of these effects it is not entirely clear how these effects operate to predispose to this condition.

There is a clear relationship between nutritional deficiency and ANUG in developing countries. This may operate by compromising the defence mechanisms to such a degree that the disease spreads more easily.

Diagnosis

The diagnosis is easily made on clinical grounds without the need to take a bacterial smear to show the fuso-spirochaetal flora. Nevertheless, it is important to take a very careful history to determine the underlying predisposing factors in each individual case.

Treatment

Treatment is divided into two stages:

1. control of the acute phase, and
2. management of the residual condition.

Control of the acute phase

This is achieved by cleaning the wound and using an antibacterial agent. The lesion is irrigated with warm water or 5-vol hydrogen peroxide solution, gently cleaned and the teeth lightly scaled. The patient is prescribed an oxygen-releasing mouthwash, such as hydrogen peroxide DPF or sodium perborate (Bocasan) DPF, to be used three times daily. The scaling of the affected teeth is completed over the next few days. This may suffice in very mild cases but most cases require an antibiotic in addition. ANUG is an anaerobic infection, thus oral metronidazole (200 mg three times daily for 3–5 days) is the first choice. It gives rapid relief of symptoms and is not prone to produce hypersensitivity reactions. Side-effects may include nausea, headaches, a metallic taste and tachycardia. It should not be prescribed in early pregnancy, if there is blood dyscrasia or in patients drinking alcohol heavily. Alcohol must be totally avoided when taking metronidazole since it precipitates nausea and vomiting. In these cases, phenoxymethyl penicillin (250 mg four times daily for 5 days) is an effective alternative. Erythromycin or tetracycline may be used if both metronidazole and penicillin are contraindicated. A 2% chlorhexidine mouthwash might also be helpful in some cases but should only be used during the short period in which mechanical oral hygiene is compromised.

It is also vital to determine the predisposing factors in each individual case and to counsel the patient on controlling these when appropriate.

Management of the residual condition

This is essential if recurrence is to be avoided. Meticulous supra- and subgingival scaling is carried out together with the removal of all predisposing local factors, such as overhanging filling margins, partially erupted teeth and food impaction.

Residual gingival deformity needs to be corrected by gingivoplasty in early cases and by inverse bevel flap procedures in all other cases. Any underlying chronic periodontitis lesion, e.g. pocketing, can be dealt with at the same time.

The maintenance of a high standard of oral hygiene is essential, therefore regular inspection and scaling should be organized.

Patients suffering unexplained recurrence should undergo medical examination and blood screening.

References

Falker, W.A. Jnr, Martin, S.A., Vincent, J.W. *et al.* (1987) A clinical and demographic and microbiologic study of ANUG patients in an urban dental school. *Journal of Clinical Periodontology* **14**, 307–314

Loesche, W.J., Syed, S.A., Laughton, B.E. and Stoll, J. (1982) The bacteriology of acute necrotizing ulcerative gingivitis. *Journal of Periodontology* **53**, 223–230

Macgregor, I.D.M. (1992) Smoking and periodontal disease. In: Seymour, R.A. and Heasman, P.A. (eds) *Drugs, Diseases and the Periodontium.* Oxford, Oxford University Press, pp. 118–119

Osuji, O.O. (1990) Necrotizing ulcerative gingivitis and cancrum oris in Ibadan, Nigeria. *Journal of Periodontology* **61**, 769–772

23

Epulides and tumours of the gingiva

Epulides

The term 'epulis' means a 'lump on the gum' and these lesions are the commonest localized enlargements of the gingiva. They are best described as chronic inflammatory hyperplasias. These can be fibrous epulides, pyogenic granulomata or giant-cell granulomata, the first two being much more common than the third.

Fibrous epulis (fibro-epithelial polyp)

This usually arises from an interdental papilla and is a firm, pink nodule of varying shape (*Figure 23.1*). They usually associate with a source of chronic irritation such as calculus or the rough edge of a restoration. Similar lesions can occur on the cheek as the result of cheek biting or related to the margin of an ill-fitting denture (denture granuloma).

Histologically the lesion consists of hyperplastic connective tissue covered by stratified squamous epithelium.

These lesions should be treated by excision with care to remove any irritating factor. The whole lesion should be placed in formal saline fixative and sent for histological confirmation of the diagnosis.

Pyogenic granuloma

The pyogenic granuloma usually arises from the interdental papilla. It appears as an elevated, pedunculated or sessile mass with a

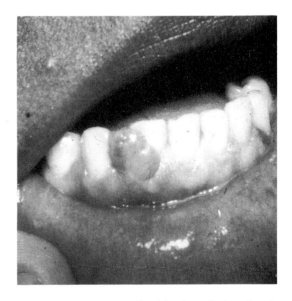

Figure 23.1 A fibrous epulis arising from the interdental papilla between 32| of a 35-year-old woman

smooth or lobulated surface (*Figure 23.2*). It is deep red or reddish-purple in colour and the surface may be ulcerated. It also has a tendency to bleed either spontaneously or on provocation with slight trauma. It may develop rapidly to a variable size and then remain stable for an indefinite period.

The lesion appears to result from local irritation but in some cases there may be a hormonal conditioning factor such as in the lesions occurring in pregnancy (pyogenic

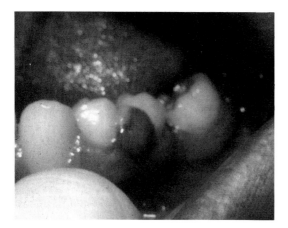

Figure 23.2 A pyogenic granuloma arising from the interdental papilla between⌐45 of a 15-year-old boy

granulomata of pregnancy) and at puberty (Chapter 6).

Histologically, the overlying stratified squamous epithelium is usually thin and atrophic but may show signs of hyperplasia in some parts of the lesion. The connective tissue contains vast numbers of endothelium-lined vascular spaces and proliferation of endothelial cells and fibroblasts. There is a moderately intense infiltration of polymorphonuclear neutrophil leucocytes (PMNs), lymphocytes and plasma cells with high numbers of PMNs at the surface of the lesion particularly when ulceration is present.

The lesion should be carefully excised with care to remove all affected tissue and any local irritating factor. Lack of care in these respects can lead to recurrence of the lesion. The whole lesion should be placed in formal saline fixative and sent for histological confirmation of the diagnosis.

Giant-cell epulis

The giant-cell epulis or granuloma is usually found growing from the gingival margin between teeth anterior to the permanent molars and its development may be related to the resorption of the deciduous molars (*Figure 23.3*). The lesion is rounded, soft and purplish-red in colour. It may grow rapidly in its early stages and tends to bleed easily.

Histologically, the connective tissue consists of numerous multinucleated giant-cells (macrophage polykaryons) and plump spindle-

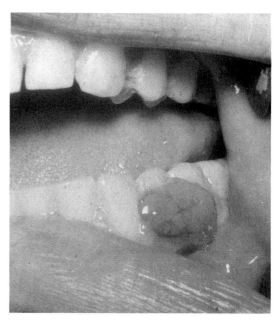

Figure 23.3 A giant-cell epulis arising from the interdental and buccal gingiva between⌐45 of a 15-year-old boy

shaped cells in a loose fibrous stroma. It is covered by stratified squamous epithelium.

A giant-cell granuloma of the jaw may erode through the outer alveolar plate and appear as a gingival swelling. This should be distinguished from the epulis by radiological investigation.

The treatment is total excision of the lesion along with the basal tissue from which it arose. The alveolar bone at the base of the lesion should also be curetted thoroughly. Histological confirmation of the diagnosis is essential and the lesion must be immediately placed in formal saline fixative for this purpose.

Neoplasms of the gingiva

True benign or occasionally malignant neoplasms may arise from the gingival or periodontal tissue and may sometimes resemble an epulis.

Epithelial neoplasms

Squamous-cell papilloma

The squamous-cell papilloma usually appears as a warty nodule with a white surface if

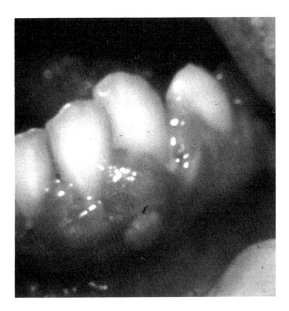

Figure 23.4 A squamous cell papilloma on the gingiva between ⎿23 in a 40-year old woman

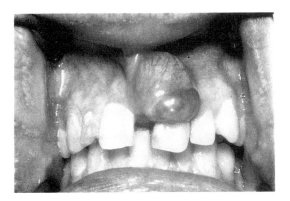

Figure 23.5 A benign true fibroma beneth the gingival and alveolar muvosa related to⎿1 in a 25-year old woman. The tumour has caused displacement at ⎿1

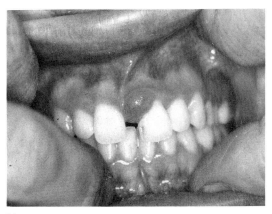

(a)

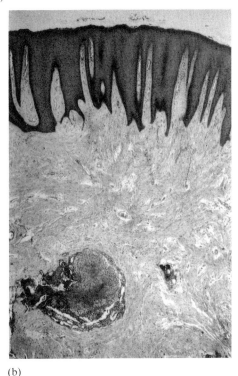

(b)

Figure 23.6 (*a*) A tumour of dental tissue origin, resembling an epulis, arising from the mesial interdental and buccal gingiva related to⎿1 in a 16-year-old girl. (*b*) Photomicrograph of a low-power view of a histological section of the above lesion. It shows the features of an adenomatoid odontogenic tumour

keratinized and a pink one if not (*Figure 23.4*). It may be related to the common wart of the skin and be due to infection with human papilloma virus (HPV).

The whole lesion should be excised and submitted for histological examination to confirm the diagnosis.

Squamous-cell carcinoma

These tumours may occasionally occur on the gingiva but are more common on other parts of the oral mucosa such as the tongue, lips, buccal mucosa, floor of the mouth or alveolar mucosa. Carcinoma of the gingiva usually presents as an ulcerated lesion with rolled edges but it may sometimes have a exophytic or verrucous type of growth. Any fast growing lesion or ulcer which fails to heal should be regarded with suspicion; 95% of oral cancer occurs after the age of 40 and it becomes more common with increasing age. Gingival carcinomas are closely related to the underlying bone and rapidly invade the periosteum and bone. Metastasis is common and early diagnosis is essential if treatment is to have any chance of success. Suspicious lesions should be quickly referred to a specialist oral surgeon and oral pathologist to confirm the diagnosis by biopsy and institute treatment.

Connective-tissue neoplasms

Benign and occasionally malignant neoplasms arising in the connective tissue can sometimes involve the gingival tissues. They may present as firm masses which stretch the overlying mucosa and may displace adjacent teeth. They may also sometimes resemble epulides. Suspicious lesions should be referred to a specialist oral surgeon and oral pathologist for definitive diagnosis.

These neoplasms may include benign fibromas (*Figure 23.5*) and myxomas and their equivalent malignant sarcomas.

Lymphoid neoplasms

Lymphomas such as Hodgkin's and non-Hodgkin's lymphoma may produce deposits beneath the oral mucosa including the gingiva. In addition deposits from a leukaemia may seed in the gingiva and multiply (*see* Chapter 6). All such cases should be quickly referred to specialists for these conditions.

Dental tissue neoplasms

Tumours of odontogenic origin may be found in the jaws and occasionally arise from dental epithelial remnants in the periodontium, such as the epithelial rests of Malassez, and occur in the periodontium or gingiva. Those in the gingiva may resemble epulides and those within the bone may expand the alveolar plate and produce a gingival swelling. They include adenomatoid odontogenic tumours, squamous odontogenic tumours and calcifying epithelial odontogenic tumours. Careful radiographic examination is necessary in these cases and they should be referred to a specialist oral surgeon and oral pathologist for definitive diagnosis and treatment. The clinical appearance and histology of an adenomatoid odontogenic tumour of the gingiva are shown in *Figure 23.6a,b*.

24

Occlusion

The term 'occlusion' applies to any contact between the mandibular and maxillary teeth in any position of the mandible. The occlusion is therefore of importance to restorative and prosthetic dentistry as well as to orthodontics and periodontics. Unfortunately each of these specialties has been concerned with a particular aspect of occlusion and has developed its own beliefs and vocabulary, leading to confusion. Many of the concepts valuable to prosthetics or orthodontics may be irrelevant or even contrary to an understanding of the role of occlusal relationships and occlusal stresses in periodontics. Many of the ideas still in current use were developed before knowledge of the neurophysiology of the masticatory system had been acquired and therefore represent a static view of occlusion in which anatomical stereotypes are important. The idea of malocclusion as expressed by Angle's classification of this generation. The concept of 'balanced occlusion' in which bilateral cuspal contacts are made in lateral excursions may well be important in prosthetics but under certain circumstances can be contrary to periodontal health. Health of the tooth-supporting tissues does not depend primarily on the conformity of the occlusion to any particular anatomical stereotype. However, occlusal stresses can play an important role in periodontal pathology (Chapter 8).

Three important aspects of masticatory function need to be considered:

1. During normal mastication teeth are separated by the food bolus and make contact at the end of the chewing cycle and during swallowing. It has been estimated that the total duration of tooth contact in a 24 hour period is 17.5 minutes made up of 9 minutes chewing contact and 8.5 minutes swallowing contact. Therefore normal functional tooth-to-tooth contact is occasional and transient and by itself unlikely to cause damage.

2. The activity of the masticatory system is largely under the control of the trigeminal nerve nucleus which, subject to the control of the higher centres, operates various forms of reflex activity. These constitute a feedback mechanism which protects the various tissues of the masticatory system, including the periodontium. For example, the presence of a hard object such as a piece of bone or nut in the bolus of soft food stimulates proprioceptors in the periodontal ligament which by reflex activity causes the jaw to open. In this way stress on the teeth and supporting tissues is controlled, unless the higher centres dictate that a conscious effort be made to crack the nut.

3. All the tissues of the masticatory system except the teeth have considerable powers of adaptation and bone, connective tissue and epithelium are in a state of constant activity and renewal. The masticatory system is not a rigid system; like other vital tissues it is immensely flexible and allows a range of environmental changes to be absorbed without damage.

Excessive occlusal stress

Attempts to define the word 'excessive' in most situations tend to beg the question. Excessive occlusal stresses are those which exceed the limits of tissue adaptation and therefore cause occlusal trauma. Occlusal trauma is the damage to the supporting tissues when subject to excessive occlusal stresses. Forces generated during mastication depend largely on the consistency of the food. Peak pressures on an adult molar have been estimated at 0.4–1.8 kg, but because of the powers of adaptation of the periodontal tissues it is impossible to define excessive occlusal stress in precise numerical terms.

Excessive stresses appear to be engendered by:

1. Abnormal or parafunctional activity.
2. Dental treatment.
3. Occlusal disharmony.
4. Destruction of the periodontal tissues by disease, i.e. chronic periodontitis.

These factors are frequently interrelated.

Parafunction

Parafunctional activity is outside the range of functional activity. It is usually habitual and the patient is often unaware of such habits during which contact may be made between the upper and lower teeth as in clenching and grinding, between the teeth and the soft tissues, cheeks, lips and tongue or between the teeth and some foreign body, e.g. pencil, pipe, etc. These habits may be associated with psychological factors, e.g. anxiety, anger, frustration, or with occupational or recreational activity.

Bruxism

The most common tooth-to-tooth habits are clenching and grinding, i.e. bruxism. A large proportion of patients with periodontal disease indulge in this habit. Many patients are aware of clenching their teeth when under stress during the day but few people are aware of a night grinding habit unless complained of by someone else. It has been estimated that during clenching or grinding the individual might impose a load of over 20 kg on a tooth over periods of 2.5 seconds at a time. This is far in excess of normal functional stresses and causes 'flow' within the viscoelastic periodontal ligament and distortion of the alveolar bone, from which the tissues are slow to recover. Furthermore, the excessive load tends to affect the proprioceptive nerve endings which are either overridden or set at a higher tolerance level, thereby impairing the protective reflex mechanism. Muscle activity becomes abnormal and the habit is perpetuated. Such disturbed muscle activity may also interfere with temporomandibular joint function. Bruxism is the most usual cause of advanced attrition in the Western world.

In the absence of gingival inflammation or periodontal destruction the supporting tissues may adapt to the load or breakdown of primary occlusal trauma. Where there is inflammatory periodontal disease the tissues usually similarly adapt. In early to moderate periodontitis the adaptive response is the same but in advanced periodontitis the rate of disease progress may be accelerated by the fusion of the marginal inflammatory and the intra-alveolar 'trauma' lesions (Chapter 8).

There are two causes of bruxism – nervous tension and occlusal interference. These two factors often act together so that an occlusal interference in an anxious person may provoke bruxism, whereas in a relaxed individual interference may be adapted to.

Diagnosis of bruxism

There may be a definite history of bruxism but as stated many patients are unaware of parafunction. A number of signs help in its detection:

1. Advanced attrition is the most obvious clue, also wear facets which could be produced only in extreme positions of mandibular movements.
2. Increased tooth mobility patterns which are not commensurate with the amount of attachment loss or degree of gingival inflammation.
3. The presence of widened periodontal ligament spaces seen in radiographs.
4. Hypertonicity of the muscles of mastication.
5. Temporomandibular joint discomfort.

Dental treatment

One of the most common causes of excessive occlusal stress in the partially dentate patient is the badly designed partial denture. Many abutment teeth suffer abnormal loading because the stress is either greater than normal or applied in an abnormal direction. The tooth used as an abutment for a free-end saddle denture is particularly vulnerable, especially when clasps without occlusal rests are used. As the denture sinks into the soft tissues, lateral and distal forces are imposed on the abutment teeth. In most cases oral hygiene is poor and the combined effect of gingival inflammation under the denture and excessive occlusal loads make loss of abutment teeth more than likely. In denture design axial loading of abutment teeth is imperative and where soft-tissue support is necessary this should be spread over as large an area as possible.

Orthodontic treatment can cause excessive occlusal stress in two ways. Large forces can cause rapid tooth movement and damage to the supporting tissues. If the alveolar plates of bone are thin they may be perforated; thus, tipping a lower incisor forward against a thin labial plate may produce a dehiscence. Slow orthodontic movement allows tissue adaptation and less likelihood of trauma. Tooth movement can also produce occlusal disharmonies with harmful results.

Failure to contour the cusps of restorations or to check the occlusion in both intercuspal and functional positions can produce cuspal interference. Unfortunately modern dental amalgams set rapidly and leave little time for careful occlusal adjustment. Failure to replace a lost tooth can result in drifting of other teeth with resultant disharmonies.

Occlusal disharmony

Functional harmony is a very important attribute of the healthy masticatory system, with all parts of the unit – muscles, ligaments, temporomandibular joints – working smoothly together. *Occlusal disharmonies are tooth contacts which interfere with smooth closing movement along any pathway into intercuspal position.* A common mistake is to assume that malocclusions are always associated with occlusal disharmonies. So flexible is the tooth eruption mechanism that even gross tooth malalignment does not necessarily produce cuspal interference; rather it is external interference with the fully erupted dentition which produces disharmony. Badly executed dentistry can create interferences but the most common cause is tooth loss. After tooth extraction neighbouring teeth may tip and drift and opposing teeth overerupt until a new position of stability is reached. Thus after extraction of the lower first molar the second and third molars tip mesially and lingually and the distal cusps of these teeth come into interfering contact with upper molar cusps. Moreover, because of the tilt, plaque may be allowed to collect on the mesial and lingual aspects of these teeth producing gingival inflammation and pocketing.

Effects of occlusal interference

1. The path of closure of the mandible may alter to avoid the interference. This may put an excessive load on other teeth, e.g. occlusal interference between molar cusps may produce a path of closure forward of the normal pathway and forward posturing of the mandible so that the upper incisors become overloaded (*Figure 24.1b*). This may result in drifting of the incisors which is more likely when there is already loss of tooth support caused by periodontal disease.
2. If there is no adaptation to the interference, the involved teeth make contact in what is called an *initial* or *premature* contact from which a slide carries the mandible into the position of maximum intercuspation (*Figure 24.1a*). This may produce excessive stress on those teeth involved directly as well as on those teeth indirectly stressed at the end of the slide. Drifting and occlusal trauma may result.
3. The interference may also initiate parafunctional habits.

The diagnosis of occlusal trauma

A number of clinical features point to the presence of occlusal trauma. A diagnosis should be based not on the presence of only one but several features together.

1. *Tooth mobility* is affected by the load on the tooth and its duration, by the proportion of

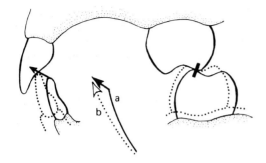

Figure 24.1 An interference between posterior teeth may produce (*a*) a slide from the initial contact into the intercuspal position, or (*b*) forward posturing of the mandible so that it closes through a forward path

tooth invested in supporting tissue and by the morphology of the root(s). It is also affected by inflammation of the attachment apparatus. Increased tooth mobility may be a sign of occlusal trauma or of hyperfunction, i.e. increased loading of the tooth without evidence of tissue breakdown. Assessment of mobility (outside the laboratory) is entirely subjective, teeth being given a score from 0 to 3 (Chapter 11). It can be detected by having the patient grind the teeth from side to side while the operator rests his fingers on the facial surfaces of the teeth. It is more usually tested for by pressing the blunt end of an instrument against one side of the tooth while a finger rests on the tooth under examination and a neighbouring tooth which acts as a fixed point.

2. Tooth wear which appears to be greater than one might expect in a patient of that age and which cannot be attributed to any special diet or deficiency in tooth mineralization.

3. The migration of one or more teeth; this is usually seen in the anterior segment often related to (i) loss of posterior support and/or (ii) an abnormal path of closure due to tooth interference between posterior teeth (*Figure 24.1*). Where bone loss due to periodontal disease has taken place tooth migration can be rapid and a common cause of patient alarm. Food impaction may occur following tooth drifting and breaking of interproximal contacts.

4. Operators with a sensitive ear may be able to detect that the percussion note of an affected tooth is dull rather than resonant.

5. There may be hypertrophy and hypertonicity of the muscles of mastication, most obviously of the masseters. This is detected by palpation but sometimes can actually be seen, especially in the bruxist patient.

6. Signs of temporomandibular pain dysfunction syndrome with jaw deviation, joint clicking, discomfort and even pain due to muscle spasm.

7. Radiographic evidence (together with mobility) offers evidence of occlusal trauma. The signs are:
   (a) Widening of the periodontal space.
   (b) Funnel-like or crescentic resorption of the alveolar crest around a tooth.
   (c) Loss of definition of the lamina dura; this is an unreliable sign as other factors including root morphology affect the radiographic appearance of the socket wall.

8. Tooth sensitivity may be associated with both occlusal trauma and pulp pathology brought about by excessive loading. Sometimes patients have an awareness of a discrepancy in their occlusion, a positive occlusal sense, and a patient may be able to point to the tooth involved.

Occlusal analysis

This is an analysis of static jaw relationships as well as of the relationships of the teeth during mandibular movements. A large number of articulators have been designed to replicate jaw movement but each of them has its limitations and the almost inevitable errors in bite registration and model mounting frequently nullify the accuracy of the articulator. A more fundamental criticism of mechanical aids is that they simply cannot reproduce the flexibility of vital tissues. However, fully adjustable articulators are necessary in carrying out complex restorative procedures. In a periodontal analysis study models are useful but careful oral examination is essential.

The examination of static jaw relations should include a record of the teeth in the arch, tooth alignment and such tooth deviations as tilting, overeruption and plunger cusps. Inter-arch examination records the Angle's classification, overbite, overjet, gross malocclusions such as crossbite and any details of cusp to fossa relationships which appear abnormal.

The examination of functional relationships is a great deal more difficult and can be carried out properly only with experience and great attention to detail. The starting point for this examination has been the subject of much debate. The intercuspal position (ICP) as the end point of functional movement would appear to be the natural starting point for analysis but it is not a fixed position and may well be the end point of a habitual mandibular closing path which compensates for and therefore masks the disharmonies we are trying to detect. The only fixed and reproducible position is the retruded contact position (RCP) where the jaw rotates around its hinge axis. Although some people swallow in RCP, it is an abnormal and strained position in most people. However, it is useful because of its reproducibility.

The essential requirement for recording RCP is to have the patient sitting in a relaxed position. Some operators even go as far as hypnotizing the patient! With the dental chair slightly reclined and the patient sitting comfortably the operator puts one hand on the patient's chin with the thumb resting on the incisal edge of the lower incisors. The patient is instructed to relax the jaw and allow the operator to move it freely up and down. When the muscles relax the mandible can be rotated around its hinge axis without discomfort and when the thumb is removed the jaw can come together in RCP. Once the patient has learned the feel of this position he or she can reproduce it at will and allow the operator to register with coloured bite papers or soft occlusal indicator wax a number of contact relations. Sometimes muscle tension is so great that closing pathways cannot be altered in this way and a bite-guard may be needed as an aid to overcome abnormal muscle patterns of activity.

An initial cusp contact in centric relation can be detected by placing coloured paper or indicator wax over the upper posterior teeth, guiding the patient into tooth contact in RCP and then sliding from there into complete closure (ICP). The direction of the slide can be observed and the point of initial contact will be marked on the teeth or seen by perforations in the indicator wax. Similarly, tooth contacts in working and non-working sides during lateral excursions, and tooth contacts in protrusive movement can be defined. These techniques can be learned only by practical experience.

It should be possible to link signs of occlusal disharmony such as drifting, mobility and faceting with the site of an occlusal disharmony and an associated slide. Thus a premature contact in RCP between the distal slope of an upper molar cusp will produce a forward slide so that the lower incisors come forward against the upper incisors.

Occlusal adjustment

Adjustment can be carried out by (i) selective grinding, (ii) restorative dentistry, (iii) orthodontics. Whatever technique is used the objectives remain the same:

1. To direct occlusal forces along the long axis of the tooth and as far as possible reduce lateral components of force.
2. To distribute forces over as many teeth as possible in maximum intercuspation and to establish 'group function' during lateral and protrusive movements by creating simultaneous gliding contacts between working teeth.
3. To establish bilateral contact between posterior teeth in RCP and a sagittal movement of no more than 1 mm between RCP and ICP.
4. And thereby eliminating the signs and symptoms of occlusal disharmony.

Selective grinding (Schuyler, 1935)

The greatest danger of selective grinding is that it can be indiscriminate. One is faced with a bewildering array of coloured dots and smudges and multiple perforations in the occlusal wax. Before any tooth grinding is carried out the consequences of any adjustment must be determined. Central to this analysis is the location of cuspal inclines which act as centric stops or supporting cusps in maximum interdigitation and thus maintain the vertical dimension of the face (*Figure 24.2*). Selective grinding is carried out with a handpiece and diamond stones and should proceed in a methodical manner.

1. Elimination of gross occlusal disharmonies which are obvious to the eye, such as plunger cusps, malposed and extruded teeth, discrepancies in marginal ridge height. Where there is a widened buccolingual diameter caused

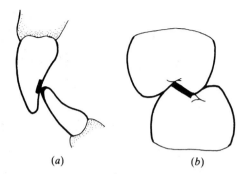

(a)   *(b)*

Figure 24.2 Centric stops (*a*) on incisors and (*b*) on posterior teeth

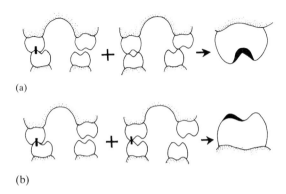

(a)

(b)

Figure 24.3 Correction of interferences between posterior teeth in RCP. If there is no interference in lateral excursions, the fossa is ground as in (*a*). If there is interference in lateral excursions, the cusp is ground as in (*b*)

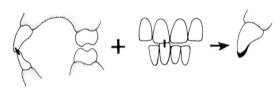

Figure 24.4 Correction of interference between incisors in protrusive movements. The adjustment should not disturb the centric stop

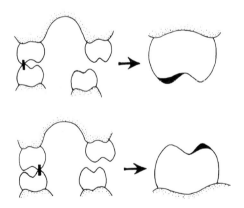

Figure 24.5 Correction of working side interference according to the BULL rule

by attrition the diameter can be reduced. Keeping the positions of supporting cusps in mind these obvious sources of occlusal disharmony can be corrected to a considerable degree as a first step.

2. Correction of prematurities in RCP. These may be divided into two groups, with or without prematurities in lateral excursions. These situations and their corrections are shown in *Figure 24.3*.

3. Correction of protrusive disharmonies. The contact between incisors and canines should be a smooth glide into the edge-to-edge position with as many anterior teeth as possible in contact. In adjustment of protrusive contact it is essential to remember that the incisal edge (or close to it) of the lower incisors is a centric stop (*Figure 24.4*). One of the most common mistakes is the reduction of an incisal edge obviously above the line of the rest of the incisors in order to achieve an improved appearance. The almost inevitable result is overeruption of the reduced tooth with recreation of the interference and consequent aggravation of the problem.

4. Correction of disharmonies in lateral excursions (*Figures 24.5* and *24.6*). The objective of this adjustment is group function on the working side and disarticulation of the non-working side. Non-working side contacts (in prosthetics called balancing contacts) are frequently associated with advanced periodontal destruction and TMJ dysfunction. A premature contact between buccal cusps in working movement and position is corrected by grinding the buccal cusp of the upper tooth, while a lingual cusp contact is corrected by grinding the lingual cusp of the lower tooth. This is the so-called BULL rule (*Figure 24.5*).

Correcting a non-working side contact can be a problem as the contact is frequently

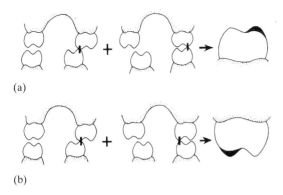

(a)

(b)

Figure 24.6 The correction of a lateral movement in the non-working side depends upon the relationships of the interfering cuspal inclines in other excursions. In (*a*) the buccal cusp of the lower tooth is in interfering contact in two positions, while in (*b*) the palatal cusp of the upper tooth is in interfering contact in two positions and is therefore the one to be corrected

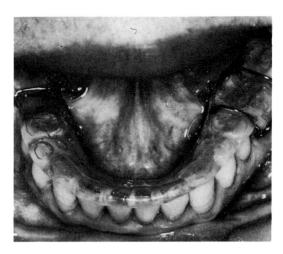

Figure 24.7 Bite-guard with occlusal coverage

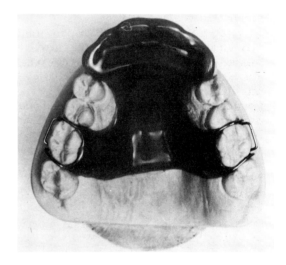

Figure 24.8 Bite-guard with anterior bite plate

between the buccal incline of the palatal cusp of the upper tooth and the lingual incline of the lower buccal cusp, i.e. supporting cusps. It is almost impossible to avoid cutting these surfaces and the adjustment will depend upon the form of contact made by these surfaces in other positions (*Figure 24.6*). If a cuspal incline is in premature contact in both working and non-working positions, this can be adjusted. On other occasions very precise adjustment of the cuspal incline is needed so that the cusp tip, as the centric stop, is retained, thus avoiding over-eruption. If grinding a centric stop is unavoidable the occlusion will need to be supervised in case there is resultant tipping of involved teeth which would create a further interference.

Finally the adjusted surfaces are polished smooth. Not infrequently the patient remarks on an improvement in the feel of the occlusion. After some weeks mobility and other features of occlusal disharmony should reduce if the adjustment has been carried out correctly.

Treatment of bruxism

The first step in the control of any parafunctional habit must be discussion with the patient. Frequently once the individual becomes aware of a habit and the damage that it can do, he or she can bring it under some degree of daytime control.

If occlusal disharmonies play a role in provoking or aggravating a clenching or grinding habit, selective grinding should help to relieve the parafunction. However, the psychological substrate of stress will remain and apart from reassuring the patient that the dental problems can be controlled, attempts to alleviate psychological problems have no place in dental treatment. Further dental treatment involves the use of bite-guards aimed at limiting the effects of excessive occlusal stress.

There are basically two forms of bite-guard, both of which are made in acrylic: (i) the occlusal shield which fits over the occlusal surfaces, incisal edges and facial and lingual tooth convexities (*Figure 24.7*) and (ii) the anterior bite plate (*Figure 24.8*).

Where attrition is severe or where there has been collapse of the posterior segments so that the free-way space is increased, the occlusal shield can be useful, especially in cases where there has been considerable periodontal destruction. Usually it is fitted over the teeth of the jaw in which there is most periodontal destruction. The occlusal surface must be flat and highly polished so that the teeth in the opposing jaw can skid across the surface without impedance. The thickness of the bite-guard must be adjusted so that the freeway space is not encroached upon, otherwise muscle tension will be intensified rather than diminished. 'Opening the bite' can be a dangerous procedure which may accelerate periodontal destruction. Sheikholeslam *et al.* (1993) have shown that where there are signs of craniomandibular disorders, i.e. headaches, neck or TMJ pain, in patients with nocturnal bruxism, full arch maxillary plane occlusal splints remove or relieve the symptoms. Alas, symptoms recur on discontinuing the use of the splint.

Where there is an obvious bruxism habit with symptoms of muscle spasm and where the lower anterior teeth are well supported by bone, a bite-guard with an anterior bite plate is extremely useful. This disengages the posterior teeth, thus eliminating any cuspal interference and interrupting the reflex activity which causes muscle spasm. It is also useful where the freeway space is small. The anterior bite plate may be used as an initial form of control of bruxism in the appropriate case and then if necessary the occlusal shield can be used for long-term control, in which case it can also be used as a splint. Depending on the habit pattern the bite-guard is worn at night or during the day, and any necessary adjustments are made until the minimal thickness compatible with comfort and efficiency is obtained. Patients with bite-guards must adhere to a strict oral hygiene regime and avoid sugar between meals.

References

Schuyler, C.H. (1935) Fundamentals in the correction of occlusal disharmony, natural and artificial. *Journal of the American Dental Association* **22**, 1193–1202

Sheikholeslam, A., Holmgren, K. and Rise, C. (1993) Therapeutic effects of the maxillary plane occlusal splint in signs and symptoms of craniomandibular disorders in patients with nocturnal bruxism. *Journal of Oral Rehabilitation* **20**, 473–482

25

Splinting

When the periodontal tissues are no longer capable of withstanding the stresses of function, teeth become mobile. This mobility can interfere with function. In many cases treatment of the periodontal lesion and occlusal adjustment, if necessary, is all that is required to strengthen the supporting tissues, reduce mobility and re-establish function. When such local treatment fails to achieve these ends, further tooth support is needed (Lindhe and Nyman, 1977).

A splint is a device for supporting weakened tissues. It serves two purposes: (i) provides rest where wound healing is in process and (ii) permits function where the tissues alone cannot perform adequately.

There has been a great deal of debate about the role of splinting in periodontal treatment, largely because the role of the splint has been misunderstood. A splint does not make loose teeth tight. A splint controls mobility when the splint is in place and when the splint is removed the tooth mobility becomes manifest again. Only the removal of disease and subsequent healing can achieve a real reduction in tooth mobility.

The aim of splinting teeth is: (i) to protect the tooth-supporting tissues during the healing period after an accident or following surgery and (ii) to bring into function teeth which cannot be used to eat efficiently or in comfort without artificial support.

If splinting is carried out incorrectly it may make firm teeth loose, as for example when a loose first premolar is linked to a stable second premolar, overloading the latter tooth and producing two loose teeth.

There are many types of splint, temporary and permanent, fixed and removable, but every splint should meet certain requirements:

1. It should incorporate as many firm teeth as is necessary to reduce the extra load on individual teeth to a minimum.
2. It should hold the teeth rigid and not impose torsional stresses on any incorporated teeth.
3. It should extend around the arch, so that anteroposterior forces and faciolingual forces are counteracted.
4. It should not interfere with the occlusion. If possible, gross tooth disharmonies should be eliminated before the application of the splint.
5. It should not irritate the pulp.
6. It should not irritate the soft tissues, gingivae, cheeks, lips or tongue.
7. It should be designed so that it can be kept clean. Interdental embrasure spaces should not be blocked by the splint.

Temporary and provisional splints

Temporary splints are used to assist healing after injury or after surgical treatment. They should be reasonably easy to apply to mobile teeth and also easy to remove after healing has taken place. They should not be left in place for longer than 2 months. If adequate stabilization has not taken place in that time a more

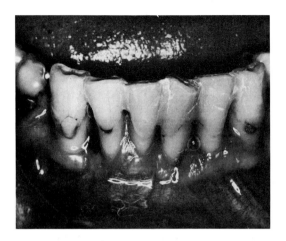

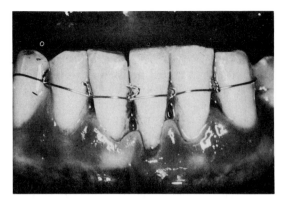

Figure 25.2 Wire splint placed prior to covering with acrylic resin

Figure 25.1 Emergency splint made with composite filling material

permanent form of splinting is necessary. Most temporary splints do not involve destroying tooth tissue.

Composite filling materials can be acid-etched to the surface of mobile teeth and linked together. This is the simplest form of temporary splinting and one which is especially useful in emergencies (*Figure 25.1*).

The wire and acrylic splint (Figure 25.2) is also fairly easy to apply and is frequently used for the stabilization of incisors. It is stronger and more reliable than the composite filling splint. Usually the teeth from canine to canine, or first premolar to first premolar, are included in the splint. A length of 0.002 inch stainless-steel wire is looped around the teeth with the lingual arch wire just incisal to the cingula. The ends of the wire are twisted together distal to the last tooth included. The interdental wires are looped around both lingual and facial arch wires and twisted tight so that the arch wire is pulled tight around the teeth just apical to the contact point. After any necessary adjustment in position the arch wire and interdental wires are finally tightened, their ends trimmed and tucked out of the way into embrasure spaces. A thin mix of quick-set acrylic is run over the wire, care being taken to avoid blocking out embrasure spaces. When set the acrylic is trimmed smooth and polished so that it is comfortable to the soft tissues.

Orthodontic bands may also be used, especially in posterior segments where they

are not obvious; 0.005 inch stainless-steel bands are fitted to the teeth to be splinted and welded together. Alternatively, the splint can be fabricated on a model and cemented into position. The edges of the bands must be contoured and polished to reduce plaque retention and avoid soft-tissue irritation.

Acrylic bite-guards already described for the treatment of bruxism may also be used as splints. The splint should cover the occlusal surface of the teeth and extend 1–2 mm over the facial surfaces of the teeth. In order to obtain adequate stability and rigidity in the upper jaw considerable palatal coverage is needed and in the lower jaw the lingual acrylic needs to be brought well down in the lingual vestibule without impeding muscle activity. The occlusal surface must be designed to allow free excursion of the mandible with no greater than 1 mm increase in vertical dimension in the molar regions. Very careful adjustment of the occlusion in the mouth is essential otherwise opposing teeth will be subject to excessive stress.

The intracoronal splint can be regarded as a semi-permanent rather than temporary splint and many consist of either a continuous intra-coronal bar, or sections of wire in the so-called A-splint.

1. *The continuous intracoronal bar.* A transverse groove, 2–3 mm wide, is cut in the lingual surface of anterior teeth coronal to the cingulum, or in the occlusal surface of posterior teeth. The groove is made about

1.5 mm deep and slightly undercut. A stainless-steel wire is bent to fit the groove which is filled with self-curing acrylic and the wire quickly pressed home. After the acrylic has set it is shaped and polished.

Alternatively, a gold bar may be cast to fit the preparation and cemented in place. As occlusal pressures may push anterior teeth away from the bar, it is advisable to improve retention by making pin-hole preparations in the base of the groove, but even with this added retention it is not advisable to splint upper anterior teeth in this way. The horizontal-pin splint represents a variation of the continuous intracoronal bar. It is strong and well retained but can be used only where some pulp recession has taken place.

A form of continuous intracoronal bar which is used to stabilize a posterior segment consists of MOD amalgam fillings placed in the teeth to be stabilized and then subsequently linked by a bar cemented with acrylic into a channel cut through the amalgams.

2. *The Rochette splint.* Acid-etch composite materials provide an opportunity for splinting without radical tooth preparation. An impression of the teeth to be splinted is taken and a chrome-cobalt splint, fitting the lingual surface of these teeth, is constructed. The lingual tooth surfaces are dried and etched and the splint is glued into position with the composite material.

If carefully prepared and in good occlusal balance, this form of splinting provides excellent stability and may be regarded as a semi-permanent splint.

Permanent splints

Permanent splints may be fixed or removable.

Fixed splints

Fixed splints provide the most reliable form of immobilization but do require considerable tooth preparation, skill and time. They consist of linked inlays or crowns.

Linked inlays are self-descriptive. Inlays which fit into dovetail preparations in the lingual surfaces of anterior teeth may be displaced if an excessive anterior force is exerted on any individual tooth. In the posterior region a series of linked MOD inlays with occlusal coverage can make a satisfactory and permanent splint.

Linked crowns provide the most reliable form of immobilization and support (Nyman and Ericsson, 1982; Lindhe and Nyman, 1979). The splint is extremely strong, holds the teeth rigidly and is the most aesthetically satisfying and unobtrusive type of splint. If teeth are missing the multiple abutment fixed bridge may be used to replace these teeth and to stabilize a segment or a complete arch. This type of splint allows one to modify the form of the teeth and in fact provides one of the most satisfactory methods of occlusal rehabilitation. This splint is difficult to make and requires a great deal of chairside time and skill. Considerable tooth preparation is necessary and there is often the possibility of pulpal involvement. Alternatively, telescope crowns soldered together may be used. These are fitted over gold copings which are cemented onto the teeth. The telescope superstructure may be fixed with temporary cement so that it may be removed periodically for inspection and cleaning.

One modification of the linked crown splint is the multiple pinlay splint which reduces tooth-tissue loss to a minimum. Three parallel pin-holes are made in each tooth to be splinted. Usually six teeth are incorporated into the splint and paralleling eighteen pin-holes presents some difficulty. Pin retention is not as good as that provided by inlays or crowns, therefore this appliance can only be used with success where functional forces are not acting to separate the appliance from the tooth, as they might be where upper incisors are under some occlusal stress. This factor restricts the application of the pinlay splint to the lower incisors.

Removable splints

The removable splint does not involve cutting tooth tissue, it is easier to construct than a fixed splint and can be altered or discarded at will. Like all removable appliances the splint may act as a plaque-retention factor and source of gingival irritation unless oral hygiene is good.

The most common type of splint is the lingual coverage splint which is essentially a

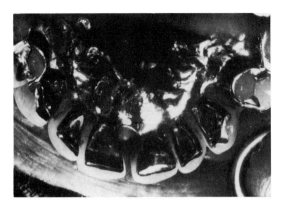

Figure 25.3 Removable splint in chrome-cobalt with lingual coverage for incisor teeth

partial denture in chrome-cobalt with extensions covering the lingual surfaces of the teeth to be protected (*Figure 25.3*). The continuous clasp splint is a variation in which support is reinforced by a labial arch bar.

Designing splints provides the opportunity for considerable ingenuity but the choice of splint should reflect patient need rather than the artistic aspirations of the operator. Many forms of splint are complex, difficult to execute and costly and are justified only when a good prognosis is likely. Where the prognosis is doubtful a simple form of splint is indicated. If the prognosis is poor the removable chrome-cobalt lingual coverage splint allows for the addition of weak teeth as they are lost.

References

Lindhe, J. and Nyman, S. (1977) The role of occlusion in periodontal disease and the biological rationale for splinting in the treatment of periodontitis. *Oral Science Reviews* **10**, 11–43

Lindhe, J. and Nyman, S. (1979) A longitudinal study of combined periodontal and prosthetic treatment of patients with advanced periodontal disease. *Journal of Periodontology* **50**, 163–169

Nyman, S. and Ericsson, I. (1982) The capacity of reduced periodontal tissues to support fixed bridgework. *Journal of Clinical Periodontology* **9**, 409–414

26

Dental implants and peri-implantology

This account is merely meant to be an introduction to this subject from the periodontal standpoint, and not to be a comprehensive account which can be obtained from a specialist text devoted to this subject.

The successful development of titanium endosseous implants over the last two decades has made it possible to place these with a degree of predictability not previously attainable (Lang and Wilson, 1992). It was first shown that titanium implants could achieve a bone-to-implant contact (Brånemark et al., 1969) and this was demonstrated in undecalcified ground sections by Schroeder et al. (1976). They referred to this contact as functional ankylosis but Brånemark et al. (1977) later created the term 'osseointegration' which they referred to as a direct structural and functional connection between the bone and the surface of a load bearing implant.

Titanium is a highly reactive metal which spontaneously forms an oxide layer in contact with air and this layer is almost resistant to further corrosion. This protects it against chemical attacks in biological tissues and gives it excellent biocompatible properties. Also functional loading of implants transfers masticatory forces to the jawbone and for this reason the stiffness of the implant should be similar to that of bone. Titanium approaches this more closely than other materials (Brånemark et al., 1969). The implant requires retention to achieve ankylotic anchorage and this is usually in the form of screw threads (Brånemark et al., 1985) and perforations (Sutter et al., 1988) and also micro-retentions

in the form of plasma coatings (Schroeder et al., 1976). This provides resistance to shearing forces essential to successful osseointegration (Carlsson et al., 1988).

Successful osseointegration appears to require 3–6 months of quiescence prior to any post-operational loading (Brunski, 1988). This can be achieved with two-stage or one-stage techniques. In the two-stage technique (Brånemark et al., 1977) the implant fixtures are submerged under the mucosal tissues at the time of the installation and this has been claimed to be necessary for success by the advocates of this technique. Recently, however, it has been shown that the non-submerged implants using a one-stage technique integrate equally well provided that they are not subjected to any loading during the osseointegration period (Lang and Wilson, 1992; Albrektsson et al., 1986). Probably the most critical aspect in achieving success is the preparation of the implant bed. Drilling in bone generates considerable heat which can result in bone necrosis. Therefore it is essential to use low drilling speeds (i.e. under 800 rpm) (Schroeder et al., 1988) and abundant irrigation with chilled sterile saline to minimize injury. The sequential use of drills of increasing diameter also helps to minimize thermal trauma. There must be a minimal gap between the prepared site and the implant which is achieved by the careful use of matched precision drills in the chosen implant system.

If stability is achieved new bone will grow and replace damaged bone resulting in an intimate bone-to-implant contact with a gap of

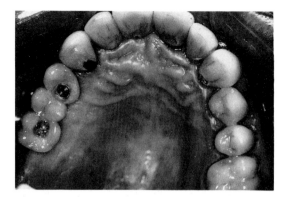

Figure 26.1 Two Brånemark osseointegrated implants in the position of 64| acting as two of the abutments of a full arch bridge. (By courtesy of Mr C. Waterman)

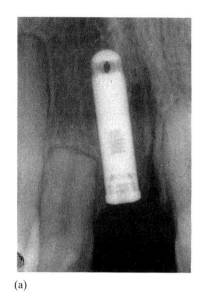

(a)

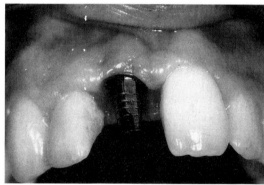

(b)

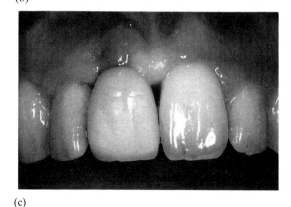

(c)

Figure 26.2 A Calcitek hydroxyapatite coated osseo-integrated dental implant used as the support to replace missing 1| . (a) A radiograph of the implant in position in the alveolar bone following stage 1. The 1| was lost due to trauma. Root resorption can be seen on 2|; (b) the superstructure in position (stage 2); (c) jacket crown tried in prior to glazing and placement. (By courtesy of Professor R. Watson)

about 20 μm or less (Schenk and Willenegger, 1977; Carlsson *et al.*, 1988). If an implant lacks primary stability healing will occur by fibrous replacement of the damaged bone.

The head of the implant fixture penetrates through the crest of the alveolar bone and relates to the gingival or alveolar mucosa. Once the implant head penetrates the mucosa, at the second operation in the two-stage technique or at the first operation in the one-stage technique, a tight soft tissue collar will form around it. This consists of fibrous tissue with fibres running parallel to the long axis of the implant (Listgarten and Lai, 1975) and an epithelial cuff. The junctional epithelium attaches to the implant surface by hemidesmosomes and a basal lamina as with natural teeth (Gould *et al.*, 1981).

Only a few total edentulous and partially edentulous patients will benefit from dental implants and these must be carefully selected both on clinical grounds and the patient's wishes after they have been fully informed about everything necessary to make an informed judgment. Successful implants may need a team approach with co-operation between oral surgeons, periodontologists, restorative and prosthetic dentists (Lang and Wilson, 1992). Any dentist or dental specialist carrying out any part of this work needs to have undergone a lengthy course of postgraduate academic and practical training in the subject. Oral surgeons or periodontologists will easily be able to acquire the necessary surgical skills but will need to acquire considerable restorative and prosthetic knowledge, skills and experience if they wish to carry out the full treatment.

Implants can be considered for stabilizing a full lower or upper denture. The use of anterior mandibular implants is probably the commonest use (Lang and Wilson, 1992). They can also be used in the partially edentulous mouth to act as abutments for bridgework (*Figure 26.1*) or as single tooth replacements (*Figure 26.2*). A very careful clinical assessment has to be made to plan any of these procedures (Bahat and Handelsman, 1992). A careful evaluation of the prognosis of the existing dentition must precede any decisions on partial cases. If implants are clinically indicated, regardless of the implant system used, success mainly depends on the patients' health and co-operation, the design of the prosthesis and the amount and quality of the bone at the implant site. All of these factors need very careful assessment and this involves comprehensive clinical and radiographical examinations of the soft tissue and bony anatomy. Relationships of the proposed implants with vital structures such as the inferior dental canal, maxillary sinus and floor of the nose must be carefully assessed. Adequate radiographs are necessary to assess these relations as well as to assess the amount and quality of the supporting bone (Iacono and Livers, 1992). These may include panoral, lateral and occlusal views. Manual examination also is necessary in conjunction with this to assess the width of the available bone and the presence of undercuts and exostoses.

Since the long term future of remaining natural teeth must be assured, there should not be any caries or periodontal activity on any of the remaining teeth and the patient must be willing to carry out all the necessary preventive measures to avoid this in the future. All necessary periodontal and restorative treatment must have been successfully completed on the remaining natural teeth. Periodontal stability is of critical importance because the bacterial flora associated with active disease can spread from adjacent natural teeth to the implant resulting in peri-implant infections (*see below*).

It is extremely important to relate the final position of the artificial teeth of a full denture in edentulous cases or the abutment teeth of a bridge in a partially edentulous case to the position of the implant fixtures before these are decided upon. The final occlusion is of critical importance and this is best determined by making up a planning appliance which acts as a stent for determining the eventual positions of the implant fixtures. The occlusion of the natural teeth must be in balance in all functional positions before any implant work is planned and any necessary occlusal equilibration must be undertaken prior to implant planning.

No details will be given here of the basic techniques since these are best obtained from books solely devoted to this subject or books where specialist authors write separate chapters on this subject. A good detailed account from a periodontal standpoint can be found in the implant section of Wilson, Kornman and Newman (1992) *Advances in Periodontics*.

Numerous implant systems are available but most clinicians in these field limit themselves to one or two systems. They include the Brånemark (Nobel Pharma), Astra (Astratec) and IMZ (General Medica) systems which are all two-stage and Bonefit and ITI (Straumann Institute) which are one-stage.

Peri-implant infections

Since the superstructure of dental implants share the same environment as the teeth and are surrounded like them by a gingival cuff, it is to be expected that bacterial plaque will form on their surfaces. In edentulous mouths the flora associated with the natural teeth is absent and therefore they appear to accumulate plaque less readily than implants in dentate mouths. This suggests that the presence of natural teeth may influence the composition of the subgingival flora around implants (Apse *et al.*, 1989). It seems likely that the early colonization of implants by putative periodontal pathogens could be more frequent in patients with poorly controlled periodontal disease on adjacent teeth. These teeth may therefore serve as a reservoir for potentially pathogenic bacteria to colonize adjacent implant surfaces.

The development of the bacterial flora of implants in edentulous mouths has been studied for up to 180 days after placement (Mombelli *et al.*, 1988). They showed that 80% of the cultivable bacteria were Gram-positive cocci in all sites but one. In this one site, which did show signs of clinical failure at day 120 including bleeding on probing, increased probing depth and pus formation, there was a decrease in the number of cocci, an increase in the number of rods and an appearance of spirochaetes. These changes were never seen in healthy sites. Further studies over 5 years (Mombelli and Mericske-Sterne, 1990) in 18 edentulous implant patients have shown that a predominantly Gram-positive coccal flora persisted around healthy implant sites over this period. Gram-negative rods such as *Fusobacterium nucleatum* and *Prevotella intermedia* were found in 9% of the samples but *Porphyromonas gingivalis* and spirochaetes were never seen at the healthy sites. Most other studies of successful implants over recent years have shown a similar pattern (Rams *et al.*, 1984; Lekholm *et al.*, 1986; Mombelli *et al.*, 1987; Apse *et al.*, 1989; Bower *et al.*, 1989; Quirynen and Listgarten, 1990). However, one recent study (Mombelli *et al.*, 1987) compared samples from 5 patients with successful implants supporting overdentures for more than a year with those from 7 patients with clinically failing implants which had probing depths exceeding 5 mm, suppuration and radiological loss of alveolar bone. *P. gingivalis*, *P. intermedia*, *F. nucleatum* and other putative periodontal pathogens were cultured and spirochaetes, fusiform bacteria, motile and curved rods were commonly seen by dark field microscopy in samples from failing sites. In contrast, the healthy sites maintained a predominantly Gram-positive coccal flora. There was also a 20-fold lower bacterial count in the healthy as compared with the failing sites.

In animals ligature-induced disease has been produced around dental implants and has been shown to be clinically, radiologically and microbiologically similar to ligature induced periodontitis (Brandes *et al.*, 1988). All of these studies would seem to indicate that implant failures after osseointegration have taken place (i.e. after 4–6 months) are most likely due to bacterial infection rather than an effect of occlusal overload.

Monitoring of implant sites and diagnosis of possible implant failure

Dental implants should be regularly monitored by careful clinical and radiological measurements for signs of possible implant failure (Bahat and Handelsman, 1992; Iacono and Livers, 1992). Probing depths are best measured from a fixed reference point such as the occlusal surface or incisal edge of implant retained crowns or the occlusal edge of the implant head in implants retaining dentures. They may be more accurately measured with constant pressure, electronic probes such as the Florida disk probe (see Chapter 12). Radiographs should be very carefully localised so that a constant bite block, film position and tube angulation is achieved (see Chapter 12) so that serial radiographs can be compared and measured (Hollender and Rockler, 1980). Comparability of serial radiographs can also be checked by measuring the distance between the implant screw threads on each radiograph. Careful measurements can then be made of the distance from an identifiable and reproducible point on the neck of the implant to the crest of the alveolar bone. Any change in attachment level in sequential clinical measurements should be verified and if confirmed should be regarded as possible evidence of loss of implant support. Any measurable change in the position of the alveolar bone level in respect to the implant on radiographs should be regarded as stronger evidence of loss of implant support. Gingival inflammation, bleeding on probing and the presence of calculus should also be noted.

In addition, paper point samples of the bacterial flora in the peri-implant sulcus may be taken and placed into anaerobic transport medium for anaerobic bacterial culture. Samples could also be taken for darkground microscopy (see Chapter 13). The presence of or an increase in the numbers of black-pigmented anaerobes or spirochaetes could be taken as a possible indication of impending peri-implant infection (Mombelli *et al.*, 1987).

Finally, in the future the measurement of proteolytic enzymes in peri-implant sulcus fluid (PISF) may be of possible diagnostic value. In this regard, the total enzyme activity and enzyme concentration of several host derived proteinases, cathepsin B, elastase and dipeptidyl peptidase (DPP) IV and a bacterial protease, trypsin-like protease, in 30 second paper strip PISF samples have been shown to significantly correlate with increased attachment and bone loss around osseointegrated dental implants (Eley, Cox and Watson, 1991). PISF samples are very easy to obtain and if these relationships were shown to be predictive in a longitudinal study of dental implants then one or more of these proteases could be used as a diagnostic test of possible impending implant failure as described in Chapter 13. This would, of course need confirmation from the other clinical and radiological measurements described above.

Treatment of implant sites

In many ways the treatment of dental implant sites is similar to that of natural teeth since the aim is to prevent the development of a pathogenic bacterial flora which would lead to resorption of supporting bone. Careful oral hygiene with soft toothbrushes and dental floss should be carefully taught. Specially designed interproximal brushes that can penetrate into the peri-implant crevice can also be used. Metallic scalers cannot be used with dental implants because they would damage the titanium surfaces of the implant and for this reason good plaque control is also necessary to prevent calculus formation. Specially designed plastic scalers can be used to remove soft deposits but these are ineffective for calculus removal. Recently plastic tips have also been produced for ultrasonic scalers for use with implants. However, if calculus does form it is usually impossible to remove with these instruments. In this case the calculus should be very carefully chipped away with curettes taking extreme care not to damage the surface. During maintenance visits the implants can be polished with a rubber cup and non-abrasive polishing paste. Regular applications of antiseptic agents such as 0.2% aqueous chlorhexdine have also been shown to be beneficial in addition to mechanical oral hygiene in some cases.

If peri-implant infections do occur then these need to be treated with the appropriate systemic antimicrobials such as metronidazole with or without adjuvant amoxycillin (Van Winkelhoff *et al.*, 1989) and this treatment has been shown to be effective in most cases. It has also been shown to eradicate black-pigmenting Gram-negative anaerobic rods and spirochaetes from subgingival implant sites (Duckworth *et al.*, 1987). Local applications of local deposit metronidazole or minocycline into the peri-implant pocket would produce a very high local concentration of these drugs and could be used as an alternative treatment.

References

Aebrektsson, T., Zarb, G., Worthington, P. and Eriksson, A.R. (1986) The long-term efficacy of currently used dental implants: A review and proposed criteria of success. *International Journal of Oral Maxillofacial Implants* **1**, 11–25

Apse, P., Ellen, R.P. Overall, C.M. and Zarb, G.A. (1989) Microbiota and crevicular fluid collagenase activity in the osseointegrated dental implant sulcus. A comparison of sites in edentulous and partially edentulous patients. *Journal of Periodontal Research* **24**, 96–105

Bahat, O. and Handelsman, M. (1992) Presurgical treatment planning and surgical guidelines for dental implants. In: Wilson, T.G.Jr., Kornman, K.S. and Newman, M.G. (eds) *Advances in Periodontics. Parts IV Implant Dentistry.* Chicago, London: Quintessence Publishing Company, pp. 323–340

Bower, R.C., Radney, N.R., Wall, C.S. and Henry, P.J. (1989) Clinical and microscopic findings in edentulous patients 3 years after incorporation of osseointegrated implant-supported bridgework. *Journal of Clinical Periodontology* **16**, 580–587

Brandes, R., Beamer, B., Holt, S.C. *et al.* (1988) Clinical-microscopic observations of ligature-induced 'periimplantitis' around osseointegrated implants. *Journal of Dental Research* **67**, 287

Brånemark, T-I., Breine, U., Adell R. *et al.* (1969) Intraosseous anchorage of dental prostheses. Experimental studies. *Scandinavian Journal of Plastic Reconstructional Surgery* **3**, 81–100

Brånemark, T-I., Breine, U., Adell, R. *et al.* (1977) Osseointegrated implants in the treatment of the edentulous jaw. Experience from a 10 year period. *Scandinavian Journal of Plastic Reconstructional Surgery* **11** (Suppl. 16), 1–132

Brånemark, P.I., Zarb, G.A. and Aebrektsson, T. (1985) *Tissue-integrated prostheses: Osseointegration in clinical dentistry.* Chicago, Quintessence

Brunski, J.B. (1988) The influence of force, motion and related quantities on the response of bone to implants. In: Fitzgerald, R.Jr. (ed.) *Non-Cemented Total Hip Arthroplasty.* New York: Raven Press, pp. 7–21

Carlsson, L., Röstlund, T., Albrektsson, B. and Albrektssòn, T. (1988) Removal torques for polished and rough titanium implants. *International Journal of Oral Maxillofacial Implants* **3**, 21–24

Duckworth, J., Brose, M., Avers, R. *et al.* (1987) Therapeutic implications of the bacterial pathogens associated with dental implants. *Journal of Dental Research* **66**, 114

Eley, B.M., Cox, S.W. and Watson, R.M. (1991) Protease activities in peri-implant sulcus fluid from patients with permucosal osseointegrated dental implants. Correlation with clinical parameters. *Clinical Oral Implant Research* **2**, 62–70

Gould, T.R.L., Brunette, D.M. and Westbury, L. (1981) The attachment mechanism of epithelial cells to titanium *in vivo. Journal of Periodontal Research* **16**, 611–616

Hollender, L. and Rockler, B. (1980) Radiographic evaluation of osseointegrated implants of the jaws. *Dentomaxillofacial Radiology* **9**, 91–95

Iacono, V.J. and Livers, H.N. (1992) Special radiographic techniques for implant dentistry. In: Wilson, T.G.Jr, Kornman, K.S. and Newman, M.G. (eds) *Advances in Periodontics. Part IV Implant Dentistry*. Chicago, London: Quintessence Publishing Company, pp. 341–375

Lang, N.P. and Wilson, T.G.Jr (1992) Choice of implant systems and clinical management. In: Wilson, T.G.Jr, Kornman, K.S. and Newman, M.G. (eds) *Advances in Periodontics. Part IV Implant Dentistry*. Chicago, London: Quintessence Publishing Company, pp. 341–345

Lekholm, U., Ericsson, I., Adell, R. and Slots, J. (1986) The condition of the soft tissues at tooth and fixative abutments supporting fixed bridges. *Journal of Clinical Periodontology* **13**, 588–562

Listgarten, M.M. and Lai, C.H. (1975) Ultrastructure of the intact interface between an endosseous epoxy resin dental implant and the host tissues. *Journal of Biologie Buccale* **3**, 13–28

Mombelli, A., Buser, D. and Lang, N.P. (1988) Colonization of osseointegrated titanium implants in edentulous patients. *Oral and Microbiological Immunology* **3**, 113–120

Mombelli, A. and Mericske-Sterne, R. (1990) Microbiological features of stable osseointegrated implants used as abutments for overdentures. *Clinical and Oral Implant Research* **1**, 1–7

Mombelli, A., Van Oosten, M.A., Schürch, E.Jr and Lang, N.P. (1987) The microbiota associated with successful or failing osseointegrated titanium implants. *Oral and Microbiological Immunology* **2**, 145–151

Quirynen, M. and Listgarten, M.M. (1990) The distribution of bacterial morphotypes around natural teeth and titanium implants. *Clinical and Oral Research* **1**, 8–12

Rams, T.E., Roberts, T.W., Tatum, H. and Keyes, P.H. (1984) Subgingival bacteriology of peridontally healthy and disease human dental implants. *Journal of Dental Research* **63**, 200

Schenk, R. and Willenegger, H. (1977) Zur Histologie der primären Knochenheilung. Modifikationen und grenzen der Spaltheilung in Abhängigkeit von der Defektgrösse. *Unfallheilk* **80**, 155–160

Schroeder, A., Pohler, O. and Sutter, F. (1976) Gewebsreaktion auf ein Titan-Hohlzylinderimplantat mit Titan-Spritzchichtoberfläche. *Schweizerische Monatsschrift fur Zahnheilkunde* **86**, 713–727

Schroeder, A., Sutter, F. and Krekeler, G. (1988) *Orale Implantogie. Allgemeine Grundlagen unt ITI-Hohlzylindersystem*. Stuttgart, New York: Georg Thieme

Sutter, F., Schroeder, A. and Buser, D. (1988) The new concept of ITI hollow-cylinder and hollow-screw implants: Part 1. Engineering and design. *International Journal of Oral Maxillofacial Implants* **3**, 161–172

Van Winkelhoff, A.B., Rodenburg, J.P., Goené, R.J. *et al.* (1989) Metronidazole plus amoxycillin in the treatment of *Actinobacillus actinomycetemcomitans* associated periodontitis./ *Journal of Clinical Periodontology* **16**, 128–131

27

The relationship between periodontal and restorative treatment

Dental restorations should be designed both to minimize plaque accumulation at the gingival margin and to avoid physical injury to the periodontal tissues. The main areas where restorative dentistry and periodontics interrelate are as follows:

- The relationship between dental restorations and gingival margins.
- The occlusal relations of dental restorations.
- The support from the periodontium for partial dentures or fixed bridgework.
- The consequences of gingival recession.
- Crown lengthening for cast restorations.
- Periodontal/pulpal infections.
- Dental implants.

1. The relationship between dental restorations and gingival margins

Dental caries usually attack smooth enamel surface, interproximally and buccal or lingual cervically, immediately coronally to the gingival margin. The enamel carious lesion tapers towards the amelodentinal junction and then spreads laterally along the junction. In this way it involves a greater area of dentine and may result in it progressing subgingivally towards the alveolar crest (*Figure 27.1*). Breakdown of the unsupported enamel may then result in damage to the attached junctional epithelium.

When the tooth is restored the margin of the restoration often has to extend slightly subgingivally in order to eliminate the caries and

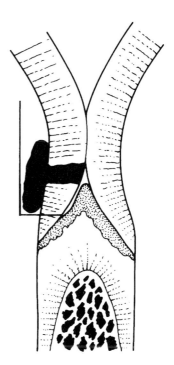

Figure 27.1 Restoration of interproximal caries. Caries below contact area extending into dentine and spreading along amelodentinal junction. The resultant restoration extends subgingivally with pocket formation

unsupported enamel (*Figure 27.1*). Whatever restorative material is used, amalgam, composite, glass ionomer, gold or porcelain, the junctional epithelium fails to adhere to its surface and a pocket results. A further important factor in this process is the restorative

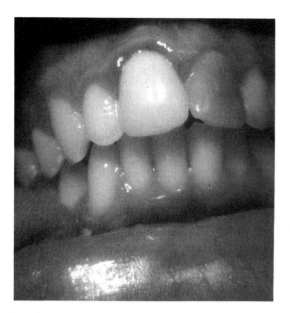

Figure 27.2 Porcelain jacket crown on 1| extending subgingivally. Severe localized gingivitis is present associated with this restoration

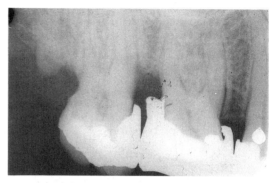

Figure 27.3 A bite-wing radiograph showing grossly overhanging amalgam restorations associated with severe gingivitis. There is also evidence of horizontal bone loss between 76| and the retained root of 8|

margin itself, since even apparently perfect margins accumulate plaque at this site. The lack of protective seal from the junctional epithelium results in the pocket becoming colonized by the bacteria found in subgingival plaque. Thus all subgingival restorations, even those judged clinically sound, will cause gingivitis of some degree extending at least to the margin of the restoration (*Figure 27.2*). This situation could eventually promote the development of chronic periodontitis.

Obviously if the restorative margin is poor then much more damage may result. Deficient or overhanging margins become completely covered with plaque over their whole complex surface and are impossible to clean (*Figure 27.3*). Therefore, they are a potent source of gingival irritation and result in severe gingivitis and frequently progression to periodontitis (*see* Chapter 4).

Clinical considerations

In view of these problems a cavity margin should not extend subgingivally except when absolutely necessary for caries removal (Reeves, 1991). Major precautions should also be taken to avoid deficient or overhanging

cervical margins. Furthermore, all restorations with deficient or overhanging cervical margins should be removed and replaced by satisfactory ones.

Amalgam restorations

Careful cavity preparation should avoid any unnecessary cervical extension. Class II preparations should be fitted with a tightly fitting and appropriately adapted matrix band and this should be firmly wedged cervically. If the cervical floor of the restoration is at or below the cement–enamel junction the proximal surface will be concave. In this situation a conventionally shaped wedge will fail to adapt the matrix to the cervical floor (*Figure 27.4*). A carefully contoured wedge should be used to adapt the matrix (Eli *et al.*, 1991). The cervical margin should be carefully checked with a fine explorer immediately the matrix is removed so that any small excesses can be trimmed with a fine instrument.

Composite and glass ionomer restorations

A wide range of composite filling and veneering materials are now available for anterior and posterior teeth. In posterior teeth they should only by used for small restorations. Glass ionomers are used to restore buccal and lingual cervical cavities and as a secondary base material for composite restorations. Both types of restoration should ideally be placed using a rubber dam since they are very moisture sensitive.

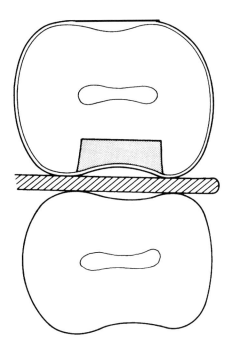

Figure 27.4 Section through a Class II cavity at the level of the cervical floor. It shows how a conventional wedge may fail to adapt the matrix to a proximal furrow on the tooth

Careful cavity preparation should avoid any unnecessary cervical extension. Matrices should be very carefully adapted, placed and wedged to avoid cervical excess. Any thin excess should be carefully fractured away after the material has fully set to leave a good tooth-restoration junction. When necessary, composites can be carefully contoured and trimmed with fine diamond stones and abrasive discs specially made for this purpose. The cervical margin should be carefully assessed with a probe and dental floss before accepting the restoration as satisfactory. Excesses with this material will not adhere to the tooth and plaque will rapidly form between its inner surface and the tooth. This actively promotes the development of secondary caries, gingivitis and periodontitis.

Very great care indeed should be taken with the use of composite as a veneer material on anterior teeth for aesthetic purposes. Its use must be fully justified since the potential for gingival damage is great. If it is decided appropriate to use this technique then sufficient tooth substance must be removed labially to accommodate the veneer without over contouring. The use of a rubber dam is mandatory. The cervical margin should be placed level with the gingival margin and the material must be very carefully contoured to avoid it acting as a plaque trap. It must be possible to clean the margin effectively with a toothbrush.

Gold and porcelain restorations

Careful cavity preparation should avoid any unnecessary cervical extension. The margins must be very precise and a very accurate full arch master impression should be taken along with a full arch impression of the opposing arch and appropriate bite registration. Supragingival placement of margins makes it much easier to take an accurate impression. The restoration must precisely fit the margins without any deficiency or excess. This depends both on the skills of the dentist and the dental technician.

Periodontal care of teeth with subgingival restorations

There will be a tendency for buccal or lingual subgingival restorations to stimulate gingival recession which may expose their cervical margin. Perhaps in this instance the gingiva knows what is good for it! The effects on the gingiva can be reduced interproximally by the regular use of floss, taking it down to just below the margin of the restoration. Obviously, any excess material at the margin will prevent this procedure. Buccally and lingually, the use of Bass technique brushing will be effective only providing the bristles of the brush can reach the cervical margin of the restoration. Regular subgingival scaling should also be carried out. These areas should be regularly checked by periodontal probing and when appropriate, radiographs to watch for any loss of attachment.

Ideally, surgical pocket elimination should be carried out to expose the margin and produce a physiological sulcus. However, this is only possible if a sufficiently deep periodontal pocket is present with the alveolar bone margin 4 mm apical to the restorative margin. If this is attempted for situations with a lesser distance the procedure is only temporarily successful in exposing the margin (Van der Velden, 1982). This is because during repair,

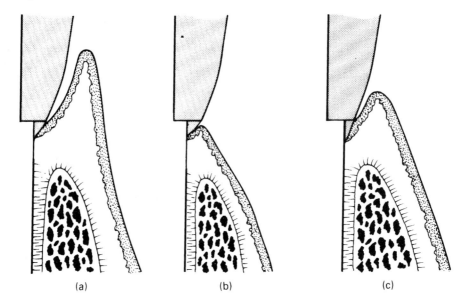

(a)   (b)   (c)

Figure 27.5 An apically repositioned flap used to expose margin of subgingival restoration with a restoration-to-bone distance less than 4 mm. (*a*) Before surgery; (*b*) after healing of surgery; (*c*) months later when gingival regeneration is complete. The gingival margin has migrated coronally to cover the restorative margin again

following the surgery, the gingiva will gradually reform its physiological form and relationships and will extend coronally so that its margin is 4 mm above the bone margin (*Figure 27.5*). If a deeper pocket is present then pocket elimination surgery using as appropriate gingivectomy or an apically repositioned flap will be successful in exposing the margin.

Crown margins

There is a strong case for supragingival margins on crowns, provided the crown length is sufficient for retention. If not, a crown lengthening procedure should be considered (*see below*). Supragingival margins greatly simplify impression taking, provision of temporary crowns, the inspection of the final restoration and its cementation. Most importantly the crown margins are accessible for cleaning.

The only possible exception to this rule is the buccal aspects of visible anterior teeth for aesthetic purposes. In this situation, the labial margin only of the crown is extended to a maximum of 0.5 mm (i.e. just) into the gingival crevice (*Figure 27.6*). Obviously, there must be complete gingival health before the provision of any crown is considered. Provided

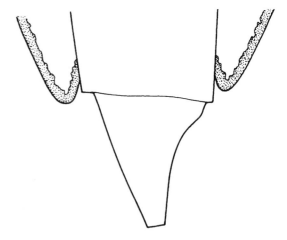

Figure 27.6 Section through an anterior crown preparation for a bonded porcelain-metal crown. The palatal finishing line is located supragingivally. The buccal finishing line is located just within the gingival crevice for aesthetic reasons. The interdental finishing line joins these two points

the labial surface consists of highly glazed porcelain, has a precise fit and is reachable by Bass technique toothbrushing then little harm should result. Good plaque control is essential to maintain this situation and it should be remembered that gingivitis in this area is very unsightly.

2. The occlusal relations of dental restorations

All dental restorations should be in a balanced occlusion in the functional intercuspal, protrusive, retruded and lateral positions. If this is not achieved then occlusal trauma lesions may result (Chapter 24). In addition, the contact areas should be correctly restored to avoid food impaction and drifting of adjacent teeth.

With plastic restorations such as amalgam these relationships must be checked and corrected by carving before the material reaches its final set. Composites in posterior teeth are more difficult to deal with and this is one of their disadvantages. The intercuspal occlusion can be roughly produced by placing a cling-film membrane over the occlusal surface so that the patient can bite on this. Since this impedes light curing, the patient can only close on this material and grind immediately after placement the composite and then open again to allow curing. This is also difficult with a rubber dam in position, which is essential to avoid moisture contamination. Therefore, composites involving the occlusal surface are usually only roughly shaped before curing and then need grinding into shape and occlusion using occlusal registering paper or wax. This is far from ideal since it destroys the original surface of the composite and makes it impossible to achieve good occlusal contouring. These problems can be overcome by using composite inlays, which are fabricated on models outside the mouth. Their initial fit and occlusion depend on the accuracy of the impressions and bites but their marginal seal is no better than that of conventional composites because they are luted in with composite acid etched to the enamel surface. Their life is therefore similar to conventional composites.

With caste gold or fused porcelain or bonded metal-porcelain restorations the correct occlusion depends on the accuracy of the models and bite registration and the skill of the dental technician. If all these functions are carried out correctly then no adjustments should be necessary at the fitting stage and the restoration(s) should be in balance in the intercuspal and functional lateral, protrusive and retruded positions (Chapter 24). Great care should also be taken to restore the correct contact area(s) with adjacent teeth. This requires accurate impressions of the arch with the restoration(s) and the opposing arch and accurate bite registration using a face bow when necessary and functional wax bites in order to place the models correctly on an articulator.

3. The support from the periodontium for partial dentures or fixed bridgework

When teeth are lost and replaced by dentures or bridges, the occlusal forces applied to the prosthesis are transmitted to the remaining supporting teeth. Obviously, the greater number of teeth lost, the larger are the forces applied to the remaining teeth. In addition, chronic periodontitis can significantly reduce the support of teeth which are therefore less able to resist occlusal forces placed upon them and more particularly additional forces placed upon them by prostheses.

It is essential that all periodontal disease is successfully treated before any prosthetic work, fixed or removable, is undertaken. If periodontal health cannot be achieved and advanced periodontitis persists then the prognosis for the remaining dentition and any prosthesis will be extremely poor. In some situations with advanced chronic periodontitis, transitional dentures may have to be provided as part of a planned transition to a full denture. However, these dentures are never stable and always to some extent reduce the life of the remaining dentition.

The aim of any prosthesis is to spread the occlusal load of missing teeth to as many remaining teeth as possible and to avoid overloading any supporting teeth. In periodontally controlled mouths, the choice usually lies between a tooth supported, skeleton, chrome cobalt partial denture and a fixed bridge. The tendency is to restrict the use of bridgework to short edentulous spans, where the abutment teeth have good periodontal support and health and to use dentures for patients with greater numbers of missing teeth and consequently fewer abutment teeth. The design of a chrome cobalt denture aims to distribute the occlusal load to as many supporting teeth as possible using occlusal rests. It also aims to minimize the stress on abutment teeth by reciprocating the forces placed upon them by retention clasps. In addition, it aims by its skeleton design, where possible, to leave uncovered the gingival margins of supporting teeth and thus to reduce its plaque retentiveness and to avoid gingival trauma. However, chrome cobalt dentures can still overstress abutment teeth if the edentulous span is long and particularly where there is a free end saddle. In these situations, tilting and rocking of abutment teeth can occur and this can reduce their functional life. In addition, the movements of a free end saddle may cause gingival and mucosal trauma. These tendencies can be minimized by a wide distribution of occlusal loads and careful reciprocation of clasps.

These forces are much more damaging with poorly designed acrylic partial dentures. Teeth with reduced periodontal support may be rocked by ill-fitting clasps and denture components and considerable gingival trauma may be caused by tissue coverage and denture movement. These dentures are also plaque retentive and will cause gingival irritation if not kept scrupulously clean.

A period of periodontal adaption will follow the placement of a new partial denture and the result will greatly depend on its design.

The problems described above may be overcome by the provision of bridgework. This is, however, extremely expensive and very demanding on clinical and technical expertise. A 15-year longitudinal study of 108 bridges made in 102 patients made by senior students in a Norwegian dental school was carried out by Valderhaug *et al.* (1993). They found that the amount of plaque was similar on crowned and control teeth but marked gingivitis was seen more frequently in crowned teeth with subgingival margins. A slight increase in mean pocket depth was seen with crowned teeth but not in control teeth although no differences could be detected in bone levels. There was also a steady increase in secondary caries around the abutment teeth from 3.3% at the 5th year to 12% at the 15th year. These findings make it clear that abutment crowns should have supragingival margins wherever possible; oral hygiene and diet should be continually monitored as should periodontal and caries status.

The amount of support provided by abutment teeth is crucial in the success of a bridge. This is usually based on Ante's law which proposes that in a fixed bridge the attached root surface area of the abutment teeth should be equal to or greater than the equivalent root surface area of the teeth to be replaced. The blanket application of this 'law' places great restraint on the use of bridges in subjects with reduced periodontal support. However, provided that periodontally healthy conditions are first produced and then maintained, it has been shown that satisfactory function can be achieved with bridges of a cross-arch design supported by teeth with markedly reduced periodontal support (Nyman and Lindhe, 1979; Nyman and Ericsson, 1982). In many of these cases successful bridges were produced with the support of as little as 16% of the presumed root area of the teeth replaced. However, these bridges involved the whole arch and took maximum advantage of cross arch support. Such bridges can also take advantage of the increased clinical crown length of treated periodontally involved teeth with attachment loss. This allows the preparation of abutments with good retention form and also allows for the provision of supragingival margins when aesthetics allows.

These sorts of bridges are probably preferable to partial dentures in cases with reduced periodontal attachment especially where there is tooth mobility. This is because the full arch fixed bridge has greater rigidity and provides a more favourable distribution of function to the remaining teeth. Moreover, the mechanoreceptors within the periodontal ligament restrict by feedback the force generated by the muscles of mastication, and thereby limit the occlusal forces on the bridge.

However, as already stated, there are three important constraints on this sort of work. First, it is extremely expensive which puts it out of reach of most patients in this category. Secondly, and most importantly, it will only be successful if existing periodontal disease is first effectively treated and then maintained both by immaculate oral hygiene and regular 3-monthly subgingival scaling. Thirdly, this work is extremely demanding on the clinical expertise of the dentist and the technical expertise of the dental technician. This is because all of the abutment crowns must fit perfectly with

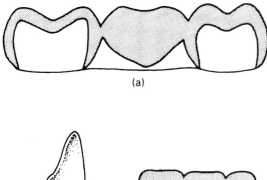

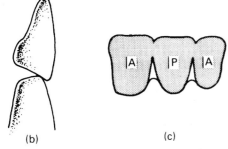

Figure 27.7 (*a*) A 'bullet-shaped' posterior pontic. This has wide interproximal spaces to allow easy passage of floss and a point contact with the ridge; (*b*) An anterior single ridge lap pontic (buccolingual view). It laps the labial ridge but remains clear palatally; (*c*) Labial view of diagram of anterior supporting crowns and pontic. The pontic (P) has wide interproximal spaces to allow the easy passage of floss to clean the proximal surface of the abutments (A) and the undersurface of the pontic

superb leak-free margins which are easy to clean and the whole occlusion must be in balance in the functional intercuspal, retrusive, lateral and protrusive positions.

Pontic design

Pontics should be designed so that the interproximal cleaning of the abutment teeth can be effectively carried out. This means that it must be possible to thread dental floss through the interproximal space between the abutments and the pontic(s). It should also be possible to pass floss under the inner surface of the pontic to clean the surface adjacent to the bridge mucosa. If such a design is provided then floss can be threaded through using a floss threader or by using superfloss with its stiffened end. It can then reach the proximal surfaces of both abutments and the undersurface of the pontic.

The ideal design for a posterior pontic is the so-called bullet-shaped pontic (*Figure 27.7a*). This has a point contact with the ridge mucosa

and is shaped to produce wide interproximal spaces to allow floss access. Its occlusal surface is also somewhat narrowed in comparison to a corresponding natural tooth in order to reduce the occlusal loads placed upon it. This design is not possible for anterior pontics because of aesthetic considerations. These usually have a single ridge-lap design, slightly lapping over the labial aspect of the ridge (*Figure 27.7b*). However, the undersurface should slope upwards from the labial edge so that it passes clear of the ridge surface palatally. The undersurface should be smooth and slightly convex for easy cleaning. The anterior-posterior dimensions of the labial aspect should resemble the tooth it is replacing but should also have wide enough interproximal spaces to allow good floss access (*Figure 27.7c*).

4. The consequences of gingival recession

Gingival recession resulting either from developmental bony dehiscences, periodontal disease or periodontal surgery exposes the root surface (Chapters 8 and 18). Trauma from toothbrushing can result in abrasion and acids from foods and drinks erosion. These processes may quickly remove the surface cementum and progressively the root dentine to produce abrasion/erosion cavities. These can occur on buccal and lingual surfaces but are much more common buccally. These cavities are often periodically sensitive to hot and cold stimuli and become retentive of food debris. These cavities or unaffected exposed root surfaces may also become carious if conditions for this are present and this will necessitate restorative treatment. Abrasion cavities also need restoring if progressive loss of dentine is taking place or if there is persistent sensitivity. These cavities are usually restored with glass ionomer materials using the newer dentine bonding agents. These materials are moisture sensitive and the work is best carried out using a rubber dam. These restorations need to be very carefully placed if a good marginal seal and smooth edge-free margins are to be achieved. Failure to do this will lead to restoration failure and gingival irritation. Obviously, further trauma and erosion need to be avoided by correct oral hygiene training and dietary advice.

5. Crown lengthening for cast restorations

Since the subgingival placement of restorative margins is undesirable, crown lengthening will have to be considered if the clinical crown is too short to achieve a retentive preparation (Allen, 1983). This is usually a problem with full crown preparations on molar teeth but can also affect other teeth. Crown lengthening would usually need to be carried out with an apically repositioned flap as it is extremely important to preserve the full amount of keratinized attached gingiva. The only possible exception to this would be where the problem is caused by gingival hyperplasia when a gingivectomy could be considered. Soft tissue surgery alone will not achieve the objective unless there is sufficient periodontal pocketing and/or gingival hyperplasia to expose the desired amount of clinical crown. Furthermore, tooth exposure will only be permanent if the bone–gingival margin distance is kept to approximately 4 mm. Therefore, in all other cases marginal bone will also have to be reduced, usually by 1–2 mm, to achieve the desired length of clinical crown.

Where these procedures are carried out, crown preparation should be delayed for at least 20 weeks until the position of the gingival margin is stable (Wise, 1985). This is particularly important with anterior crowns when aesthetics are important.

6. Periodontal/pulpal infections

There may be communication between the pulp and periodontal ligament (*Figure 27.8*) via

- Dentinal tubules
- Lateral and accessory root canals
- The apical foramen
- Cracks and fracture lines
- Iatrogenic perforations

These may sometimes give rise to:

- Pulpal disease with secondary periodontal involvement
- Periodontal disease with secondary pulpal involvement
- Combined lesions where coincidental periodontal and pulpal origin lesions have merged.

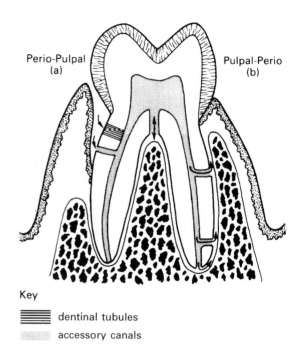

Key

▤ dentinal tubules

▨ accessory canals

Figure 27.8 Pathways between the pulp and the periodontium (*a*) perio-pulpal via dentinal tubules and accessory canals; (*b*) pulpal-perio via accessory canals and apical foramen

Pulpal disease with secondary periodontal involvement

Infection from the pulp may pass into the periodontal ligament space through the apical foramen or through lateral canals (Hiatt, 1977). Lateral canals are most common in the apical third of the root but may also occur less commonly in the middle and coronal thirds. In addition, lateral canals are relatively common in the furcation areas of multirooted teeth (*Figure 27.8*).

Infection passing from the pulp into the apical periodontium via the apical foramen or lateral canals in the apical third usually produces an apical granuloma or abscess. Infection usually tracks through the bone to form a subperiosteal abscess which drains into the vestibule. A very small percentage of apical abscesses, less than 1%, drain via the periodontal ligament to discharge from the gingival margin. This route is, however, more likely if infection passes via a lateral canal in the coronal or middle third of the root. This is also very likely if the infection passes via a

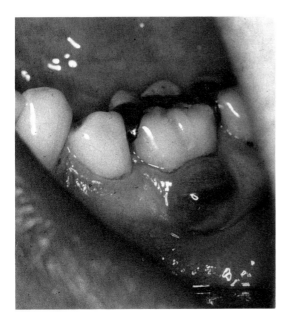

Figure 27.9 An abscess in the furcation area of the lower molar with pus discharging from the gingival margin in a girl of 19 years of age. The condition was associated with a primary pulpal infection and drained into the periodontium via accessory furcation canals. The condition resolved following successful endodontic treatment

lateral canal in the furcation area of a molar tooth (*Figure 27.8*) and in this situation it may simulate periodontal furcation infection (*Figure 27.9*). Fortunately, this is most likely to occur in a young patient with no signs of periodontal disease elsewhere in the mouth and is therefore less likely to deceive.

Infection may also pass from the pulp to the periodontal ligament space via fracture line due to trauma or iatrogenic perforations which may occur during endodontic treatment or post preparation (Tidmarsh, 1979). This also may lead to discharge of pus from the gingival margin and could lead to misdiagnosis of a lesion of periodontal origin.

Periodontal disease with secondary pulpal involvement

Gingival recession may expose dentinal tubules to irritation from the oral involvement and lead to hypersensitivity. It can also lead to abrasion and erosion. However, secondary and peritubular dentine formation in these instances usually minimizes pulpal irritation.

Within periodontal pockets the root surface is exposed to bacteria and their products. Scaling and root planing will remove diseased cementum and expose the dentine tubules, which may transmit irritants (*Figure 27.8*). However, secondary dentine formation usually protects the pulp from irreversible damage.

Periodontal pockets may also involve lateral canals in the coronal and middle thirds of the root and the furcation area and infection could pass via these communications into the pulp (*Figure 27.8*). Finally, teeth with advanced chronic periodontitis could pass secondary infection from the pocket to the pulp via lateral canals in the apical third or the apical foramen.

Combined lesions

In these cases there is no clear indication from the history or examination of a primary causal link with chronic periodontitis or pulpal disease. A true combined lesion is the result of the fusion of two separate lesions, one marginal periodontal and the other pulpal. The pulpal lesion spreads to the periodontium via apical foramen or lateral canals and both lesions enlarge and merge together.

Diagnosis

The correct diagnosis of these conditions involves a careful history of the onset and development of the symptoms and signs followed by a careful clinical examination. This should be backed up by the appropriate radiographs and vitality tests. It is much more difficult to get a clear history from a chronic periodontal–pulpal lesion than immediately after an acute episode.

Clinical examination

One should be alerted to the possibility of a periodontal–pulpal lesion by discoloured clinical crowns, pus discharge from the gingival margin buccally or palatally or from the furcation area between the molar roots and by deep localized pocketing uncharacteristic of the mouth as a whole.

When a primary pulpal lesion spreads to the periodontal ligament and thence to the previously healthy marginal periodontium, it usually spreads along a narrow pathway. When this area is carefully probed it reveals a localized narrow pocket in an otherwise healthy mouth. The pocket contains pus but no plaque or calculus. The age of the patient may also give a clue to its origin since pulpal disease is more common in the young than periodontitis. In particular, the discharge of pus from the furcation area of a single molar in a young patient with an otherwise healthy mouth is very suggestive of a primary pulpal lesion (*Figure 27.9*).

Vitality testing

The response of the pulp to vitality testing depends on an intact nerve supply, whereas pulpal vitality may be maintained with an intact blood supply alone. Testing may be carried out electrically, thermally or by using a bur in a cavity within a non-anaesthetized tooth. None of these tests are infallible and both false positives and negatives may occur. They are particularly likely in heavily filled, multirooted molar teeth.

Radiography

Careful long-cone paralleling radiographs should be taken of the suspected tooth. Where appropriate, radiographs of the rest of the mouth may also be needed. The radiographs of the suspected tooth should show an undistorted view of both the apical and marginal periodontium. The radiographs should be checked for widening of the apical periodontal space, apical or lateral areas of radiolucency, furcation radiolucency and the presence, extent and pattern of marginal bone loss. It should be remembered that the furcation radiolucency can be either pulpal or periodontal in origin.

Treatment

Pulpal disease with secondary periodontal involvement

The pulpal disease will have progressed to partial or total necrosis and endodontic treatment should be commenced immediately. If drainage of pus from the gingival margin is not rapidly controlled by mechanical cleaning of the pulp chamber and root canals then a course of an appropriate antibiotic should be

given. This is best based on a sample of pus which is sent to a microbiology laboratory for antibiotic sensitivity testing. However, as speed is the essence in these cases, treatment can usually be started with amoxycillin provided that the patient is not hypersensitive to penicillin. If the infection is rapidly controlled by these measures then the involved marginal periodontium may regenerate and successful endodontic treatment will lead to a return to full periodontal health. However, if the infection is allowed to become chronic the healing is much less predictable. This is because the chronic infection can cause pathological changes to occur on the root surface with the cementum becoming infected and necrotic. This leads to a downgrowth of junctional epithelium along the changed root surface which leads to the establishment of a deep chronic periodontal pocket. For this reason, rapid diagnosis and treatment of the primary pulpal disease in these cases are essential for a successful outcome. Chronic lesions will need both endodontic and periodontal treatment including periodontal surgery. The outcome of the periodontal treatment of such lesions is doubtful.

Periodontal disease with secondary pulpal involvement

An assessment of the prognosis of the tooth in terms of its remaining alveolar bone support should be made before further treatment is planned and instituted.

Lesions of periodontal origin are invariably chronic. An assessment should first be made of the state of the pulp and it should be ascertained whether the pulpal disease is reversible or irreversible, i.e. whether the pulp is hyperaemic or necrotic. If the pulp is necrotic then endodontic treatment should be carried out first. If, on the other hand, the pulp appears to be still vital but hypersensitive then periodontal treatment should be carried out first to see whether the reduction in the source of irritation will lead to pulpal recovery.

The periodontal lesion should be first treated by careful, meticulous subgingival scaling and root planing. The condition of the rest of the mouth should be taken into account in the overall treatment plan. Meticulous oral hygiene must be established. The periodontal lesion will invariably require periodontal surgery and the precise technique employed will depend upon the depth of the pocket and pattern of bone resorption (Chapters 16 and 17).

The outcome can be difficult to determine in cases associated with advanced periodontitis and all cases should receive·regular maintenance treatment.

Combined lesions

If the prognosis is reasonable both periodontal and endodontic treatment is carried out as outlined above. The endodontic treatment should be carried out first. The periodontal treatment invariably includes periodontal surgery in these cases. The outcome of treatment is uncertain in cases associated with advanced periodontitis.

7. Dental implants

Osseointegrated dental implants and their clinical implications have been discussed in Chapter 26. They require very careful design and great clinical and technical expertise. They also require careful maintenance to prevent peri-implant disease. All of this is covered in Chapter 26.

References

Allen, E.P. (1993) Surgical crown lengthening for function and aesthetics. *Dental Clinics of North America* **37**, 163–180

Eli, I., Weiss, E., Kozlovsky, A. and Levi, N. (1991) Wedges in restorative dentistry: principles and applications. *Journal of Oral Rehabilitation* **18**, 257–264

Hiatt, W.H. (1977) Pulpal periodontal disease. *Journal of Periodontology* **48**, 598–609

Nyman, S. and Ericsson, I. (1982) The capacity of reduced periodontal tissues to support fixed bridgework. *Journal of Clinical Periodontology* **9**, 409–414

Nyman, S. and Lindhe, J. (1979) A longitudinal study of combined periodontal and prosthetic treatment for patients with advanced periodontitis. *Journal of Periodontology* **50**, 163–169

Reeves, W.G. (1991) Restorative margin placement and periodontal health. *Journal of Prosthetic Dentistry* **66**, 733–736

Tidmarsh, B.G. (1979) Accidental perforation of the roots of teeth. *Journal of Oral Rehabilitation* **6**, 235–240

Van der Velden, U., (1982) Regeneration of the interdental soft tissue following denudation procedures. *Journal of Clinical Periodontology* **9**, 455–459

Valderhaug, J., Ellingsen, J.E. and Jokstad, A. (1993) Oral hygiene, periodontal condition and carious lesions in patients treated with dental bridges. A 15-year clinical and radiographic follow-up study. *Journal of Clinical Periodontology* **20**, 482–489

Wise, W.D. (1985) Stability of the gingival crest after surgery and before anterior crown placement. *Journal of Prosthetic Dentistry* **53**, 20–23

Further reading

Nevins, M. (1993) Periodontal considerations in prosthodontic treatment. In: Yukna, R.A., Newman, M.G. and Williams, R.C. (eds) *Current Opinion in Periodontology*. Philadelphia: Current Science, pp. 151–156

Wilson, R.D. (1992) Restorative dentistry. In: Wilson, T., Kornman, K. and Newman, M. (eds) *Advances in Periodontics*. Chicago: Quintessence, pp. 226–244

Index

297